Overlapping Pain and Psychiatric Syndromes

Overlapping Pain and Psychiatric Syndromes

Global Perspectives

EDITED BY MARIO INCAYAWAR, MD, MSC, PHD

DIRECTOR, RUNAJAMBI INSTITUTE
MONTREAL, QUEBEC, CANADA
FORMER HENRY R. LUCE, PROFESSOR IN BRAIN, MIND,
AND MEDICINE: CROSS-CULTURAL PERSPECTIVES, PITZER,
CLAREMONT MCKENNA, AND HARVEY MUDD COLLEGES,
CLAREMONT, CALIFORNIA, USA

SIOUI MALDONADO-BOUCHARD, MSC, PHD

RESEARCH ASSOCIATE
RUNAJAMBI INSTITUTE
MONTREAL, QUEBEC, CANADA

MICHAEL R. CLARK, MD, MPH, MBA

HONORARY EDITOR
JOHNS HOPKINS UNIVERSITY
BALTIMORE, MARYLAND, USA

OXFORD
UNIVERSITY PRESS

Oxford University Press is a department of the University of Oxford. It furthers
the University's objective of excellence in research, scholarship, and education
by publishing worldwide. Oxford is a registered trade mark of Oxford University
Press in the UK and certain other countries.

Published in the United States of America by Oxford University Press
198 Madison Avenue, New York, NY 10016, United States of America.

Library of Congress Cataloging-in-Publication Data
Names: Incayawar, Mario, editor. | Maldonado-Bouchard, Sioui, editor. |
Clark, M. R. (Michael R.), editor.
Title: Overlapping pain and psychiatric syndromes : global perspectives /
[edited by] Mario Incayawar, Sioui Maldonado-Bouchard, Michael R. Clark.
Other titles: Overlapping pain and psychiatric syndromes
Description: New York, NY : Oxford University Press, [2020] |
Includes bibliographical references and index.
Identifiers: LCCN 2020016047 (print) | LCCN 2020016048 (ebook) |
ISBN 9780190248253 (hardback) | ISBN 9780190248277 (epub) |
ISBN 9780190248284 (online)
Subjects: MESH: Chronic Pain—complications | Chronic Pain—therapy |
Mental Disorders—diagnosis | Mental Disorders—therapy
Classification: LCC RB127 (print) | LCC RB127 (ebook) |
NLM WL 704.6 | DDC 616/.0472—dc23
LC record available at https://lccn.loc.gov/2020016047
LC ebook record available at https://lccn.loc.gov/2020016048

9 8 7 6 5 4 3 2 1

Printed by Integrated Books International, United States of America

To Lise Bouchard, PhD—a wife, a scholar, a colleague, a wonderful star. Without her love, support, and company, I would have been at a loss in life.

CONTENTS

During the past two decades, Mario Incayawar, the senior editor of this impressive volume assessing the current state of knowledge in the overlapping clinical domains of pain and psychiatric syndromes, has established a reputation as an innovative thinker and steady contributor to the fields of cultural psychiatry and pain medicine, with a particular focus on the indigenous Quichua population of the Andean mountain region of South America. During these years, he founded and is the director of the Runajambi Institute for the Study of Quichua Culture and Health, based in the Andean community, working closely with Lise Bouchard and Sioui Maldonado-Bouchard. Between them, they bring the perspectives of clinical medicine, psychiatry, anthropology, linguistics, neuroscience, and genetics to the elucidation of the complex interactions between chronic pain and psychiatric disorders. Each of them has contributed insightful chapters to this volume, which includes 29 chapters written by international scholars on a wide range of topics relating to overlapping chronic pain and psychiatric disorders.

In his clearly written chapter reviewing the epidemiological literature on the co-occurrence of chronic pain and psychiatric illness, Jan Jaracz points out that both pain and depression are among the most prevalent conditions clinicians encounter in medical practice. The presence of depression in people with chronic pain is significantly higher than that in the general population, and this proportion is even higher in patients attending specialty clinics. Pain exerts a negative impact on the effects of treatment, including a poorer outcome in multiple domains of quality of life. Moreover, pain increases the economic burden resulting from psychiatric disorders. Psychiatric comorbidities, particularly depression and anxiety, are common in people suffering from pain, and conversely, painful symptoms are common in persons with major depression, anxiety disorders, and other psychiatric disorders. Patients with these comorbidities experience a serious, negative impact on their daily activities and on their family, social, and working lives.

Major depression and low back pain are two leading causes of years lost due to disability. The presence of both conditions is related to greater disability, increased medical care use, more severe life events, and poorer treatment response, in comparison to the presence of either condition alone. Chronic pain predicts psychiatric comorbidities. Anxiety and/or depression with pain impairs recovery from depression and predicts poorer analgesic outcomes, greater pain intensity, interference with daily activities, and greater medical care expenditures than either pain or depression, or anxiety, alone. The younger the age at pain onset, the greater the pain intensity and the greater the likelihood of an accompanying psychiatric illness. There is also increased risk for suicide in patients with pain, correlated with the presence of depression and substance use.

In his chapter on the assessment and monitoring of patients with chronic pain and co-occurring substance use and abuse, Jon Streltzer emphasizes that substance abuse complicates pain management and that treatment of pain with long-term opioids, particularly in high doses, is associated with substantial medical comorbidity, unintentional overdoses, and death. Recent estimates suggest that the prevalence of substance use disorders in the chronic pain population in the United States is between 20 and 40%.

Pain is a common medical problem in older people. In their chapter on pain and comorbid psychiatric illnesses in elderly people, Mellar P. Davis and John L. Shuster, Jr. emphasize that chronic pain is often associated with anxiety, depression, and frailty. Poor self-rated health is strongly associated with pain severity in elderly people, and pain-related interference with daily activities leads to depression. Basic activities of daily living, such as social isolation and basic education only, play a role as mediatory factors between depression and pain in elderly people. More than 20% of elderly Americans use analgesic medications on a daily basis. Depression accompanying pain decreases pain tolerance and lowers pain threshold.

This volume includes numerous chapters that contribute valuable clinical and theoretical perspectives to the understanding of the complex interactions between chronic pain and psychiatric disorders. Illustrative clinical case examples are included in many of the chapters, as are intriguing suggestions for further research. Clearly, as these chapters demonstrate, the study of chronic pain and psychiatric disorders is a challenging and rapidly expanding field, attracting physicians, social scientists, demographers, and neuroscientists alike to the unanswered questions.

Ronald Wintrob, MD

Clinical Professor of Psychiatry and Human Behavior, Brown University, Providence, RI, USA

Chronic pain seldom presents alone. Pain patients frequently have comorbid psychiatric conditions, and those suffering from mental illness often experience pain. Pain conditions and psychiatric disorders have customarily been understood and treated as different and separate clinical entities, to the detriment of patients' well-being. This book responds to the significant gap that exists in understanding the overlapping pain and psychiatric syndromes. Pain and comorbidities with other nonpsychiatric clinical conditions, such as diabetes and hypertension, have been covered to some extent elsewhere.

This book studies the complex and striking relationships between pain and psychiatric disorders. It is tailored to support a broad cross-section of health professionals and academicians, including pain practitioners, psychiatrists, neurologists, anesthesiologists, rheumatologists, primary care and family physicians, psychologists, nurses, social workers, physical therapists, health administrators, and policymakers, among others.

Research in the field of chronic pain and psychiatric comorbidity is sparse, and scholarship in this area is extremely limited. Reflecting these deficiencies, health practitioners have little knowledge of overlapping pain and psychiatric syndromes, and they feel poorly prepared to manage them effectively. Similarly, medical trainees receive minimal or no training at all on this clinical issue. Academic medical programs around the world have an urgent need to integrate knowledge brought by current developments in the social sciences, neurosciences, genetics/epigenetics, pain medicine, and psychiatry related to pain and psychiatric comorbidity. This volume hopes to respond and contribute to the previously mentioned gaps and unmet needs.

The inspiration for preparing this book comes from the clinical experiences of Mario Incayawar in the Andes of South America. As a young physician, he received mostly illiterate Inca patients, who presented almost exclusively with somatic symptoms. It was exceptional to have a patient who complained about psychological symptoms. However, he was aware that patients disclosed spontaneously and frequently psychological issues to their trusted traditional healers. Noting this disparity, he conducted a study of *Jaki*, a culture-bound syndrome highly prevalent in the Andes. In working with 50 *Jaki* patients referred to him by traditional healers, he was able to show that among those patients, 82% made the Western psychiatric diagnosis of depression, 44% somatoform disorders, and 40% anxiety disorders. It is worth noting that those patients presented both somatic (e.g., migratory pain, headaches, muscle pain, fatigue) and abundant psychological symptoms (e.g., sadness, worries, insomnia, feeling of rejection, fear, ideas of persecution, and suicidal ideation, among others). It appeared that with a proper, culturally sensitive interview, the Inca patients expressed psychological symptoms like any other human group and that their stoical demeanor was dependent on the quality of the doctor–patient relationship. The lesson learned from the Andes is that psychiatric patients suffered from pain and pain patients often experienced psychiatric symptoms.

We made a significant effort to cover prominent pain and psychiatric conditions and important regions of the world. The chapters are original contributions from recognized world experts in the field of pain and psychiatry. The contributors came from Canada, the United Kingdom, Quichua Nation, India, Romania, Poland, Germany, France, South Korea, and the United States.

Many colleagues and friends generously contributed to this book. Mario Incayawar is deeply grateful to Dr. Sioui Maldonado-Bouchard for enthusiastically welcoming the idea for this book and for her commitment to this challenging academic project. Similarly, Dr. Maldonado-Bouchard is truly thankful to Dr. Incayawar for this unique opportunity, which has allowed her to learn greatly about pain and psychiatry comorbidities and also the value of patience and perseverance. The patience, understanding, and support we received from Ms. Andrea Knobloch, Senior Editor, Medicine, Oxford University Press, is greatly appreciated. With her flexible and highly professional assistance, she has greatly facilitated the successful completion of our book.

We want to express our gratitude to all our Inca patients in the Andes who helped us understand the intriguing relationship between pain and psychiatric disorders. Their integrative, pluralistic worldview, medical system, and theory of illness and disease paved the way for the development of this book. Our heartfelt appreciation goes to our contributors. Their outstanding and diligent work effectively kindled and rekindled the fire.

Mario Incayawar, MD, MSc, PhD
Director, Runajambi Institute, Montreal, Quebec, Canada
Sioui Maldonado-Bouchard, MSc, PhD
Research Associate, Runajambi Institute, Montreal, Quebec, Canada
February 11, 2020

CONTRIBUTORS

Benjamin L. Berey, PhD
Post-doctoral Fellow
Brown University
Providence, RI, USA

Sophie Bergeron, PhD
Full Professor
Department of Psychology
Université de Montréal
Montréal, QC, Canada

**Dinesh Bhugra, CBE, MA, MSc,
MBBS, DSc(Hon), PhD, FRCP,
FRCPE, FRCPsych, FFPHM,
FRCPsych(Hon),FHKCPsych(Hon),
FACPsych(Hon),FAMS(Singapore),
FKCL, MPhil, FAcadME, FRSA,
DIFAPA**
Professor Emeritus
Mental Health & Cultural Diversity,
    IoPPN
Kings College
London, UK

Lise Bouchard, MA, PhD
Director of Research
Runajambi Institute
Québec, Canada

Marike Bredow-Zeden, DMD
Department of Oral and Maxillofacial
    Surgery/Plastic Surgery
University of Greifswald
Greifswald, Germany

Julia Brillante, PsyD
Child Clinical Psychology
    Postdoctoral Fellow
NewYork-Presbyterian Hospital/
    Columbia University Medical
    Center
New York, NY, USA

**Santosh K. Chaturvedi, MD,
FRCPsych**
Senior Professor
Department of Psychiatry
National Institute of Mental Health &
    Neurosciences
Bangalore, India

Martin D. Cheatle, PhD
Associate Professor
Department of Psychiatry
Perelman School of Medicine,
    University of Pennsylvania
Philadelphia, PA, USA

Michael R. Clark, MD, MPH, MBA
Chair, Psychiatry & Behavioral Health
Inova Health System
Falls Church, VA, USA
Professor, Psychiatry & Behavioral
  Sciences
George Washington University School
  of Medicine & Health Sciences
Washington, DC, USA

Anne Corbett, BSc, MRes, PhD
Senior Lecturer in Dementia
  Research
Exeter University
Exeter, UK

Ashley F. Curtis, PhD
Assistant Professor
Departments of Psychiatry and
  Psychological Sciences
University of Missouri
Columbia, MO, USA

Janie Damien, BSc
Graduate Student
Université de Sherbrooke
Québec, Canada

**Mellar P. Davis, MD,
FCCP, FAAHPM**
Director of Palliative Services
Geisinger Medical Center
Danville, PA, USA

Geetha Desai, MD, DNB, PhD
Professor
Department of Psychiatry
National Institute of Mental Health
  and Neuro Sciences (NIMHANS)
Bengaluru, India

**Dan L. Dumitrascu, MD,
AGAF, RFF**
Professor
Iuliu Hatieganu University of
  Medicine and Pharmacy
Cluj-Napoca, Romania

**Renée El- Gabalawy, MA, PhD,
CPsych**
Assistant Professor & Clinical
  Psychologist
Departments of Anesthesiology,
  Perioperative and Pain Medicine &
  Clinical Health Psychology
University of Manitoba
Manitoba, Canada

Usef Faghihi, PhD
Assistant Professor
Department of Mathematics and
  Computer Science
Université du Québec à
  Trois-Rivières
Québec, Canada

Kara B. Fehling, PhD
Clinical Psychologist
NYCBT
New York, NY, USA

Simmie L. Foster, MD, PhD
Depression Clinical Research
  Program
Department of Psychiatry
Massachusetts General Hospital
Harvard Medical School
Boston, MA, USA

Tessa M. Frohe, PhD
Post-doctoral Fellow
University of Washington
Seattle, WA, USA

Maël Gagnon-Mailhot, BA
Research Assistant & Graduate
  student
Université de Sherbrooke & Bishop's
  University
Quebec, Canada

Ana B. Goya Arce, PhD
Post-Doctoral Fellow
Department of Anesthesiology,
  Perioperative and Pain Medicine
Stanford University
Stanford, CA, USA

Bernard L. Harlow, MPH, PhD
Professor
Department of Epidemiology
Boston University School of
  Public Health
Boston, MA, USA

Miriam J. Haviland, MSPH
Doctoral Student, Epidemiology
Department of Epidemiology
Boston University School of
  Public Health
Boston, MA, USA

J. Gregory Hobelmann, MD, MPH
Chief Medical and Clinical Officer
Ashely Addiction Treatment
Adjunct Faculty, Johns Hopkins
  Department of Psychiatry and
  Behavioral Sciences
Baltimore, MD, USA

Pamela L. Holens, MEd, MA, PhD
Associate Professor, Department of
  Clinical Health Psychology
Clinical Director and Psychologist,
  Winnipeg Operational Stress
  Injury Clinic
University of Manitoba
Manitoba, Canada

Mario Incayawar, MD, MSc, PhD
Director, Runajambi Institute
Quichua (Inca) Nation
Medical Director, Cross-Cultural
  Clinic for Pain and Psychiatry
Former Henry R. Luce, Professor in
  Brain, Mind and Medicine: Cross-
  Cultural Perspectives
Pitzer, Claremont McKenna, and
  Harvey Mudd Colleges
Claremont, CA, USA

Anjana Jagpal, MA
Graduate Assistant
Department of Psychology
DePaul University
Chicago, IL, USA

Jan Jaracz, MD, PhD
Professor
Department of Psychiatry
Poznań University of Medical
  Sciences
Poznań, Poland

Sang Won Jeon, MD
Associate Professor
Department of Psychiatry, Kangbuk
  Samsung Hospital
Sungkyunkwan University School of
  Medicine
Seoul, Republic of Korea

Daniel B. Kay, PhD
Assistant Professor
Department of Psychology
Brigham Young University
Provo, UT, USA

Yong-Ku Kim, MD, PhD
Professor
Department of Psychiatry
College of Medicine
Korea University
Seoul, Korea

Stefan Kindler, MD, DDS
Consultant
Department of Oral and Maxillofacial
    Surgery/Plastic Surgery
University of Greifswald
Greifswald, Germany

Amy Kranzler, PhD
Assistant Professor
Montefiore Medical Center/Albert
    Einstein College of Medicine
Bronx, NY, USA

Sioui Maldonado-Bouchard, MSc, PhD
Medical Student, Université de
    Montréal School of Medicine
Montreal, Quebec, Canada
Research Associate
Runajambi Institute
Quichua (Inca) Nation
Québec, Canada

Serge Marchand, PhD
Scientific Director, Professor,
    Investigator
FRQS, Université de Sherbrooke,
    Centre de recherche du CHUS
Québec, Canada

Katherine T. Martucci, PhD
Assistant Professor
Center for Translational Pain
    Medicine
Department of Anesthesiology
Duke University School of Medicine
Durham, NC, USA

Elizabeth A. McCallion, MS
Graduate Student/Psychology Intern
University of New Mexico/VA Palo
    Alto Health Care System
Albuquerque, NM, USA

Christina S. McCrae, PhD
Director, MizZzou Sleep
    Research Lab
Professor, Department of Psychiatry,
    School of Medicine
University of Missouri
Columbia, MO, USA

Christopher Paul, MD
Assistant Professor
Department of Anesthesiology
University of Arkansas for Medical
    Sciences
Little Rock, AR, USA

Vincent Pelland, MD
Resident, Family Medicine
Centre Intégré Universitaire de Santé
    et de Services Sociaux de l'Estrie—
    Centre Hospitalier Universitaire
    de Sherbrooke (CIUSSS de
    l'Estrie-CHUS)
Québec, Canada

Rachel Roy, BA (Hons)
Research Coordinator for Clinical
    Research Network within SPOR
    Chronic Pain Network
University of Manitoba
Manitoba, Canada

Djea Saravane, MD, MSc, PhD
Head of Integrated Medicine and
    Pain Clinic in Mental Health,
    Autistic Spectrum Disorders,
    Polyhandicap and Rare Genetic
    Handicap
Advisor, Vesalius Foundation
Barthelemy Hospital—Etampes
Essonne, France

Edward A. Selby, PhD
Associate Professor
Department of Psychology
Rutgers, The State University of
New Jersey
New Brunswick, NJ, USA

John L. Shuster, Jr., MD, FAPM
Psychiatrist, VA Tennessee Valley
Health System
Clinical Professor of Psychiatry,
Vanderbilt University
Medical Center
Nashville, TN, USA

Jordana L. Sommer, BA (Hons), MA
Graduate Student, Department of
Psychology
Research Associate, Department of
Anesthesiology, Perioperative and
Pain Medicine
University of Manitoba
Manitoba, Canada

**Mihaela Fadgyas Stanculete, MD,
MSc, PhD**
Senior Lecturer
Department of Neuroscience,
Psychiatry
Iuliu Hatieganu University of
Medicine and Pharmacy
Cluj-Napoca, Romania

Jon Streltzer, MD
Professor Emeritus of Psychiatry
John A. Burns School of Medicine
University of Hawaii
Honolulu, HI, USA

Judith A. Strong, PhD
Research Professor
Department of Anesthesiology
University of Cincinnati College of
Medicine
Cincinnati, OH, USA

John A. Sturgeon, PhD
Assistant Professor
Department of Anesthesiology and
Pain Medicine
University of Washington School of
Medicine
Seattle, WA, USA

Nicole K. Y. Tang, DPhil, CPsychol
Reader, Department of Psychology
Director, Warwick Sleep and
Pain Lab
University of Warwick
Coventry, UK

Blake H. Tearnan, PhD
Renown Medical Center
Rehabilitation Hospital
Reno, NV, USA

Cynthia O. Townsend, PhD, ABPP
Clinical Director, Pain
Rehabilitation Center
Assistant Professor, Department of
Psychiatry and Psychology
Mayo Clinic
Phoenix, AZ, USA

Donald R. Townsend, PhD, DBSM
Diplomate American Board of Sleep
Medicine
Founder, Insomnia Expertz, PLLC
Phoenix, AZ, USA

Susan T. Tran, PhD
Assistant Professor
Department of Psychology
DePaul University
Chicago, IL, USA

Glenn J. Treisman, MD, PhD
Eugene Meyer III Professor of
    Psychiatry and Medicine
Department of Psychiatry and
    Behavioral Sciences
Johns Hopkins University School
    of Medicine
Baltimore, MD, USA

Channing Twyner, MD
Assistant Professor
Department of Anesthesiology
University of Mississippi
    Medical Center
Jackson, MS, USA

Kevin E. Vowles, PhD
Professor of Clinical Health
    Psychology
School of Psychology
Queens University Belfast
Belfast, Northern Ireland, UK

James Weisberg, PhD
Associate Professor
Pain Psychologist
Division of Pain Medicine
Department of Anesthesiology and
    Perioperative Medicine
University of Alabama at
    Birmingham
Birmingham, AL, USA

Ronald Wintrob, MD
Former Chair, World Psychiatric
    Association—TPS
Clinical Professor of Psychiatry and
    Human Behavior
Brown University
Providence, RI, USA

Katie Witkiewitz, PhD
Regents' Professor
Department of Psychology
University of New Mexico
Albuquerque, NM, USA

Ipek Yalcin, PhD, PharmD
Research Director
Institut des Neurosciences Cellulaires
    et Intégratives
Centre National de la Recherche
    Scientifique UPR3212
Université de Strasbourg
Strasbourg, France

Jun-Ming Zhang, MD, MSc
Professor and Vice Chair for
    Research
Department of Anesthesiology
University of Cincinnati College of
    Medicine
Cincinnati, OH, USA

Min Zhuo, PhD
Professor
Department of Physiology
University of Toronto
Ontario, Canada

PART I

The Nature of Pain and Psychiatric Comorbidity

The Need to Fathom Overlapping Pain and Psychiatric Syndromes

MARIO INCAYAWAR ■

A CLINICAL CONUNDRUM

The health practitioner at the bedside of a patient suffering from chronic pain and a psychiatric comorbid condition is facing a true clinical conundrum. The comorbidity is frequent yet poorly understood, the diagnosis is difficult, and the treatment that follows is less than appropriate. Pain conditions and psychiatric disorders have customarily been understood and treated as different and separate clinical entities, to the detriment of patients' well-being. Fathoming the overlapping pain and psychiatric disorders should be in the interest of everybody, including doctors, nurses, pain specialists, psychiatrists, social workers, psychologists, hospital administrators, and health policymakers. The benefits of increased awareness should translate to decreased patients' suffering/stigma, increased patients' engagement, less cost to society, better quality health care, and more personalized, patient-centered medical care.

NEEDLESS SUFFERING IN PAIN AND MENTAL ILLNESS

Burden of Mental Illness

The global burden of mental illness and pain is immense. Worldwide, mental illness accounts for about 23% of the total disease burden, and the need for mental health services and support systems is growing. It is estimated that there are some 500 million people in the world suffering from mental illness. The number of identified cases is probably an underestimation because of the difficulties of mental health workers in making a psychiatric diagnosis of patients from other cultures.[1] Beyond the suffering associated with the psychiatric condition itself, there is the additional suffering due to lost productivity, family disruption, accidents, stigma, discrimination, premature death, and limited access to mental health services.

Teenagers are one particularly vulnerable group. It is well known that the median age for the onset of any mental disorder is about 14 years.[2] Nevertheless, mental illness in young people goes unrecognized and untreated.[3]

The inequality in access to mental health services is an immense challenge globally. In an international mental health survey conducted in 14 countries in the Americas, Europe, the Middle East, Africa, and Asia, 35 to 50% of serious psychiatric conditions in developed countries were untreated in the year before the interview. In developing countries, 76 to 85% of serious cases received no treatment.[4] As McKenzie, Patel, and Araya pointed out, mental health services in the developing world "are often greatly under-resourced, under strain, and leave most people with mental health problems with no care."[5] Even in developed countries such as Canada, only 7.2% of the health care budget is dedicated to mental health. According to a team of leading global mental health researchers, the overwhelming majority of patients with mental disorders in the world "are not being provided with even the basic mental health care that we know they should and can receive."[6]

In the United States, one in five adults, roughly 45 million people, suffer from mental illnesses, including major depression, anxiety, and less common disorders such as schizophrenia and bipolar disorder. The economic burden is immense, accounting for more than $300 billion in disability-associated costs per year, loss of work productivity, divorce, accidents, and accidental drug overdoses. Major depressive disorders alone accounted for $173.2 billion in 2005 and $210.5 billion in 2010.[7] The global economic burden of mental disorders was estimated to be US $8.5 trillion in 2010; it will double by 2030.[8] Compounded to this extraordinary burden related to mental illness are the societal costs of pain comorbidity.

Burden of Pain

The burden of pain across the globe is expected to be massive; unfortunately, the precise societal cost is unknown. Scattered data are available that give us a glimpse of the problem. In New Zealand, 82% of the population reported a life-disrupting pain experience.[9] An international survey conducted by the World Health Organization showed that 22% of primary care patients in 14 countries reported persistent pain.[10] Almost three decades ago, the US Department of Health and Human Services reported that pain caused 40 million medical visits per year, costing the country more than $100 billion annually in health care expenditure and lost productivity.[11] Later, according to the Institute of Medicine's 2011 report titled *Relieving Pain in America—A Blueprint for Transforming Prevention, Care, Education, and Research*, 116 million American adults were reported to suffer from chronic pain, which is more than the total affected by heart disease, cancer, and diabetes combined, and which costs the country $635 billion each year.[12] Unquestionably, pain is widespread around the world, and its importance as a global public health problem has been recognized by the World Health Organization.[10] It is necessary to highlight that pain is the most common complaint bringing people to a physician's office.[13]

Despite being pain a serious public health issue worldwide, inadequate treatment of pain is highly prevalent. Pain undertreatment has been documented among children, elderly patients, patients with cancer, surgical patients, and ethnic minority groups, among others.[14–18] Because of the recognition of this worldwide neglect, pain has been declared a fundamental human rights issue.[19]

The economic burden of pain and psychiatric disorders in the United States, based on the data given previously, could safely be estimated to be about $1 trillion dollars each year. The global burden of overlapping pain and psychiatric syndromes is certainly massive, and the consequent human suffering is heartbreaking.

Epidemiology of Overlapping Pain and Psychiatric Syndromes

Very little is known and research is scarce on the overlapping of pain and psychiatric syndromes. In one of the first studies on this topic published in 1983, Reich et al. reported that 98% of chronic pain patients reviewed by the University of California Davis Medical Center pain board had an Axis I psychiatric disorder, and 37% had an Axis II diagnosis. Those patients in pain with psychiatric comorbidities appeared to have lower improvement rates.[20] It is worth noting that Veterans Administration patients in the United States, who were being treated for chronic pain, were found to be two to three times more likely to be diagnosed with psychiatric comorbidities, including post-traumatic stress disorder (PTSD), bipolar disorder, anxiety or adjustment disorder, major depression, and personality disorders.[21]

What we know better is the separate epidemiology of mental disorders and pain. As stated in this book by Professor Jaracz in Chapter 2, the prevalence of chronic pain in the general population ranges from 19 to 33%, with higher rates in elderly people. In the case of major depression, the estimated lifetime prevalence is 11 to 14%. However, the prevalence of depression in persons with chronic pain is about 21%, and the proportion increases to 52 to 85% among patients visiting specialist clinics. Equally, at least 50% of patients with depression report painful symptoms. For more epidemiological information on pain and psychiatric comorbidity, see Chapter 2. Nonetheless, the nature of the overlap between pain and psychiatric syndromes has been largely overlooked by health professionals and biomedical researchers.

SCOPE OF THE OVERLAP

There is a wide overlap of chronic pain conditions and psychiatric disorders. Yet, most doctors, medical students, and other health professionals are unaware of it or are poorly equipped to manage it adequately. Most of the patients suffering from chronic pain syndromes will experience concomitantly one or several mental illnesses. Similarly, most patients affected by a mental illness experience pain. The scope of the overlap of pain and psychiatric disorders is broad. It appears that almost any psychiatric condition, including personality disorders, is in some way related to pain, and also the reverse: that chronic pain goes along with psychological suffering.

This book covers a wide range of psychiatric illnesses related to diverse chronic pain conditions. It studies this upsetting relationship among diverse groups such as adults, women, children, teenagers, and elderly people. The mental disorders covered include anxiety disorders, depressive disorders, PTSD, substance use and abuse, alcohol abuse, malingering, suicide, bipolar disorder, schizophrenia, sleep disorders, catastrophizing, somatization, personality disorders, self-injury, autism, intellectual disability, dementia, and a unique culture-bound syndrome of the Andes, called *Jaki*. Among the pain syndromes covered in this book are temporomandibular joint disorder, headache, abdominal pain, chest pain in teens, fibromyalgia, irritable bowel syndrome, cancer pain, vulvodynia, and urogenital pain. It also reviews the cultural dimension of overlapping pain and psychiatric disorders. It closes with a chapter on the potential of artificial intelligence in helping to address the clinical challenges of comorbid chronic pain and psychiatric disorders.

STIGMA, SHAME, AND SUFFERING

Stigma and shame are ubiquitous among patients suffering from mental illness or chronic pain, or both concomitantly. Stigma in society and within a health care organization underlies patients' avoidance or delay in seeking help and is a barrier to quality medical care.[22] Stereotypical negative views about mental illness become a mark of disgrace that affects patients in multiple ways. Despite decades-long efforts to educate the public, mental illness is still associated with negative beliefs of dangerousness, incompetence, and permanence. With the frequent mass shootings in the United States, the media wrongly portrays this violence as closely related to mental illness. Increasingly, citizens view mental illness as threatening. Numerous repercussions of stigma have been reported, including discrimination, unemployment, poor self-esteem, higher illness severity, poor adherence to care, and reduced global functioning. Higher stigma scores were found associated with higher severity of a mental disorder, higher unemployment, and poorer quality of life.[23]

In an interesting survey conducted at the Medical University of Vienna with 101 pain and psychiatric patients, the researchers found that 60% of them believed that most people would not allow a psychiatric patient to take care of their children, most young women would be reluctant to date a man who has been treated for a mental illness and most employers would pass over the application of a psychiatric patient in favor of another applicant, 50% thought that most people think less of a person who has been in a mental hospital, and over 50% of all participants believed that the general population thinks that psychiatric patients are "less intelligent, less trustworthy and that their opinion is taken less seriously by others."[24] In this study, "the fear of being stigmatized was more severe among somatoform pain patients as compared to patients suffering from epilepsy or dissociative disorders."

For patients suffering from chronic pain, the ordeal is similar; their perception that their pain experience is subjective ("not measurable or not objective") is a source of significant shame and distress. For Goldberg, the historical roots of stigma toward pain in society and within the medical setting are based on the 19th- and 20th-century ideas of mechanical objectivity and somaticism.[25]

As stated by Goldberg, ameliorating stigma is an ethical imperative. It is safe to assume that patients suffering from comorbid pain and psychiatric syndromes are more at risk for stigmatization than patients affected by other conditions, such as pulmonary, hematological, and cardiac diseases, among others. There is a need for research on stigma in this particular group of patients, who suffer from a dual burden of chronic pain and a mental disorder. Similarly, there is a need for educational programs to control stigma inside and outside the medical setting. Too many patients are enduring needless distress caused by the stigmatization of their pain or mental illness.

BIAS, DISPARITIES, AND INEQUITIES

Cross-cultural interactions can cause serious miscommunication with important clinical consequences.[26] In this era of globalization and worldwide migrations, the danger of miscommunication between ethnically discordant doctors and patients is imminent. Psychiatrists and pain medicine practitioners should be aware of their value system and be attentive to ethnic and racial biases, discrimination and disparities in care, and the spread of health inequities, which is ethically unacceptable.

In a study in the New England region of the United States, Bates found high expressiveness of pain among Latino patients, even among those who were adjusting well to their pain and considered they had a happy life. Interestingly, the researcher found that many American staff nurses believed their expressiveness to be inappropriate, especially in men. Referring to a male patient, one nurse said, "He starts to yell when I apply the alcohol swab—even before I put in the needle for the I.V. He looks so macho but he acts like a baby."[27]

When interactions between ethnically or culturally discordant doctors and patients unfold well, they are treated as "good" patients. In the United States and the United Kingdom, doctors appear to expect low expression of emotions and pain in their patients. In an interesting observation made in Britain by Bond, he says, "Any observant visitor to a hospital ward in Britain will become aware, sooner or later, that ability to endure pain with little or no complaint is admired and regarded as a highly desirable behavior. Pain sufferer's stoicism is rewarded with admiration, sympathy, and more material expressions of approval, notably the administration of pain-relieving medicines. In contrast, when patients are found overexpressive they will be viewed as complainers. Those patients who whine in pain, especially if regarded as excessive or unnecessary are punished by expressions of disapproval, both verbal and practical, in the form of withholding analgesics or the administration of placebo substances."[28] Thus, understanding patients' cultures and also being aware of psychiatrists' and pain practitioners' values, beliefs, and attitudes or biases related to pain, psychiatric disorders, and treatment choices are clinically useful.

Health professionals' stereotypical views about certain groups of patients or unconscious biases against them could result in disparities in access to care and quality of services, or could eventually become plain discrimination.[29] Bias and health disparities are widely present in multicultural societies. There is quite rich literature on ethnic minorities and disparities and inadequate treatments provided for a wide range of conditions. An entire book was recently published by Incayawar and Todd on the undertreatment of pain in diverse populations.[29] For example, African American and Latino patients in the United States seem two to three times more likely to receive inadequate pain treatment as Anglo-Americans.[18] In a recent postpartum pain management study with 9900 women, Hispanic women were 61% more likely to report pain scores of 5 or higher (out of 10), and black women were more than twice as likely to report high pain scores than white women. Despite reporting and experiencing higher pain severity, African American and Hispanic women were significantly less likely to receive an opioid prescription at discharge than white women.[30]

The practitioner should also be aware of the disparities in the prevalence of pain and psychiatric disorders among social and ethnic groups and their special needs. It is reasonable to anticipate that bias and disparities could be present and even be more severe among chronic pain patients who concomitantly suffer from a mental illness. The failure to consider bias and disparities in medical practice could eventually result in health inequities and social injustice.

THE FUTURE: PERSON-CENTERED AND PRECISION MEDICINE

The field of overlapping pain medicine and psychiatric disorders is brimming with possibilities. Recent advances in neurobiology, neurosciences, genetics, pharmacogenetics, epigenetics, psychotherapy, and even digital health, including telemedicine, electronic health records development, artificial intelligence, and machine learning, will translate into better quality medical care, more individualized medicine, and reduction of the societal burden of pain research and mental illness. It is encouraging that recently the National Institutes of Health launched a funding program on chronic pain comorbidities named "Research on Chronic Overlapping Pain Conditions" (Funding Opportunity Announcement Number PA-18-939). This book presents a spectrum of exciting new developments in research and clinical practice that will greatly benefit the practitioner who is willing to offer to their patients person-centered quality care.

Digital Medicine

New digital technologies, such as robotics, machine learning, and artificial intelligence, are already helping to improve health care service delivery to multiple organizations. Recently, the Department of Health and Human Services of North Carolina announced the implementation of a patient intake platform to screen new patients for social determinants of health. The digital platform is capable of sending in real-time alerts and analyses to clinicians and program administrators to quickly and reliably help link patients with the services they need. It is expected that the advance of digital technologies, machine learning, and the associated powerful algorithms will help clinicians in their daily clinical work and eventually allow them to offer more time and have a more humane encounter with their patients. Digital technologies should help practitioners to spend less time seeing their computer screens and more time looking at their patients while conducting a clinical interview.

Pharmacogenetics

Another field that promises to deeply transform clinical treatment in pain and psychiatry is pharmacogenetics and epigenetics. There is an agreement that health and disease are the outcomes of complex genes and environment interactions. This natural process is mediated by the DNA sequence and by epigenetic modifications that regulate the transcriptional capacity of genes.

Pharmacogenetics allows us to explore how patients from diverse cultural and ethnic backgrounds respond differently to medicines, including medicines used to control pain or treat mental disorders.[31–34] A recent study on clozapine underuse in treatment-resistant schizophrenia highlights the relevance of the ethnic dimension of psychopharmacology. The so-called Duffy-null or rs2814778 genotype is frequent among people of African descent. This genotype, more commonly known as *benign ethnic neutropenia*, causes confusion among physicians. The administration of clozapine is suspended prematurely because of the presence of neutropenia. Patients of African descent who are suffering from treatment-resistant schizophrenia are literally deprived of a helpful medicine. Now, the rs2814778 genotyping is being proposed as a pharmacogenetic test that could improve doctors' management of clozapine.[35,36]

Turning to pain, carbamazepine is an anticonvulsant molecule frequently used to treat trigeminal neuralgia and bipolar disorder. However, patients carrying the HLA B*15:02 variant of the HLA B complex gene (human leukocyte antigen) could develop a severe, even fatal skin rash called Stevens-Johnson syndrome/toxic epidermal necrolysis. People of Han Chinese ethnicity carry this gene variant and should not be administered carbamazepine. Although not well understood, cytotoxic T cells and natural killer cells appear to release granulysin that destroys cells in the skin and mucous membranes. The death of these cells causes the blistering and peeling that is characteristic of Stevens-Johnson syndrome. The US Food and Drug Administration recommends that all patients of Asian descent be tested for an HLA-B gene variant before initiating therapy to avoid carbamazepine-induced Stevens-Johnson syndrome/toxic epidermal necrolysis. Literacy in pharmacogenetics of psychotropics and medicines used in pain medicine could certainly help develop a practice of effective personalized medicine and precision psychiatry.[37]

Epigenetics

Epigenetic processes, including DNA methylation, microRNAs, and histone tail modifications, among others, affect gene expression without altering the DNA sequence. Epigenetics allows us to make the link between external environmental forces such as physical (e.g., diet, toxins, infections, exposure to chemical products) or psychosocial (e.g., early-life negative events, trauma, prenatal exposures to maternal mental illness or pain, social interactions) and genes.[38] Experiences, such as traumatic stress, do not alter the DNA sequence but can modify its functioning, leading to either enhanced or silenced expression of specific genes. Those epigenetic changes could affect the inner workings of genes, the production or inhibition of complex proteins, and consequently the emergence of disease and particular pharmacological treatment responses to pain and psychiatric medication.[34,39,40] A wonderful example, offered by nature, of epigenetics at play comes from honeybees. Genetically identical *Apis mellifera* larvae will develop into a fertile queen following feeding with a special diet of the royal jelly or will become a sterile honeybee worker with a regular diet. This nutritional manipulation induces DNA methylation that changes the expression of genes, produces a phenotype shift, and causes the final development of a queen.[41] Furthermore, epigenetic-wise interventions based on receiving positive social support may have the potential to blunt the negative effects of perilous genes and protect us against developing a mental disorder or chronic pain later in life.[42] Future epigenetic studies will trace the imprints of experience on our DNA and allow us to understand more about our environment and our vulnerabilities or resilience to pain and mental illness.

Education and Training

The education of future pain and psychiatric professionals is brimming with possibilities, too. Although the coverage of pain management and the care of the mentally ill is still weak in medical schools, pain fellowship programs are not only teaching students to examine, diagnose, and treat chronic pain (administrating regional nerve blocks and the pharmacological management of acute and chronic pain in both outpatient and inpatient settings) but also adding to their treatment armamentarium psychosocial therapies, including cognitive behavioral therapies. Young generations of mental health professionals and pain practitioners will be trained in a more person-centered approach to medical care.[43] In the mid-term, the education and training of doctors and other health professionals on overlapping pain and mental illness could adopt a "pan-omics" medical approach whereby multiple layers of biological data on an individual patient are explored. The layers that could be included in understanding the nature of a disease, as described by Eric Topol, are genomics, transcriptomics, proteomics, metabolomics, microbiomics, epigenomics, and exposomics.[44] The exposome will take into consideration all agents, physical and psychosocial, to which an individual patient has been exposed.

There is a great need to fathom overlapping pain and psychiatric syndromes. The physicians of the future will be doctors who consider their patients as human beings (i.e., not focusing just on patients' diseased organ or biological system) embedded in their physical and social environments. They will provide person-centered care, a biologically individualized/personalized therapy, and in so doing will practice a more precise medicine and psychiatry.

REFERENCES

1. Mackin P, Targum SD, Kalali A, Rom D, Young AH. Culture and assessment of manic symptoms. *Br J Psychiatry*. 2006;189:379–380.
2. Kessler RC, Berglund P, Demler O, Jin R, Walters EE. Lifetime prevalence and age-of-onset distributions of DSM-IV disorders in the National Comorbidity Survey Replication. *Arch Gen Psychiatry*. 2005;62(6):593–602.
3. Friedman RA. Uncovering an epidemic: Screening for mental illness in teens. *N Engl J Med*. 2006;355(26):2717–2719.
4. Demyttenaere K, Bruffaerts R, Posada-Villa J, et al. Prevalence, severity, and unmet need for treatment of mental disorders in the World Health Organization World Mental Health Surveys. *JAMA*. 2004;291(21):2581–2590.
5. McKenzie K, Patel V, Araya R. Learning from low-income countries: Mental health. *Br Med J*. 2004;329(7475):1138–1140.

6. Patel V, Saraceno B, Kleinman A. Beyond evidence: The moral case for international mental health. *Am J Psychiatry.* 2006;163(8):1312–1315.

7. Greenberg PE, Fournier AA, Sisitsky T, Pike CT, Kessler RC. The economic burden of adults with major depressive disorder in the United States (2005 and 2010). *J Clin Psychiatry.* 2015;76(2):155–162.

8. Trautmann S, Rehm J, Wittchen H-U. The economic costs of mental disorders. *EMBO Rep.* 2016;17(9):1245–1249.

9. James FR, Large RG, Bushnell JA, Wells JE. Epidemiology of pain in New Zealand. *Pain.* 1991;44(3):279–283.

10. Gureje O, Von Korff M, Simon GE, Gater R. Persistent pain and well-being: A World Health Organization study in primary care. *JAMA.* 1998;280(2):147–151.

11. US Department of Health and Human Services. *Management of Cancer Pain.* AHCPR Publication No. 94-0592. Rockville, MD: US Dept. of Health and Human Services, Public Health Service, Agency for Health Care Policy and Research; 1994.

12. Institute of Medicine (US) Committee on Advancing Pain Research Care and Education. *Relieving Pain in America: A Blueprint for Transforming Prevention, Care, Education, and Research.* Washington, DC: National Academies Press; 2011.

13. Osterweis M, Kleinman A, Mechanic D. *Pain and Disability: Clinical, Behavioral, and Public Policy Perspectives.* Washington, DC: National Academy Press; 1987.

14. Todd KH, Deaton C, D'Adamo AP, Goe L. Ethnicity and analgesic practice. *Ann Emerg Med.* 2000;35(1):11–16.

15. Bonham VL. Race, ethnicity, and pain treatment: Striving to understand the causes and solutions to the disparities in pain treatment. *J Law Med Ethics.* 2001;29(1):52–68.

16. Cleeland CS, Gonin R, Baez L, Loehrer P, Pandya KJ. Pain and treatment of pain in minority patients with cancer. The Eastern Cooperative Oncology Group Minority Outpatient Pain Study. *Ann Intern Med.* 1997;127(9):813–816.

17. Ng B, Dimsdale JE, Rollnik JD, Shapiro H. The effect of ethnicity on prescriptions for patient-controlled analgesia for postoperative pain. *Pain.* 1996;66(1):9–12.

18. Todd KH, Samaroo N, Hoffman JR. Ethnicity as a risk factor for inadequate emergency department analgesia. *JAMA.* 1993;269(12):1537–1539.

19. Brennan F, Carr DB, Cousins M. Pain management: A fundamental human right. *Anesth Analg.* 2007;105(1):205–221.

20. Reich J, Tupin JP, Abramowitz SI. Psychiatric diagnosis of chronic pain patients. *Am J Psychiatry.* 1983;140(11):1495–1498.

21. Sandbrink F. What is special about veterans in pain specialty care? *Pain Med.* 2017;18(4):623–625.

22. De P, Pozen A, Budhwani H. Is perceived stigma in clinical settings associated with poor health status among New York City's residents of color? *Med Care.* 2019;57(12):960–967.

23. Quenneville AF, Badoud D, Nicastro R, et al. Internalized stigmatization in borderline personality disorder and attention deficit hyperactivity disorder in comparison to bipolar disorder. *J Affect Disord.* 2020;262:317–322.

24. Freidl M, Spitzl SP, Prause W, et al. The stigma of mental illness: Anticipation and attitudes among patients with epileptic, dissociative or somatoform pain disorder. *Int Rev Psychiatry.* 2007;19(2):123–129.

25. Goldberg DS. Pain, objectivity and history: Understanding pain stigma. *Med Humanit*. 2017;43(4):238–243.
26. Bouchard L. A linguistic approach for understanding pain in the medical encounter. In: Incayawar M, Todd KH, eds. *Culture, Brain, and Analgesia: Understanding and Managing Pain in Diverse Populations*. New York, NY: Oxford University Press; 2013:9–19.
27. Bates MS. *Biocultural Dimensions of Chronic Pain: Implications for Treatment of Multi-ethnic Populations*. Albany, NY: State University of New York Press; 1996.
28. Bond MR. The suffering of severe intractable pain. In: Kosterlitz HW, Terenius LY, Merskey H, Dahlam K, eds. *Pain and Society: Report of the Dahlem Workshop on Pain and Society, Berlin 1979, November 26–30*. Weinheim, Germany: Verlag Chemie; 1980:53–62.
29. Incayawar M, Todd KH. *Culture, Brain, and Analgesia: Understanding and Managing Pain in Diverse Populations*. New York, NY: Oxford University Press; 2013.
30. Badreldin N, Grobman WA, Yee LM. Racial disparities in postpartum pain management. *Obstet Gynecol*. 2019;134(6):1147–1153.
31. Lee A, Gin T, Oh TE. Opioid requirements and responses in Asians. *Anaesth Intensive Care*. 1997;25(6):665–670.
32. Ng CH, Lin KM. *Ethno-Psychopharmacology: Advances in Current Practice*. Cambridge, UK: Cambridge University Press; 2008.
33. Lin KM, Poland RE, Wan YJ, Smith MW, Lesser IM. The evolving science of pharmacogenetics: Clinical and ethnic perspectives. *Psychopharmacol Bull*. 1996;32(2):205–217.
34. Incayawar M, Todd KH. Culture, pharmacogenomics, and personalized analgesia. In: Incayawar M, Todd KH, eds. *Culture, Brain, and Analgesia: Understanding and Managing Pain in Diverse Populations*. New York, NY: Oxford University Press; 2013:403–411.
35. Legge SE, Pardiñas AF, Helthuis M, et al. A genome-wide association study in individuals of African ancestry reveals the importance of the Duffy-null genotype in the assessment of clozapine-related neutropenia. *Mol Psychiatry*. 2019;24(3):328–337.
36. Dinardo CL, Kerbauy MN, Santos TC, et al. Duffy null genotype or Fy (a-b-) phenotype are more accurate than self-declared race for diagnosing benign ethnic neutropenia in Brazilian population. *Int J Lab Hematol*. 2017;39(6):e144–e146.
37. Hirschtritt ME, Besterman AD, Ross DA. Psychiatric pharmacogenomics: How close are we? *Biol Psychiatry*. 2016;80(8):e63–e65.
38. Oberlander TF, Weinberg J, Papsdorf M, Grunau R, Misri S, Devlin AM. Prenatal exposure to maternal depression, neonatal methylation of human glucocorticoid receptor gene (NR3C1) and infant cortisol stress responses. *Epigenetics*. 2008;3(2):97–106.
39. Gluckman PD, Hanson MA, Cooper C, Thornburg KL. Effect of in utero and early-life conditions on adult health and disease. *N Engl J Med*. 2008;359(1):61–73.
40. Doehring A, Geisslinger G, Lotsch J. Epigenetics in pain and analgesia: An imminent research field. *Eur J Pain*. 2011;15(1):11–16.
41. Kucharski R, Maleszka J, Foret S, Maleszka R. Nutritional control of reproductive status in honeybees via DNA methylation. *Science*. 2008;319(5871):1827–1830.

42. Kaufman J, Yang B-Z, Douglas-Palumberi H, et al. Social supports and serotonin transporter gene moderate depression in maltreated children. *Proc Natl Acad Sci U S A*. 2004;101(49):17316–17321.

43. Karp JF. Pain medicine fellows need explicit training in engaging patients in patient-centered pain management. *Pain Med*. 2012;13(8):985–986.

44. Topol EJ. Individualized medicine from prewomb to tomb. *Cell*. 2014;157(1):241–253.

2

Recognizing the Co-occurrence of Chronic Pain and Mental Illness

JAN JARACZ ■

INTRODUCTION

Chronic pain commonly co-occurs with psychiatric disorders. The close bidirectional relationship between pain and depression was discovered by artists and writers long before the publication of the first epidemiological studies. This phenomenon was persuasively demonstrated by Frida Kahlo in her 1944 painting entitled, "*La Columna Rota*" ("Broken Column"). In this self-portrait, pain is expressed by metal nails stuck into her face and whole body, while depression is expressed by tears in her eyes. On the basis of his personal experience, William Styron, in his book *Darkness Visible: A Memoir of Madness* (p. 26, Open Road media New York 2010) (first published in 1990), gave an accurate description of the co-occurrence of depression and pain; he wrote: "Mysteriously and in ways that are totally remote from natural experience, the gray drizzle of horror induced by depression takes on the quality of physical pain."

It has been showed that psychiatric disorders co-occurring with pain are frequent medical problems. Moreover, a growing body of literature has shown that psychiatric comorbidity, particularly depression and anxiety, is common in people suffering from pain and, conversely, that painful symptoms are common in persons with major depression, anxiety disorders, and other psychiatric disorders.

EPIDEMIOLOGY OF CHRONIC PAIN

Epidemiological data from a large-scale survey conducted in 15 European countries and Israel showed that 19% of 46,394 respondents had suffered from pain of moderate or severe intensity that had a serious, negative impact on their daily activities and their social and working lives. The results of this study showed that 21% of those who suffered from pain fulfilled the diagnostic criteria of depression.[1] In another telephone survey conducted in the United Kingdom, Germany, Italy, Portugal, and Spain ($N = 18, 980$), 17.1% of respondents reported having at least one painful physical condition.[2]

Similar results were obtained by Reid at al. using systematic review principles in searching and summarizing the results of 45 studies conducted in Europe. The 1-month prevalence of moderate to severe, noncancer chronic pain was 19%.[3]

Recently, Jackson et al. published a systematic review and meta-analysis of 122 publications investigating the prevalence of pain in 28 low-income and middle-income countries. The results of this study showed that the prevalence of any type of chronic pain in the general adult population was 33%. Higher rates (56%) were found in the elderly population.[4] In primary care patients, 30% of visits were related to pain.[5] This rate was significantly higher (73.5%) in the population of patients aged 65 years and older.[6]

EPIDEMIOLOGY OF DEPRESSION

The World Health Organization ranks depression as the fourth leading cause of disability worldwide,[7] and by 2020, it will probably be the second leading cause.[8]

Recent data on the epidemiology of depression from 18 high-income and low- to middle-income countries were obtained using the World Health Organization Composite International Diagnostic Interview (CIDI). This study showed that 14.6% of the population studied in 10 high-income countries and 11.1% from 8 low- to middle-income countries fulfilled lifetime diagnostic criteria of a *Diagnostic and Statistical Manual of Mental Disorders*, fourth edition (DSM-IV) major depressive episode (MDE). The 12-month prevalences of MDE have been estimated as 5.5% and 5.9% in high-income and low- to middle-income countries, respectively.[9]

In Spain, 14.3% of patients in primary care fulfilled the DSM-IV diagnostic criteria for major depression and 4.8% for dysthymia.[10]

The disability-adjusted life year (DALY) is a single measure to quantify the burden of diseases, injuries, and risk factors. Major depression and low back pain were classified as two leading causes of years lost due to disability (YLD) at the global level in 2000 and 2011. Chronic pain is a common comorbid condition associated with 20 other leading causes of YLD, including diabetes mellitus, osteoarthritis, migraine, and road injury.[11]

It is clear, therefore, that both pain and depression are among the most commonly prevalent medical conditions in medical practice.

DEPRESSION IN CHRONIC PAIN

The prevalence of depression in populations of patients with chronic pain has been a focus of interest since the 1960s. In 2003, Bair et al.[12] elaborated a review of studies examining pain and depression comorbidity. The authors identified 42 papers published between 1966 and 2002 that reported investigations conducted in different settings. They found the presence of depression in 52% (range, 1.5–100%) of patients in pain clinics and inpatient pain programs, in 56% (21–89%) of patients in rheumatology and orthopedic clinics, and in as many as 85% (35–100%) of patients of dental clinics. In primary care, 27% (5.9–46%) of patients had concomitant symptoms of depression. The occurrence of depression was higher in patients with multiple pain locations and a chronic course of pain. Furthermore, the severity of pain was also correlated with the higher prevalence of depression. The results of this study provided strong evidence that depression has a negative impact on the severity of a painful condition, its duration, and its chronicity. It can be seen that there is a significant variation in the rates of depression in different populations of patients with pain. This probably is related to the diversity of methodological approaches employed, including the methods of identification of depression and assessment of pain used. Nevertheless, this review gave clear evidence that the prevalence of depression in subjects with pain is significantly higher than that in the general population, where 12-month prevalence estimates are 6%.

The results of a large computer-assisted telephone interview survey conducted in Europe showed that 21% of respondents with chronic pain had been previously diagnosed with depression.[1]

More recent studies focusing on specific populations of patients with pain confirmed a high comorbidity with depression. In persons with chronic headache and migraine, the prevalence of depression was 2.2 to 4.0 times higher than that found in the general population.[13] The results of a meta-analysis published in 2016 by Tran et al. demonstrated that depression, together with other emotional disturbances, is also a common problem in patients with pain due to a spinal cord injury.[14]

Pain is a common medical problem in older people. The 2-year English Longitudinal Study of Aging enrolled 3654 adults who were 65 years and older. At baseline, one-third of this population (30.1%) reported moderate or severe pain. Interestingly, the presence of pain at baseline was an independent risk predictor for depression developing 2 years later (odds ratio [OR] = 1.54; 95% confidence interval [CI] = 1.19–2.0). Conversely, depression at baseline was an independent risk factor for the occurrence of pain after 2 years. Older age, female gender, lower education, poor vision, higher mobility disability, lower activities of daily living (ADLs), smoking, and a more negative interaction with family members at baseline were identified as independent predictors of depression at the 2-year follow-up.[15]

Several factors may increase the probability of the presence of depression in patients with pain. For example, basic ADLs, such as social isolation and basic education only, play a role as mediatory factors between depression and pain in elderly people.[16]

Depression is considered the strongest risk factor for suicide. An interesting review published by Hasset et al. demonstrated that chronic pain appears to be an important risk factor for suicide as well.[17] The risk for suicide was higher in almost all pain conditions, except arthritis and neuropathy. However, the risk reached statistical significance only in back pain (hazard ratio [HR] = 1.13), migraine (HR = 1.34), and psychogenic pain (HR = 1.58). The increased risk for suicide in patients with pain was also correlated with the presence of depression and substance use.

PAIN IN MAJOR DEPRESSION

In a multinational, cross-sectional telephone survey of a random sample of 18,980 people from five European countries, major depressive disorder (MDD) was diagnosed in 4.0%. A significant proportion (43.4%) of the subjects with MDD reported having at least one chronic painful physical condition. This proportion was four times higher than that in the remaining sample.[18]

The second aim of the literature review by Bair et al. was to assess the prevalence of pain in patients with depression.[12] On the basis of their review of 14 studies published between 1957 and 2003, the authors demonstrated that the mean prevalence of pain in different populations of patients with depression was 65% (range, 15–100%). The discrepancy among the results of the studies reviewed is due to the different methodological approaches used, including the diagnosis of depression, the definitions of the pain condition, and the diverse methods of pain assessment.

These observations were confirmed subsequently by several large studies. In a cross-sectional, population-based study of noninstitutionalized adults in six European countries, the frequency of reporting painful symptoms in respondents with major depression was 50%, which was almost twice that in a population without depressive symptomatology.[19] In their more recent multinational, longitudinal study, Factors Influencing Depression Endpoints Research (FINDER), Demyttenaere et al. in 2010 evaluated pain severity and the interference of pain with daily functioning in outpatients with depression during 6 months observation. Moderate to severe pain was defined as a score higher than 30 on the Visual Analog Scale (VAS). In a population of 3308 patients, 56.3% met this criterion at baseline.[20] Further evidence confirming a close relationship between pain and depression was demonstrated by Kroenke et al.[21] In their 12-month longitudinal study, it was shown that a preceding change in pain severity was a strong predictor of subsequent depression severity and, conversely, that a preceding change in depression severity was a strong predictor of subsequent pain severity. The presence of both conditions is related to greater disability, increased health care use, and a poorer treatment response compared with the presence of either condition alone. The Spanish multicenter, cross-sectional study was aimed at estimating the prevalence of pain in depressive patients (mostly with major depression and dysthymia) who were under the care of psychiatrists in their regular practice.[22] The severity of pain symptoms was evaluated at the time of the study using the VAS. Among the 3566 patients enrolled in this study, 2107 (59.1%) reported pain. In another survey, a secondary analysis of data from a Sequenced Treatment Alternatives to Relieve Depression study (STAR*D) confirmed a high prevalence of pain in 3745 depressed outpatients. As many as 77% of the patients involved in this study met the criteria for having pain.[23]

The results of these studies provide important information for practitioners, who should carefully investigate pain in depressed patients as well as depression in subjects with chronic pain in order to improve the quality of care.

The studies cited earlier provide further interesting information regarding demographic and clinical correlates of pain. The probability of the presence of pain in depressed patients is correlated with several demographic factors listed in Table 2.1.

Certain symptoms of major depression, such as anhedonia, sleep problems, depressed mood, and loss of energy,[22] as well as anxiety and melancholic features,[23] were also associated with the severity of painful symptoms. Several clinical features of depression are also correlated with pain intensity (Table 2.2).

Table 2.1 DEMOGRAPHIC CORRELATES OF PAIN IN
DEPRESSED PATIENTS

	Factor	References
1	Being female	18, 20, 22
2	Having fewer years of education	23
3	Being unemployed	18, 20, 23
4	Being older	20, 22

Painful symptoms in depression constitute a group of nonhomogenous phenomena, challenging a careful differential diagnosis. Frequently, pain in depression is a manifestation of a concomitant medical condition. However, it may also represent unexplained painful physical symptoms occurring during a depressive episode. In the FINDER study, it was reported that, in a group of depressed patients with moderate/severe pain, 29.9% had a current painful medical condition. Moreover, 51.1% of these patients were diagnosed with a current chronic medical condition.[20] In a Spanish study, the proportion of patients with pain, but without documented physical explanation for that pain, was estimated as 42.8%.[22]

The presence of painful symptoms has a varied clinical and economic impact on depressive patients. Depressed patients presenting with symptoms of somatization, including painful somatic symptoms, had a lower probability of correct diagnosis of depression.[24] This effect is probably seen because patients with depression and concomitant painful symptoms were more likely to concentrate on, and to report, somatic symptoms and, therefore, to use general medical services rather than visiting a mental health specialist compared with patients with depression without pain.[25] In accordance with these data, Demyttenaere et al. demonstrated that in persons with MDD and coexisting pain, rates of help-seeking for emotional symptoms were lower, and its initiation was delayed.[19] It has also been showed in a large body of literature that the presence of symptoms of pain at baseline is associated with a worse response to antidepressants[26,27] and a longer time to remission.[23,28–30] These observations were confirmed recently by Fishbain et al.[31] on the basis of the

Table 2.2 RELATIONSHIP BETWEEN PAIN INTENSITY AND CLINICAL FEATURES
OF DEPRESSION

	Clinical feature	References
1	Greater baseline severity of depressive symptoms	20, 22, 23
2	Number of concomitant medical conditions	20, 23
3	Higher body mass index (BMI)	20
4	Severity of nonpainful somatic symptoms of depression	20
5	Greater disability	21

results of an evidence-based structured review of 17 studies. Furthermore, painful symptoms in depression have a significant impact on functioning in daily activities[20] and lead to poorer outcomes in multiple domains of health-related quality of life.[26]

The presence of painful physical symptoms in depression considerably increases the economic burden related to lost work time and health care resource use compared with the presence of depression alone.[32] In addition, an additive effect of depression and painful physical symptoms on lost work days was found.[19] Gameroff and Olson[33] estimated that the medical care charges of patients with major depression, and at least moderate pain-related interference, were at least twice those for depressed patients with little or no pain-related interference. Clearly, the occurrence of pain in depression has a disadvantageous impact on clinical course, response to treatment, and economics.

PAIN AND BIPOLAR DISORDER

A growing interest in pain in bipolar disorder (BD) has been noted in recent years. It has been demonstrated that chronic multisite pain commonly co-occurs with mood disorders, particularly BD.[34] Almost half (46%) of 740 primary care patients with BD in the Washington State Mental Health Integration Program[35] received current treatment for a pain condition or reported regular pain interfering with daily functioning. A recent meta-analysis of 22 cross-sectional studies indicated that about one-fourth of individuals with BD experienced chronic pain. Compared with control subjects, the relative risk of pain in this population was 2.14 times higher.[36]

FUNCTIONAL SOMATIC SYNDROMES

The comorbidity of pain and depression is also a common problem in functional somatic syndromes such as fibromyalgia and irritable bowel syndrome (IBS).

Fibromyalgia affects 2% of the population and is more prevalent in females (3.4%) than in males (0.5%).[37] According to epidemiological data, 62 to 86% of patients with fibromyalgia meet DSM-IV diagnostic criteria for major depression. The presence of depression was associated with higher pain perception, lower quality of life, and the presence of more severe life events.[38] IBS is a frequently diagnosed gastrointestinal disorder in clinical practice. This functional disorder is characterized by, among other things, abdominal pain or discomfort associated with bowel habit alterations. Depression is one of the more common psychiatric comorbidities affecting one-third of patients with IBS, and pain is a common clinical feature.[39]

Evidence supports the hypothesis suggesting the existence of an epidemiological, clinical, and biological overlap between FM, IBS, and depression and pain.[40]

PAIN AND ANXIETY DISORDERS

Several seminal studies suggest that there is also a strong relationship between anxiety disorders and chronic pain. The results of cross-national, population-based surveys conducted in 17 countries (N = 85,088) revealed that, in patients with neck and back pain compared with those without these conditions, the pooled OR for anxiety disorders was 2.2 [95% CI = 2.1–2.4]. The highest OR (2.7) was shown for generalized anxiety disorder.[41] In a study conducted in the United States, a strong association of chronic spinal pain and anxiety disorders was reported as well.[42] In another study of 100 consecutive patients attending a pain clinic, diagnostic criteria of any anxiety disorders in the past 12 months were met by 25%, whereas 37% of this population had symptoms of major depression.[43] This finding suggests that the prevalence of anxiety disorders in patients with chronic spinal pain is six times higher than that in the general population. Interestingly, in the majority of subjects (77%), anxiety disorders preceded the onset of pain, compared with only 37% among patients with mood disorders. The presence of anxiety disorders was associated with pain intensity. The biological mechanism of this association is not fully understood.

The opposite approach was applied in a study of 416 psychiatric inpatients who were examined using a brief pain inventory. One-third of them (31%) reported substantial pain. Among the psychiatric diagnoses, the highest prevalence of pain (49%) was detected in women with post-traumatic stress disorder.[44]

Results of these studies provide relevant cues for clinicians. In the management of patients with chronic pain, the presence of comorbid anxiety disorders should be considered throughout the diagnostic process.

FINAL REMARKS

Epidemiological data provide consistent evidence of the co-occurrence of pain and psychiatric disorders. Depression in painful physical conditions and painful symptoms in depression constitute a common comorbidity. Also, a significant proportion of patients with bipolar disorder have pain complaints.

An association between chronic pain and anxiety disorders has also been well-documented. In all clinical situations, an additive adverse impact of one condition on several aspects of the other has been established. This information is very important for all those practitioners who take care of patients with pain and psychiatric disorders. To improve medical care, patients with chronic pain should be screened for comorbid psychiatric disorders, and conversely, those with psychiatric disorders should be monitored for painful symptoms. Where a dual diagnosis exists, effective models of management should be applied.

REFERENCES

1. Breivik H, Collett B, Ventafridda V, Cohen R, Gallacher D. Survey of chronic pain in Europe: Prevalence, impact on daily life, and treatment. *Eur J Pain.* 2006;10:287–333.
2. Ohayon MM, Schatzberg AF. Using chronic pain to predict depressive morbidity in the general population. *Arch Gen Psychiatry.* 2003;60:39–47.
3. Reid KJ, Harker J, Bala MM, et al. Epidemiology of chronic non-cancer pain in Europe: Narrative review of prevalence, pain treatments and pain impact. *J Curr Med Res Opin.* 2011;27:449–462.
4. Jackson T, Thomas S, Stabile V, Han X, Shotwell M, McQueen K. Prevalence of chronic pain in low-income and middle-income countries: A systematic review and meta-analysis. *Lancet.* 2015;27(385)(suppl 2):S1.
5. Hasselström J, Liu-Palmgren J, Rasjö-Wrååk G. Prevalence of pain in general practice. *Eur J Pain.* 2002;6:375–385.
6. Miró J, Paredes S, Rull M, et al. Pain in older adults: A prevalence study in the Mediterranean region of Catalonia. *Eur J Pain.* 2007;11:83–92.
7. Murray CJ, Lopez AD. Evidence-based health policy: Lessons from the Global Burden of Disease Study. *Science.* 1996;274(5288):740–743.
8. Murray CJL, Lopez AD, eds. The Global Burden of Disease: A Comprehensive Assessment of Mortality and Disability From Diseases, Injuries, and Risk Factors in 1990 and Projected to 2020. Cambridge, MA: Harvard University Press; 1996.
9. Bromet E, Andrade LH, Hwang I, et al. Cross-national epidemiology of DSM-IV major depressive episode. *BMC Med.* 2011;9:90.
10. Aragonès E, Piñol JL, Labad A, Masdéu RM, Pino M, Cervera J. Prevalence and determinants of depressive disorders in primary care practice in Spain. *Int J Psychiatry Med.* 2004;34:21–35.
11. Department of Health Statistics and Information Systems. *WHO Methods and Data Sources for Global Burden of Disease Estimates 2000–2011.* WHO, Geneva: World Health Organization; November 2013.
12. Bair MJ, Robinson RL, Katon W, Kroenke K. Depression and pain comorbidity: A literature review. *Arch Intern Med.* 2003;163:2433–2445.
13. Pompili M, Di Cosimo D, Innamorati M, Lester D, Tatarelli R, Martelletti P. Psychiatric comorbidity in patients with chronic daily headache and migraine: A

selective overview including personality traits and suicide risk. *J Headache Pain.* 2009;10:283–290.

14. Tran J, Dorstyn DS, Burke AL. Psychosocial aspects of spinal cord injury pain: A meta-analysis. *Spinal Cord.* 2016;54:640–648.

15. Chou KL. Reciprocal relationship between pain and depression in older adults: Evidence from the English longitudinal study of ageing. *J Affect Disord.* 2007;102:115–123.

16. Iliffe S, Kharicha K, Carmaciu C, et al. The relationship between pain intensity and severity and depression in older people: Exploratory study. *BMC Fam Pract.* 2009;10:54.

17. Hassett AL, Aquino JK, Ilgen MA. The risk of suicide mortality in chronic pain patients. *Curr Pain Headache Rep.* 2014;18:436.

18. Ohayon MM, Schatzberg AF. Using chronic pain to predict depressive morbidity in the general population. *Arch Gen Psychiatry.* 2003;60:39–47.

19. Demyttenaere K, Bonnewyn A, Bruffaerts R, Brugha T, De Graaf R, Alonso J. Comorbid painful physical symptoms and depression: Prevalence, work loss, and help seeking. *J Affect Disord.* 2006;92:185–193.

20. Demyttenaere K, Reed C, Quail D, et al. Presence and predictors of pain in depression: Results from the FINDER study. *J Affect Disord.* 2010;125:53–60.

21. Kroenke K, Wu J, Bair MJ, Krebs EE, Damush TM, Tu W. Reciprocal relationship between pain and depression: A 12-month longitudinal analysis in primary care. *J Pain.* 2011;12:964–973.

22. Agüera-Ortiz L, Failde I, Mico JA, Cervilla J, López-Ibor JJ. Pain as a symptom of depression: Prevalence and clinical correlates in patients attending psychiatric clinics. *J Affect Disord.* 2011;130:106–112.

23. Leuchter AF, Husain MM, Cook IA, et al. Painful physical symptoms and treatment outcome in major depressive disorder: A STAR*D (Sequenced Treatment Alternatives to Relieve Depression) report. *Psychol Med.* 2010;40:239–251.

24. Kirmayer LJ, Robbins JM, Dworkind M, Yaffe MJ. Somatization and the recognition of depression and anxiety in primary care. *Am J Psychiatry.* 1993;150:734–741.

25. Bao Y, Sturm R, Croghan TW. A national study of the effect of chronic pain on the use of health care by depressed persons. *Psychiatr Serv.* 2003;54:693–697.

26. Bair MJ, Robinson RL, Eckert GJ, Stang PE, Croghan TW, Kroenke K. Impact of pain on depression treatment response in primary care. *Psychosom Med.* 2004;66:17–22.

27. Kroenke K, Shen J, Oxman TE, Williams JW Jr, Dietrich AJ. Impact of pain on the outcomes of depression treatment: Results from the RESPECT trial. *Pain.* 2008;134:209–215.

28. Karp JF, Scott J, Houck P, Reynolds CF 3rd, Kupfer DJ, Frank E. Pain predicts longer time to remission during treatment of recurrent depression. *J Clin Psychiatry.* 2005;66:591–597.

29. Fuller-Thomson E, Battiston M, Gadalla TM, Brennenstuhl S. Bouncing back: Remission from depression in a 12-year panel study of a representative Canadian community sample. *Soc Psychiatry Psychiatr Epidemiol.* 2014;49:903–910.

30. Greco T, Eckert G, Kroenke K. The outcome of physical symptoms with treatment of depression. *J Gen Intern Med.* 2004;19:813–818.

31. Fishbain DA, Cole B, Lewis JE, Gao J. Does pain interfere with antidepressant depression treatment response and remission in patients with depression and pain? An evidence-based structured review. *Pain Med.* 2014;15:1522–1539.
32. Greenberg PE, Leong SA, Birnbaum HG, Robinson RL. The economic burden of depression with painful symptoms. *J Clin Psychiatry.* 2003;64(suppl 7):17–23.
33. Gameroff MJ, Olfson M. Major depressive disorder, somatic pain, and health care costs in an urban primary care practice. *J Clin Psychiatry.* 2006;67:1232–1239.
34. Nicholl BI, Mackay D, Cullen B, et al. Chronic multisite pain in major depression and bipolar disorder: Cross-sectional study of 149,611 participants in UK Biobank. *BMC Psychiatry.* 2014;14:350.
35. Cerimele JM, Chan YF, Chwastiak LA, Unutzer J. Pain in primary care patients with bipolar disorder. *Gen Hosp Psychiatry.* 2014;36:228.
36. Stubbs B, Eggermont L, Mitchell AJ, et al. The prevalence of pain in bipolar disorder: A systematic review and large-scale meta-analysis. *Acta Psychiatr Scand.* 2015;131:75–88.
37. Wolfe F, Ross K, Anderson J, Russell IJ, Hebert L. The prevalence and characteristics of fibromyalgia in the general population. *Arthritis Rheum.* 1995;38:19–28.
38. Aguglia A, Salvi V, Maina G, Rossetto I, Aguglia E. Fibromyalgia syndrome and depressive symptoms: Comorbidity and clinical correlates. *J Affect Disord.* 2011;128:262–266.
39. Creed F, Ratcliffe J, Fernandes L, et al. Outcome in severe irritable bowel syndrome with and without accompanying depressive, panic and neurasthenic disorders. *Br J Psychiatry.* 2005;186:507–515.
40. Goldenberg DL. Pain/depression dyad: A key to a better understanding and treatment of functional somatic syndrome. *Am J Med.* 2010;123:675–682.
41. Demyttenaere K, Bruffaerts R, Lee S, et al. Mental disorders among persons with chronic back or neck pain: Results from the World Mental Health Surveys. *Pain.* 2007;129:332–342.
42. Von Korff M, Crane P, Lane M, et al. Chronic spinal pain and physical-mental comorbidity in the United States: Results from the National Comorbidity Survey Replication. *Pain.* 2005;113:331–339.
43. Knaster P, Karlsson H, Estlander AM, Kalso E. Psychiatric disorders as assessed with SCID in chronic pain patients: The anxiety disorders precede the onset of pain. *Gen Hosp Psychiatry.* 2012;34:46–52.
44. Greggersen W, Rudolf S, Findel C, et al. Pain complaints in a sample of psychiatric inpatients. *Gen Hosp Psychiatry.* 2010;32:509–513.

3

Glial Cells and Pro-inflammatory Cytokines as Shared Neurobiological Bases for Chronic Pain and Psychiatric Disorders

JUDITH A. STRONG, SANG WON JEON, JUN-MING ZHANG, AND YONG-KU KIM ■

INTRODUCTION

In this chapter, we discuss the role of cytokines and glial cells in psychiatric and chronic pain disorders. The key points of the chapter are highlighted in Box 3.1. Cytokines are small secreted proteins that were originally defined by their roles in signaling between immune cells, but it is now known that other cell types may synthesize and respond to cytokines. In particular, neurons and glial cells release cytokines and express cytokine receptors; cytokines are one important mechanism of communication between neurons, glia, and immune cells. Long-lasting changes in properties of neurons and glia play key roles, and often very similar roles, in both psychiatric disorders and chronic pain states. Cytokines mediate some of these long-lasting changes. The broad term *cytokine* includes many subtypes, such as chemokines (originally defined by their ability to cause chemotaxis of immune cells), interleukins (originally defined by their role in signaling from one leukocyte to another), and interferons (originally defined by their role in interfering with viral replication). We will focus here on some of the better studied cytokines that have been implicated in pain and psychiatry; others have provided a more comprehensive review of additional cytokines.[1–4]

Box 3.1

KEY CONCEPTS

- Neuroinflammation (including activation of glial cells and release of cytokines) plays an important role in psychiatric disorders and chronic pain.
- An increase in molecules associated with type 1 inflammation, and decrease in type 2 anti-inflammatory mediators, have been particularly implicated in psychiatric and pain disorders.
- Cytokines and their receptors, first described in the immune system, are also produced by neurons and glial cells.
- Cytokines play key roles in communication between neurons and glia.
- Cytokines and activated glia are observed throughout the nervous system, from the peripheral nerve endings to the sensory ganglia, spinal cord, and brain.
- Many cytokines implicated in psychiatric disorders, especially depression, are also implicated in chronic pain.

Cytokines are often characterized as pro-inflammatory and anti-inflammatory, though it is perhaps more accurate to refer to these as type 1 and type 2 cytokines. Generally, in the periphery, type 1 or classical inflammation includes tissue destruction, nitric oxide production, M1 polarized macrophages, and Th1 T cells. Type 2 inflammation, which includes Th2 cells, M2 polarized macrophages, eosinophils, and the cytokines, sometimes referred to as anti-inflammatory (because they oppose type 1 inflammation), is involved with tissue remodeling, wound healing, and combatting multicellular parasites. In the context of this chapter, the type 2 inflammation is often considered "good" inflammation, but these processes may also play a pathological role, for example, in allergy and fibrosis.[5,6]

Neuroinflammation is an important concept throughout the chapter. Originally, inflammation was described as the immune response to stimuli such as pathogens or tissue damage, with the characteristic signs of heat, pain, redness, and swelling as memorized by every medical student. Acute inflammation is essential to protecting the body from pathogens and tissue damage, but chronic peripheral inflammation can be one cause of chronic pain. It is now known that many of the same immune molecules are elevated within nerve tissues in a process referred to as *neuroinflammation*, often without actual pathogens being present. In peripheral nerves, infiltration of immune cells, activation of resident immune cells, and immune-like responses of Schwann cells contribute to chronic pain conditions, including those defined as "neuropathic" (i.e., due to nerve damage).[7] In the central nervous system (CNS), microglia play the role of resident immune cells. In addition to playing a role supporting neurons in normal brain tissue, microglia are activated to help remove pathogens or other harmful molecules from the brain. However, their prolonged activation contributes to neurodegenerative diseases[8] as well as psychiatric disorders (discussed in the next section, "Role of Glia and Cytokines in Psychiatric Disorders"). Neuroinflammation in the spinal cord contributes to chronic pain states (discussed later in the section, "Preclinical Studies: Role of Glia and Cytokines in Chronic Pain"). Although the CNS has a blood–brain barrier and was long considered an immune-privileged site, infiltration of immune cells from the periphery is now known to contribute to neuroinflammation in some conditions.[8] Such neuroinflammation in the CNS is observed, for example, in chronic psychological stress, physical stress, infection, Alzheimer disease, and (as discussed in the next section) psychiatric disorders. In the peripheral sensory ganglia (dorsal root ganglia [DRG]), satellite glial cells surrounding the neuronal cell bodies share some properties with microglial cells and become activated in and contribute to various pain states.[9] Hence, at every level of the nervous system, neuroinflammation, glial cell activation, and cytokine release can occur as a normal protective mechanism or as a mediator of pathological conditions.

ROLE OF GLIA AND CYTOKINES IN PSYCHIATRIC DISORDERS

Allostasis and Neuroinflammation

Humans resist or adapt to internal and external stimuli. This process is called "allostasis," and if the allostatic load exceeds the manageable range, the "default mode," which is an existing equilibrium state, is adjusted. After the default mode is changed, even though the stimuli are lost, it is not restored to the original state.[10] According to the perspective of psychoneuroimmunology, which has rapidly developed of late, neuroinflammation is the most important element of allostasis, and various results occur depending on the degree, region, and duration of the neuroinflammatory response. In particular, the change in the default mode, while homeostasis is not maintained because of chronic inflammation, has been cited as an important underlying cause of psychiatric illness.[11] As a result, studies measuring the neuroinflammatory changes in various psychiatric disorders, such as depression, anxiety disorder, schizophrenia, and neurodegenerative diseases, have been actively conducted, and the link between physical illnesses (e.g., pain, medical conditions) and psychiatric disorders has also been interpreted in the context of neuroinflammation.

In particular, depression is the disorder most likely to result from a change in the CNS caused by the dysfunction of the immune system (Figure 3.1). Depression manifests many of the symptoms of sickness behaviors appearing in the inflamed state, and increase of the inflammatory proteins, including the pro-inflammatory cytokines and C-reactive protein (CRP), is commonly observed in patients with depression. Recent studies suggested that the abnormalities in the immune system due to internal stress (e.g., infection, inflammation, and internal psychological stressors) or external stress (e.g., painful stimuli, cold temperature, and stressful psychological environments) play an important role in the expression and continuance of depressive symptoms in vulnerable individuals.[12,13] Moreover, the cytokines can regulate activity of the two biological systems that are most closely associated with the pathophysiology of depression: the hypothalamic-pituitary-adrenal (HPA) axis and the catecholamine/sympathetic nervous system (Figure 3.2).[14]

Abnormalities of the Neuroglial Cells in Psychiatric Disorders (Depression)

The neuroglial cells account for 90% of the cells existing in the CNS and consist primarily of oligodendrocytes, astrocytes, and microglia. Such cells provide metabolic support for neurons, regulate synaptic plasticity, and act as immune cells secreting cytokines.

According to the findings of various studies in which brain autopsy was conducted in patients with depression, the number of neuroglial cells decreased in the cortex of the CNS.[15] In particular, decrease of the neuroglial cells was remarkably observed in the prefrontal and cingulate cortices. Among the neuroglial cells, the association between the astrocytes and mood disorders is known to be greater. It has been established that glial fibrillary acid protein (GFAP), a known marker of astrocytes, decreases in the cerebral cortex and limbic system of animal models and patients with depression.[16,17] In the peripheral blood, as the depressive symptoms become more severe, the expression of the marker of neuroglial cell degeneration, S100 calcium-binding protein B (S100B protein), increases, and the expression of S100B protein decreases after the administration of antidepressants.[18] The region where a change in the neuroglial cells is most clearly observed in the CNS of patients with depression is the prefrontal cortex.[19] Additionally, it has been shown that the density of astrocytes and the expression of GFAP in the amygdala and cerebellum of patients with depression decrease compared with those of patients

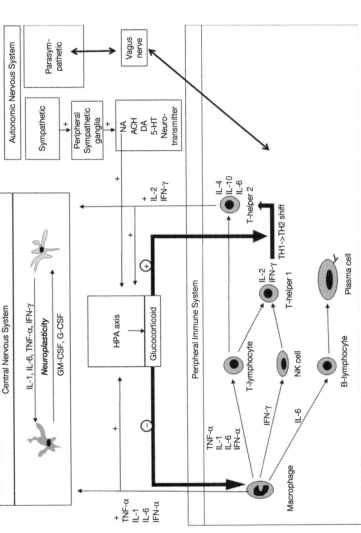

Figure 3.1. The role of the cytokine network in depression in connection with the immune system, hypothalamic-pituitary-adrenal (HPA) axis), and autonomic nerve system (ANS). The diagram shows communication between the peripheral and central cytokine system. Early innate pro-inflammatory cytokines released by macrophages (tumor necrosis factor-α [TNF-α], interleukin-1 [IL-1], IL-6, and interferon-α [IFN-α]), and later produced T-cell cytokines (IL-2 and IFN-γ) stimulate glucocorticoid secretion by acting at the HPA axis. Glucocorticoids provide negative feedback to the peripheral immune system to suppress the production of pro-inflammatory cytokines. Glucocorticoids also play an important role in causing a shift from cellular (T-helper 1 [TH1]) to humoral (TH2) immune responses. Central cytokines (IL-1, IL-6, TNF-α, and IFN-γ) secreted from astrocytes or microglia are considered to be involved in brain neuroplasticity. The ANS also regulates peripheral cytokine production. The parasympathetic nerve directly reaches the immune system, while the sympathetic nerve affects the immune system through noradrenaline (NA) secretion from the peripheral sympathetic ganglia. 5-HT = serotonin; ACH = acetylcholine; DA = dopamine; G-CSF = granulocyte colony-stimulating factor; GM-CSF = granulocyte-macrophage colony-stimulating factor.

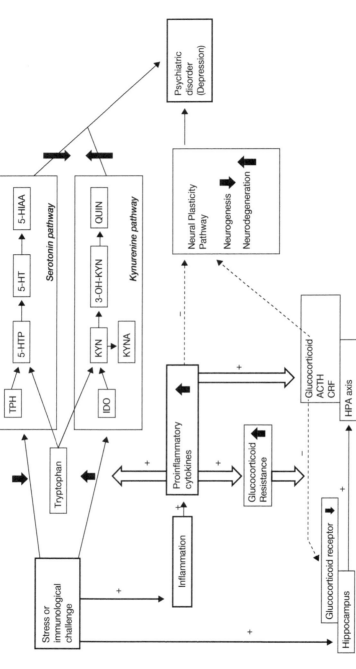

Figure 3.2. The role of pro-inflammatory cytokines in the pathogenesis of psychiatric disorders (depression). 3-OH-KYN = 3-hydroxykynurenine; 5-HIAA = 5-hydroxyindoleacetic acid; 5-HT = serotonin; 5-HTP = 5-hydroxytryptophan; ACTH = pituitary adrenocorticotropic hormone; CRF = corticotropin-releasing factor; HPA = hypothalamic-pituitary-adrenal (axis); IDO = indolamine-2,3-dioxygenase; KYN = kynurenine; KYNA = kynurenine acid; QUIN = quinolinic acid; TPH = tryptophan hydroxylase.

with schizophrenia or bipolar disorder, and the normal control group.[20,21] In some studies, however, decreases in the neuroglial cells and in the expression of GFAP are not observed in patients with depression. The reason for this seems to be that regions other than the prefrontal cortex or amygdala were examined, or the patients enrolled in the studies were too young.[22] Taken together, these findings show that the decreases of the astrocytes and their markers (GFAP, S100B, glutamate transporter) can be considered an important pathophysiology of depression. Moreover, a deficit of oligodendrocytes, in addition to a deficit of astrocytes, also plays an important role in the development of mood disorders.[23]

Role of Neuroglia and Cytokine Imbalance in Psychiatric Disorders

The main cytokines that are secreted from the microglia, T-helper 1 (Th1) lymphocytes, and M1 macrophages are pro-inflammatory cytokines accelerating inflammation, and include interleukin-1β (IL-1β), IL-2, IL-6, tumor necrosis factor-α (TNF-α), and interferon-γ (IFN-γ). Such pro-inflammatory cytokines are part of Th1 or type 1 inflammation. Pro-inflammatory cytokines increase prostaglandin E2 (PGE2) by activating cyclooxygenase-2 (COX-2) and regulate the inflammatory process by activating the inflammatory cells. In contrast, the cytokines that are mainly secreted from the astrocytes, T-helper 2 (Th2) lymphocytes, regulatory T cells (T regs), and M2 macrophages are anti-inflammatory cytokines that reduce type 1 inflammation and include IL-4, IL-5, and IL-10. Such anti-inflammatory cytokines are part of Th2 or type 2 inflammation. These cytokines maintain balance while interacting with one another, and if the inflammation becomes chronic, the pro-inflammatory cytokines increase while the anti-inflammatory cytokines decrease. The imbalance of the cytokines seems to lead to the development of various psychiatric disorders. The theory that explains this is the Th1–Th2 cytokine seesaw hypothesis, which is that the direction of inflammation progression is determined according to the relative dominance ratio of Th1 versus T2 cytokines. Here, the activation of the microglia, astrocytes, T cells, and glutamate is an important element (see Figure 3.1).[24,25]

The Th1–Th2 imbalance in the CNS affects the metabolism of tryptophan, a precursor of serotonin. Indolamine-2,3-dioxygenase (IDO) secreted from the microglia and astrocytes is a rate-limiting enzyme decomposing tryptophan into kynurenine and serotonin into 5-hydroxyindoleacetic acid (5HTT). Kynurenine 3-monooxygenase (KMO), secreted from the microglia, is a rate-limiting enzyme decomposing kynurenine into 3-hydroxykinurenine. Tryptophan-2,3-dioxygenase (TDO) and kynurenine aminotransferase

(KAT), secreted from the astrocytes, are rate-limiting enzymes decomposing tryptophan into kynurenine, and kynurenine into kynurenic acid, respectively (see Figure 3.2).[26] When the Th1 cytokines are more predominant than the Th2 cytokines in the nervous system, the neuroglial cells increase the secretion of IDO and KMO, and as a result, serotonin decreases while kynurenine increases. Here, the kynurenine is converted into quinolinic acid, an N-methyl-D-aspartate (NMDA) receptor agonist, in the microglia, thereby increasing the neurotransmission of glutamate and the influx of calcium to the cells, which makes the neuroinflammation permanent by reducing the Th2 activity of the astrocytes and accelerating the activation of the Th1 cells.[27] On the other hand, kynurenine is converted into kynurenic acid (an NMDA receptor antagonist) in the astrocytes, thereby reducing the neurotransmission of glutamate.[28]

These phenomena support the neural plasticity theory related to glutamate in psychiatric disorders such as depression and schizophrenia.[29] In particular, it is an appropriate model to understand the pathophysiology of depression in that glutamate increases in the cortex, and the degree of increase is associated with the severity of the depressive symptoms; and ketamine (an NMDA receptor antagonist) shows a strong antidepressant effect.[30] Therefore, the role of the neuroglial cells and the imbalance of the cytokines are topics that will draw further attention. Recently, in a meta-analysis comparing 822 patients with depression and 726 subjects in the control group, who had been included in 29 studies, the increases of soluble IL-2 receptor (sIL-2R), IL-6, and TNF-α were pointed out as depression trait markers.[31] In a study conducted on 47 patients with depression who had attempted to commit suicide, 17 patients with depression who had not attempted suicide, and 16 subjects in the control group, the increases of TNF-α and IL-6 and the decrease of IL-2 were suggested as a state marker of suicide attempt.[32] The increase and decrease of the cytokines appear slightly different in each study, and the reason for this may be that the duration of the disease in patients who participated in the studies varied. Among the various cytokines, the marker that has been most consistently measured is the increase of IL-6, and it has been proposed that this must be considered an indicator for evaluating the treatment effect in depression and the risk for suicide.[33]

Many studies on cytokines, however, were conducted with peripheral blood smear examination and thus failed to fully reflect the condition of the CNS. Moreover, because various confounding factors are involved, such as systemic illness, the studies had poor reproducibility and limitations on interpretation. On the other hand, most of the studies that have been conducted by obtaining samples from the CNS were small laboratory studies yielding indefinite findings. For these reasons, studies using S100B as a new marker have been attempted recently.

S100B is a peptide secreted from the neuroglial cells and is involved in the regulation of calcium homeostasis by acting as the receptor for the advanced glycation end products (RAGE) of neurons and neuroglial cells. It has effects of neuroprotection or neurotoxicity on the nerves, depending on its concentration.[33] Because S100B passes the brain–blood vessel barriers relatively easily and is detected in the peripheral blood, it is called "CRP for the brain" and is used as a clinical indicator in cerebral ischemia, cerebral hemorrhage, brain injury, and degenerative brain diseases.[34] In mood disorders, an increase of serum S100B has been shown, especially noticeable in acute depression and manic episodes, and it had a positive correlation with suicidality.[35] Increase of S100B is also observed in schizophrenia, showing positive correlations with paranoia, negative symptoms, cognitive decline, lowered treatment response, and disease duration.[36] It is known that serum S100B decreases in response to antidepressant and antipsychotic treatments.[37]

Pro-inflammatory Cytokines in Depression and Other Psychiatric Disorders

The pro-inflammatory cytokines include IL-1, IL-2, IL-6, IFN-γ, and TNF-α, while the anti-inflammatory cytokines include IL-4, IL-5, IL-10, IL-11, IL-13, and TGF-β.[14] These cytokines interact with one another to maintain balance.[38] For example, IL-10 reduces the creation of TNF, and a cytokine antagonizing the IL-1 receptor (IL-1 receptor antagonist [IL-1ra]) exists.

The cytokines created from the peripheral immune system are directly delivered to the CNS through the blood–brain barrier (e.g., by the choroid plexus, which serves as one interface between the peripheral and central immune responses[39]) and also indirectly affect the brain by causing secretion of nitric oxide and PGE2 in the blood vessels.[38] Because cytokines are also secreted from the neurons and glial cells within the brain, the changes in cytokines may cause or reflect the abnormalities in the CNS. Additionally, the cytokine receptors' high density in the hypothalamus, hippocampus, locus coeruleus, and prefrontal cortex, which are important regions for cognitive and affective functions, explains their association with psychiatric disorders, including depression.[40]

The typical pro-inflammatory cytokines, IL-1 and IL-2, increase the synthesis and circulation of serotonin, norepinephrine, and dopamine while lowering serotonin by increasing the activity of IDO, which inhibits the synthesis of serotonin by causing tryptophan to break down into the kynurenine pathway rather than the serotonin pathway.[41] In addition, norepinephrine and dopamine promote the secretion of corticotropin-releasing factor (CRF) and activate the immune response by activating the sympathetic nerves along with the pro-inflammatory cytokines, including IL-6. This process can raise the temperature of the CNS as well as the periphery, resulting in so-called sickness behavior.[41] Sickness behavior refers to the changes in behavior occurring mainly during an infection and includes fatigue, depression, anxiety, hypersomnia, loss of appetite, and poor concentration. From the finding that the pro-inflammatory cytokines increased and the anti-inflammatory cytokines decreased in the blood of patients with depression[42] and the finding that PGE2 increased in the cerebrospinal fluid,[43] the hypothesis that depression is a type of sickness behavior has been derived.

In other words, cytokines regulate the secretion of neurotransmitters in the CNS. They particularly act on the hypothalamus, playing a pivotal role in the endocrine system; regulate the activation of the HPA axis; and affect the development of various psychiatric symptoms, such as depression and anxiety. Because cytokines were recently found to promote the differentiation and remodeling of the neurons in the brain, their role in neurodegenerative diseases has also drawn attention of late. In particular, apoptosis increases in the brain of patients with chronic depression, resulting in the reduction of the volumes of the hippocampus, prefrontal lobe, and amygdala and the expansion of the cerebral ventricle, which increases the potential to develop dementia. In this process, the chronic inflammatory response is thought to be involved.[44]

Stress and Psychiatric Disorders Mediated by Neuroglia and Cytokines

Stress lowers neurogenesis in the hippocampus and causes an inflammatory response through the secretion of cytokines. When inflammation occurs, the immune system is activated, and the pro-inflammatory cytokines secreted from immune cells increase. The cytokines induce secretion of glucocorticoid by stimulating the HPA axis, and consequently, the immune function is suppressed. Cytokines are secreted from the immune cells in the brain as well as from the peripheral immune cells. Chronic stress causes the activation of microglia, and the cytokines secreted from the microglia affect neurogenesis. A recent study showed that the neurogenesis is suppressed or promoted depending on the degree of activation of microglia.[45] This means that there are cells with various functions within the microglia population, and some of them facilitate neurogenesis, while others suppress it. Inflammation and cytokines generally play the role of directly suppressing neurogenesis.[45] Pro-inflammatory cytokines, including TNF-α and IFN-α, suppress neurogenesis through the regulation of IL-1.[46,47] Moreover, the finding of a recent study that the suppression of IL-1β activation could prevent the decline of neurogenesis due to stress confirms that cytokines play an important role in suppressing neurogenesis in the brain.[48] On the other hand, the administration of medications that suppress inflammation restores or increases neurogenesis.[49] These findings support the facts that chronic stress facilitates the secretion of cytokines in the peripheral blood and microglia of the brain and that cytokines affect neurogenesis (see Figure 3.2).

Cytokine Hypothesis in Depression

Many clinical and experimental studies suggested the hypothesis that cytokine disorders due to internal or external stress play a key role in the expression and continuance of depressive symptoms in vulnerable individuals.[50]

The recent studies on the interactions between the brain and the immune system obtained several important findings regarding the association between cytokines and depression. The evidence supporting the cytokine hypothesis of depression is as follows. First, cytokine injection into experimental animals or humans caused symptoms similar to those of depression. For example, IL-2 and IFN-α, which were administered for hepatitis or cancer treatment, caused fatigue, apathy, cognitive disorders, anhedonia, helplessness, and dysphoria.[51] Likewise, when cytokines, including IL-1, IL-6, and IFN-γ, were injected into experimental animals, anhedonia, helplessness, loss of appetite, social withdrawal, psychomotor slowing, and changes in sleep/learning/memory were observed.[52] Second, in depression, increase of the pro-inflammatory cytokines with immunoregulatory functions (including IL-1, IL-6, IL-12, and TNF-α) and PGE2 was observed.[25,50,53,54] Third, the cytokines activate the HPA axis by stimulating the hypothalamic corticotropin-releasing hormone (CRH) and the pituitary adrenocorticotropic hormone (ACTH)[55,56] and make serotonin synthesis in the brain deficient by activating IDO, which metabolizes tryptophan, a precursor of serotonin, into kynurenine.[57] This supports the fact that the cytokines are closely associated with both HPA axis and catecholamine/sympathetic nervous system activation, which are most important in the pathophysiology of depression. Fourth, antidepressants suppress the secretion of cytokines in the immune cells or improve depressive symptoms by acting as antagonists of the cytokine receptors. In fact, antidepressants suppress the release of the pro-inflammatory cytokines secreted from monocytes or macrophages, act as suppressors of chemotaxis, and increase the production of anti-inflammatory cytokines.[58] In an in vitro study, antidepressants showed suppressive immune effects through the suppression of IFN-γ and the increase of IL-10 at therapeutic doses.[59] In addition, antidepressants remarkably suppressed the production of IL-1β, IL- 6, and TNF-α stimulated by lipopolysaccharide and also suppressed the production of IL-2 and IFN-γ by T cells.[60]

Initially, it was considered that the hypersecretion of cortisol through the activation of the HPA axis suppresses immune function in depression.[61] In recent studies, however, the immune cells were considered not to have been affected by cortisol increases because the function of the glucocorticoid receptor of the immune cells was suppressed in chronic stress or depression. Chronic stress and depression lead to oversecretion of pro-inflammatory cytokines, which inhibit the function of glucocorticoid receptors in immune cells.[62] As evidence for this, pro-inflammatory cytokines, including IL-1β and IL-6, activated the HPA axis by stimulating the secretion of CRH from the paraventricular nucleus of the hypothalamus and accelerated the secretion of ACTH and glucocorticoid. Additionally, IL-1 disturbed the movement of the glucocorticoid receptor from the cytoplasm to the cell nucleus and suppressed the transcription of the genes normally activated by the glucocorticoid receptor.[62;63] These findings imply that the cytokines directly regulate the function of the glucocorticoid receptor and may cause glucocorticoid resistance (see Figure 3.2). These findings strongly support the view that cytokines can be related to the pathophysiology of depression and the mechanism of action of antidepressants.

ROLE OF GLIA AND CYTOKINES IN CHRONIC PAIN

Preclinical Studies: Role of Glia and Cytokines in Chronic Pain

In discussing the role of glia and cytokines in chronic pain, many similarities to their role in psychiatric disorders discussed in the previous section will become evident. These similarities include the importance of increased type 1 cytokines and decreased type 2 cytokines (in many cases, the same cytokines) and the key role of glial activation and neuroinflammation at all levels of the sensory system.

SPINAL CORD
In the spinal cord dorsal horn, the first waystation for peripheral pain signals to enter the CNS, peripheral nerve injury rapidly leads to microglia activation and proliferation.[64–66] Although the proliferation and shape changes indicative of microglia activation in spinal cord are more marked after peripheral nerve injury than after peripheral inflammation, initiation of pain in both conditions can be inhibited by the microglia inhibitor minocycline. However, this treatment cannot reverse pain that is already established.[64,65] Experimentally, direct stimulation of sensory nerves can also activate spinal microglia.[65,67]

In addition to the sensory neurons' neurotransmitters, cytokines, including monocyte chemoattractant protein 1 (MCP-1, systemic name CCL2), IL-1β, and fractalkine, are also among the signals released from sensory neurons to activate the spinal microglia.[64-66] (Both MCP-1 and fractalkine were originally described as chemokines that recruit monocytes and T cells to sites of peripheral inflammation.) In turn, activated microglia release cytokines, including MCP-1, TNFα, IL-1β, and IL-6, that contribute to the pathological changes in the dorsal horn. Each of these cytokines has been shown to induce pain when injected into the spinal cord and to directly increase excitatory (including glutamatergic) and decrease inhibitory neurotransmission within the dorsal horn. In addition, blocking these cytokines by intrathecal injection of inhibitors or genetic manipulation reduces pain behavior in rodent models.[1,64,66,67] Brain-derived neurotrophic factor (BDNF) also plays an important role in signaling from microglia. BDNF is synthesized and released by activated microglia and can disinhibit the dorsal horn neurons to enhance pain transmission. BDNF alone, in the absence of nerve injury, can activate pain in naïve animals when applied to the spinal cord, and antagonizing it genetically or pharmacologically reduces pain.[64-67] However, recent studies indicate important gender differences. The microglia–BDNF pathway was initially described in studies of male rodents, and it is now known that, in females, microglia do not release BDNF (despite showing other signs of activation); instead, T cells may mediate some of the pain-promoting effects that are mediated by microglia in males.[68]

In the earlier section, "Role of Glia and Cytokines in Psychiatric Disorders," studies were discussed that show a reduction in astrocytes in particular brain regions may contribute to psychiatric disorders. In contrast, in pain studies, proliferation and activation of astrocytes in spinal cord contributes to chronic neuropathic or inflammatory pain in rodent models, especially to the maintenance of pain. Activated microglia affect not only neurons but also activate astrocytes, in part by releasing of TNF-α, IL-18, and MCP-1.[1,66,69] Compared with microglia, astrocytes activate more slowly and are more involved with maintenance of pain.[1,66,67] Release of cytokines, including MCP-1, is one mechanism by which activated astrocytes can cause pain.[69] By decreasing expression of glutamate transporters, astrocytes can also enhance glutamatergic transmission in the dorsal horn,[66,67] similar to the process discussed earlier that occurs in the brain regions related to depression.

An interesting example of the importance of cytokine balance is the recent study that explained why nerve injury does not lead to neuropathic pain in very young (before adolescence) rodents. Unlike the results in adults described previously, in very young animals peripheral nerve injury (or peripheral nerve stimulation to activate C-fibers) caused an increase in the anti-inflammatory cytokines IL-4 and IL-10 in spinal cord; blocking IL-10's action unmasked pain behaviors and a pro-inflammatory cytokine profile in young animals that were more similar to those observed in adults. Indeed, in this study, pain behaviors emerged, but only after a long delay, in the animals injured at a young age. In these animals, pain behavior appeared at adolescence, the age at which the adult profile of a purely pro-inflammatory cytokine profile is first observed.[70]

Peripheral Nerve

In conditions of peripheral inflammation, nociceptive sensory neurons become sensitized because of the action of multiple inflammatory mediators produced by the immune response on the nerve endings.[71] Cytokines may contribute to inflammatory pain not only by promoting the release of these inflammatory mediators but also by their direct actions on sensory neurons. Hence, direct effects of the cytokines may be observed in isolated sensory neurons in vitro, and the neurons may become more sensitive to various cytokines after injury and inflammation. These actions may be relevant not only during the normal, acute inflammatory response but also during pathological inflammatory conditions such as arthritis. Cytokine effects may be important not only at the nerve endings but also in the DRG, where the distal inflammatory signal can also lead to neuroinflammation, including macrophage invasion, around the neuronal cell bodies. Pro-inflammatory cytokines with direct excitatory effects on neurons that have been implicated in inflammatory pain conditions include TNF-α, IL-6, IL-1β, MCP-1, macrophage inflammatory protein 1α (MIP-1α, systemic name CCL3), IL-17, and growth-related oncogene/keratinocyte chemoattractant α (GRO/KC, systemic name CXCL1).[3,72] Some of the same cytokines may play a similar role in neuropathic pain conditions in which remaining intact nerve fibers may be exposed to the immune response in the injured nerve. In addition, peripheral nerve injury induces neuroinflammation in the remote DRG, locally exposing the cell bodies to some of the same cytokines as their axons.[73,74]

Dorsal Root Ganglia and Satellite Glial Cells

In the DRG (as well as the trigeminal and autonomic ganglia), specialized glial cells, the satellite glial cells (SGC), closely ensheathe the neuronal cell bodies. These cells have some properties of astrocytes and some properties of microglia, based on their function and the molecules they express.[9] They are less well understood than spinal cord glia. However, as in spinal cord, peripheral nerve injury or peripheral inflammation leads to proliferation, activation, and increased gap junction coupling of SGC.[67] SGC activation depends on sensory neuron activity.[67,75] In addition, in some conditions, particularly those related to low back pain, the DRG themselves experience local sterile inflammation—for example, when the nucleus pulposus from a nearby ruptured disk acts as an immune stimulant, or stenosis leads to DRG compression. Such conditions have been modeled in rodents by placing immune stimulants or nucleus pulposus near the DRG or by compressing the DRG.[76] In addition to the satellite glia, infiltrating and resident immune cells such as macrophages contribute to pathological changes in the DRG in pain models. The DRG do not have as strong a blood–brain barrier as is seen in the CNS.

Cytokines have been implicated in the increased sensory neuron excitability observed in rodent pain models. Many type 1 pro-inflammatory cytokines have been demonstrated to increase within the DRG in pain models, to cause pain when exogenously applied, and to increase sensory neuron excitability. These include IL-1β, TNF-α, IL-6, MCP-1, and MIP-1α.[2,7,74] As discussed earlier in the section, "Peripheral Nerve," these studies include experiments on isolated, cultured sensory neurons, indicating that many cytokines can directly affect neurons.

Molecular mediators of SGC–sensory neuron communication are less well studied than in spinal cord, and studies have focused more on purinergic signaling and cell coupling.[67,77,78] However, SGC have been shown to release TNF-α[79] and to play a role in IL-1β changes after inflammation.[78] As in the CNS, regulation of neuronal glutamate processing by SGC has been described.[78]

Local Roles of the Sympathetic Nervous System in Chronic Pain

The previous section, "Role of Glia and Cytokines in Psychiatric Disorders," highlighted the central activation of the sympathetic nervous system in psychiatric disorders such as depression. The sympathetic nervous system also plays a role in pain. Certain conditions, most notably complex regional pain syndrome (CRPS), are classified as sympathetically maintained pain, and local sympathetic blockade is one treatment.[80] Mechanisms by which the sympathetic nerves can regulate pain include abnormal interactions with sensory nerves; direct innervation of immune tissues such as thymus, spleen, and bone marrow; regulation of endothelial cells and hence immune cell extravasation; and the presence of sympathetic transmitter receptors on immune cells.[81–84] Experimentally, these mechanisms may be either pro-inflammatory or anti-inflammatory, making it difficult to predict the overall effect of widespread sympathetic activation. Of particular relevance to this chapter is a recent study[85] showing marked reduction of pain induced by local inflammation of the DRG when the local sympathetic innervation of the DRG was interrupted by cutting the gray rami to the lumbar DRGs. DRG inflammation resulted in upregulation of a number of type 1 pro-inflammatory cytokines in the DRG, including

MCP-1, IL-6, MIP-1α, and IL-1β, and downregulation of type 2 cytokines, including IL-4, while the local sympathectomy partially restored this cytokine profile toward the normal, type 2 biased profile. Hence, regulation of cytokines may be one important mechanism for sympathetic regulation of pain. Further evidence for a local pro-inflammatory role of the sympathetic nervous system in this study was the observation that the localized sympathectomy, which also removed sympathetic innervation of the hind paw, reduced paw swelling, macrophage infiltration, and pain behaviors induced by injection of complete Freund's adjuvant into the paw.

Human Studies: Role of Cytokines and Glia in Chronic Pain

Studies in humans provide evidence that some of the cytokines implicated in preclinical studies may also be important in human pain conditions. It will be evident from the previous sections that cytokines can play very localized roles, so it may not always be feasible to measure increases in blood samples, which are most easily obtained in human studies. Thus, it is perhaps not surprising that studies of blood levels of particular cytokines' association with particular pain conditions are not always consistent.[86] In a recent study of patients with CRPS,[87] researchers measured plasma levels of several cytokines and soluble cytokine receptors and found that patients fell into two clusters. Thirty-two percent of patients had a much more pro-inflammatory profile, significantly different from healthy controls, while the rest did not differ significantly from controls. Overall, CRPS patients had approximately two-fold differences from controls in numerous markers, including TNF-α, MCP-1, IL-8, and some of the soluble receptors from the IL-1 family, but these differences were driven almost entirely by much larger differences in the smaller patient cluster. Importantly, other clinical variables did not predict cluster, suggesting that measuring the cytokine profile provides information that cannot be derived from the clinical presentation. Thus, heterogeneity of patients may also account for some of the conflicting findings regarding plasma levels of particular cytokines in pain conditions. However, this study also suggests that cytokines may be useful tools for investigating and explaining heterogeneity, perhaps ultimately being used to predict and guide treatment.

Some human studies have been conducted using cerebrospinal fluid samples in a number of different pain conditions, including low back pain, osteoarthritis, and fibromyalgia.[88] In addition to elevated levels of some of the cytokines extensively discussed in this chapter, such as IL-1β, MCP-1, TNF-α, and IL-6, in several human pain conditions IL-8 was also elevated. This cytokine does not have a rodent counterpart, but rodents do have the cytokine GRO/KC

(CXCL1), which activates the same receptor and has been shown to directly affect rat sensory neurons[89] and to be elevated in a rat back pain model.[90]

Studies examining localized cytokine changes in degenerating or ruptured disks (an important cause of low back pain) have also been conducted in humans and have implicated both TNF-α and IL-1β, correlating with the severity of degeneration.[91]

TNF-α inhibitors are already in use clinically for arthritis; interestingly, one human study showed that they provided pain relief much more rapidly than they reduced joint inflammation,[92] consistent with the previously cited preclinical studies about direct roles of TNF-α in mediating the chronic pain state directly through actions on glia and neurons. In contrast are the recent failure of clinical trials using glia inhibitors; it has been suggested that one reason for the failure of preclinical studies to be borne out in humans could be the differences between human and rodent glial cells.[67] Ongoing studies of human glial cells, including their introduction into rodent models, may address this issue.

CONCLUSION

In summary, imbalance between type 1 pro-inflammatory cytokines and type 2 anti-inflammatory cytokines has been implicated in both psychiatric disorders (especially depression and anxiety) and chronic pain disorders. Many of the same cytokines have been intensively studied in both fields, especially TNF-α, IL-1β, and IL-6. An important role played by cytokines in these two classes of disorders is communication between neurons and activated glial cells, that is, in mediating neuroinflammation. These processes have been described at all levels of the nervous system, from peripheral nerve endings to the sensory ganglia and spinal cord, and up to the limbic system and cortex.

Because cytokines may act very locally, it would not be a foregone conclusion that because similar cytokines are elevated in depression and in chronic pain, these conditions must be related. However, many studies suggest a relationship.[7,93,94] For example, antidepressants are used in the treatment of chronic pain conditions; although their efficacy is often attributed to modulation of the descending pain pathway, as discussed earlier in the section, "Cytokine Hypothesis and Depression," they may also have anti-inflammatory effects in the periphery. Some chronic pain conditions are associated with elevated systemic cytokine concentrations and hence might be expected to activate "sickness behavior," as discussed previously in the section, "Pro-inflammatory Cytokines in Depression and Other Psychiatric Disorders" in the context of depression. One component of both depression and sickness behavior is a reduction in the pain threshold.[94] Depression and chronic pain are often comorbid, such that depression is associated with poorer outcomes in chronic pain conditions, and chronic pain patients are more likely to have depression. There is not a single direction of causation; having either depression or chronic pain predisposes individuals to subsequently develop the other condition. A similar relationship may pertain to anxiety and chronic pain. The search for new treatments for psychiatric disorders and for chronic pain may benefit from consideration of the many pathways and molecules that these conditions have in common.

REFERENCES

1. Mika J, Zychowska M, Popiolek-Barczyk K, Rojewska E, Przewlocka B. Importance of glial activation in neuropathic pain. *Eur J Pharmacol*. 2013;716(1–3):106–119.
2. Liou JT, Lee CM, Day YJ. The immune aspect in neuropathic pain: Role of chemokines. *Acta Anaesthesiol Taiwan*. 2013;51(3):127–132.
3. Dawes JM, McMahon SB. Chemokines as peripheral pain mediators. *Neurosci Lett*. 2013;557(part A):1–8.
4. Stuart MJ, Singhal G, Baune BT. Systematic review of the neurobiological relevance of chemokines to psychiatric disorders. *Front Cell Neurosci*. 2015;9:357.
5. Allen JE, Sutherland TE. Host protective roles of type 2 immunity: Parasite killing and tissue repair, flip sides of the same coin. *Semin Immunol*. 2014;26(4):329–340.
6. Rickard AJ, Young MJ. Corticosteroid receptors, macrophages and cardiovascular disease. *J Mol Endocrinol*. 2009;42(6):449–459.
7. Lees JG, Fivelman B, Duffy SS, Makker PG, Perera CJ, Moalem-Taylor G. Cytokines in neuropathic pain and associated depression. *Mod Trends Pharmacopsychiatry*. 2015;30:51–66.
8. Schwartz M, Deczkowska A. Neurological disease as a failure of brain-immune crosstalk: The multiple faces of neuroinflammation. *Trends Immunol*. 2016;37(10):668–679.
9. Hanani M. Satellite glial cells in sensory ganglia: From form to function. *Brain Res Brain Res Rev*. 2005;48(3):457–476.
10. Borsook D, Maleki N, Becerra L, McEwen B. Understanding migraine through the lens of maladaptive stress responses: A model disease of allostatic load. *Neuron*. 2012;73(2):219–234.
11. Kesler SR. Default mode network as a potential biomarker of chemotherapy-related brain injury. *Neurobiol Aging*. 2014;35(suppl 2):S11–S19.
12. Maes M. The cytokine hypothesis of depression: Inflammation, oxidative & nitrosative stress (IO&NS) and leaky gut as new targets for adjunctive treatments in depression. *Neuro Endocrinol Lett*. 2008;29(3):287–291.
13. Leonard BE. The immune system, depression and the action of antidepressants. *Prog Neuropsychopharmacol Biol Psychiatry*. 2001;25(4):767–780.
14. Leonard BE. The HPA and immune axes in stress: The involvement of the serotonergic system. *Eur Psychiatry*. 2005;20(suppl 3):S302–S306.

15. Sanacora G, Banasr M. From pathophysiology to novel antidepressant drugs: Glial contributions to the pathology and treatment of mood disorders. *Biol Psychiatry.* 2013;73(12):1172–1179.

16. Miguel-Hidalgo JJ, Baucom C, Dilley G, et al. Glial fibrillary acidic protein immunoreactivity in the prefrontal cortex distinguishes younger from older adults in major depressive disorder. *Biol Psychiatry.* 2000;48(8):861–873.

17. Gosselin RD, Gibney S, O'Malley D, Dinan TG, Cryan JF. Region specific decrease in glial fibrillary acidic protein immunoreactivity in the brain of a rat model of depression. *Neuroscience.* 2009;159(2):915–925.

18. Schroeter ML, Abdul-Khaliq H, Diefenbacher A, Blasig IE. S100B is increased in mood disorders and may be reduced by antidepressive treatment. *Neuroreport.* 2002;13(13):1675–1678.

19. Miguel-Hidalgo JJ, Rajkowska G. Comparison of prefrontal cell pathology between depression and alcohol dependence. *J Psychiatr Res.* 2003;37(5):411–420.

20. Altshuler LL, Abulseoud OA, Foland-Ross L, et al. Amygdala astrocyte reduction in subjects with major depressive disorder but not bipolar disorder. *Bipolar Disord.* 2010;12(5):541–549.

21. John CS, Smith KL, Van't Veer A, et al. Blockade of astrocytic glutamate uptake in the prefrontal cortex induces anhedonia. *Neuropsychopharmacology.* 2012;37(11):2467–2475.

22. Rodnight RB, Gottfried C. Morphological plasticity of rodent astroglia. *J Neurochem.* 2013;124(3):263–275.

23. Vostrikov VM, Uranova NA, Orlovskaya DD. Deficit of perineuronal oligodendrocytes in the prefrontal cortex in schizophrenia and mood disorders. *Schizophr Res.* 2007;94(1–3):273–280.

24. Kim YK, Myint AM, Lee BH, et al. Th1, Th2 and Th3 cytokine alteration in schizophrenia. *Prog Neuropsychopharmacol Biol Psychiatry.* 2004;28(7):1129–1134.

25. Myint AM, Leonard BE, Steinbusch HW, Kim YK. Th1, Th2, and Th3 cytokine alterations in major depression. *J Affect Disord.* 2005;88(2):167–173.

26. Mandi Y, Vecsei L. The kynurenine system and immunoregulation. *J Neural Transm (Vienna).* 2012;119(2):197–209.

27. Maddison DC, Giorgini F. The kynurenine pathway and neurodegenerative disease. *Semin Cell Dev Biol.* 2015;40:134–141.

28. Bay-Richter C, Linderholm KR, Lim CK, et al. A role for inflammatory metabolites as modulators of the glutamate N-methyl-D-aspartate receptor in depression and suicidality. *Brain Behav Immun.* 2015;43:110–117.

29. Tartar JL, King MA, Devine DP. Glutamate-mediated neuroplasticity in a limbic input to the hypothalamus. *Stress.* 2006;9(1):13–19.

30. Schmidt FM, Kirkby KC, Lichtblau N. Inflammation and immune regulation as potential drug targets in antidepressant treatment. *Curr Neuropharmacol.* 2016;14(7):674–687.

31. Liu Y, Ho RC, Mak A. Interleukin (IL)-6, tumour necrosis factor alpha (TNF-alpha) and soluble interleukin-2 receptors (sIL-2R) are elevated in patients with major depressive disorder: A meta-analysis and meta-regression. *J Affect Disord.* 2012;139(3):230–239.

32. Janelidze S, Mattei D, Westrin A, Traskman-Bendz L, Brundin L. Cytokine levels in the blood may distinguish suicide attempters from depressed patients. *Brain Behav Immun*. 2011;25(2):335–339.

33. Gananca L, Oquendo MA, Tyrka AR, Cisneros-Trujillo S, Mann JJ, Sublette ME. The role of cytokines in the pathophysiology of suicidal behavior. *Psychoneuroendocrinology*. 2016;63:296–310.

34. Sen J, Belli A. S100B in neuropathologic states: The CRP of the brain? *J Neurosci Res*. 2007;85(7):1373–1380.

35. Schroeter ML, Abdul-Khaliq H, Krebs M, Diefenbacher A, Blasig IE. Serum markers support disease-specific glial pathology in major depression. *J Affect Disord*. 2008;111(2–3):271–280.

36. Rothermundt M, Ahn JN, Jorgens S. S100B in schizophrenia: An update. *Gen Physiol Biophys*. 2009;28(spec no focus):F76–F81.

37. Kalia M, Costa ESJ. Biomarkers of psychiatric diseases: Current status and future prospects. *Metabolism*. 2015;64(3 suppl 1):S11–S15.

38. Kronfol Z, Remick DG. Cytokines and the brain: Implications for clinical psychiatry. *Am J Psychiatry*. 2000;157(5):683–694.

39. Devorak J, Torres-Platas SG, Davoli MA, Prud'homme J, Turecki G, Mechawar N. Cellular and molecular inflammatory profile of the choroid plexus in depression and suicide. *Front Psychiatry*. 2015;6:138.

40. Anisman H, Merali Z. Cytokines, stress and depressive illness: Brain-immune interactions. *Ann Med*. 2003;35(1):2–11.

41. Christmas DM, Potokar J, Davies SJ. A biological pathway linking inflammation and depression: Activation of indoleamine 2,3-dioxygenase. *Neuropsychiatr Dis Treat*. 2011;7:431–439.

42. Maes M, Stevens W, DeClerck L, et al. Immune disorders in depression: Higher T helper/T suppressor-cytotoxic cell ratio. *Acta Psychiatr Scand*. 1992;86(6):423–431.

43. Song C, Lin A, Bonaccorso S, et al. The inflammatory response system and the availability of plasma tryptophan in patients with primary sleep disorders and major depression. *J Affect Disord*. 1998;49(3):211–219.

44. Leonard BE, Myint A. Inflammation and depression: Is there a causal connection with dementia? *Neurotox Res*. 2006;10(2):149–160.

45. Ekdahl CT, Kokaia Z, Lindvall O. Brain inflammation and adult neurogenesis: The dual role of microglia. *Neuroscience*. 2009;158(3):1021–1029.

46. Kaneko N, Kudo K, Mabuchi T, et al. Suppression of cell proliferation by interferon-alpha through interleukin-1 production in adult rat dentate gyrus. *Neuropsychopharmacology*. 2006;31(12):2619–2626.

47. Iosif RE, Ekdahl CT, Ahlenius H, et al. Tumor necrosis factor receptor 1 is a negative regulator of progenitor proliferation in adult hippocampal neurogenesis. *J Neurosci*. 2006;26(38):9703–9712.

48. Koo JW, Duman RS. IL-1beta is an essential mediator of the antineurogenic and anhedonic effects of stress. *Proc Natl Acad Sci U S A*. 2008;105(2):751–756.

49. Monje ML, Toda H, Palmer TD. Inflammatory blockade restores adult hippocampal neurogenesis. *Science*. 2003;302(5651):1760–1765.

50. Kim YK, Suh IB, Kim H, et al. The plasma levels of interleukin-12 in schizophrenia, major depression, and bipolar mania: Effects of psychotropic drugs. *Mol Psychiatry.* 2002;7(10):1107–1114.

51. Meyers CA. Mood and cognitive disorders in cancer patients receiving cytokine therapy. *Adv Exp Med Biol.* 1999;461:75–81.

52. Dantzer R, Aubert A, Bluthe RM, et al. Mechanisms of the behavioural effects of cytokines. *Adv Exp Med Biol.* 1999;461:83–105.

53. Kim YK, Na KS, Shin KH, Jung HY, Choi SH, Kim JB. Cytokine imbalance in the pathophysiology of major depressive disorder. *Prog Neuropsychopharmacol Biol Psychiatry.* 2007;31(5):1044–1053.

54. Lee KM, Kim YK. The role of IL-12 and TGF-beta1 in the pathophysiology of major depressive disorder. *Int Immunopharmacol.* 2006;6(8):1298–1304.

55. Sapolsky R, Rivier C, Yamamoto G, Plotsky P, Vale W. Interleukin-1 stimulates the secretion of hypothalamic corticotropin-releasing factor. *Science.* 1987;238(4826):522–524.

56. Maes M, Scharpe S, Meltzer HY, et al. Relationships between interleukin-6 activity, acute phase proteins, and function of the hypothalamic-pituitary-adrenal axis in severe depression. *Psychiatry Res.* 1993;49(1):11–27.

57. Guillemin GJ, Kerr SJ, Pemberton LA, et al. IFN-beta1b induces kynurenine pathway metabolism in human macrophages: Potential implications for multiple sclerosis treatment. *J Interferon Cytokine Res.* 2001;21(12):1097–1101.

58. Neveu PJ, Castanon N. Is there evidence for an effect of antidepressant drugs on immune function? *Adv Exp Med Biol.* 1999;461:267–281.

59. Maes M, Song C, Lin AH, et al. Negative immunoregulatory effects of antidepressants: Inhibition of interferon-gamma and stimulation of interleukin-10 secretion. *Neuropsychopharmacology.* 1999;20(4):370–379.

60. Xia Z, DePierre JW, Nassberger L. Tricyclic antidepressants inhibit IL-6, IL-1 beta and TNF-alpha release in human blood monocytes and IL-2 and interferon-gamma in T cells. *Immunopharmacology.* 1996;34(1):27–37.

61. Nabriski D, Saperstein A, Brand H, et al. Role of corticotropin-releasing factor in immunosuppression. *Trans Assoc Am Physicians.* 1991;104:238–247.

62. Miller AH, Pariante CM, Pearce BD. Effects of cytokines on glucocorticoid receptor expression and function: Glucocorticoid resistance and relevance to depression. *Adv Exp Med Biol.* 1999;461:107–116.

63. Kim YK, Maes M. The role of the cytokine network in psychological stress. *Acta Neuropsychiatr.* 2003;15(3):148–155.

64. Taves S, Berta T, Chen G, Ji RR. Microglia and spinal cord synaptic plasticity in persistent pain. *Neural Plast.* 2013;2013:753656.

65. Tsuda M, Beggs S, Salter MW, Inoue K. Microglia and intractable chronic pain. *Glia.* 2013;61(1):55–61.

66. Old EA, Clark AK, Malcangio M. The role of glia in the spinal cord in neuropathic and inflammatory pain. *Handb Exp Pharmacol.* 2015;227:145–170.

67. Ji RR, Berta T, Nedergaard M. Glia and pain: Is chronic pain a gliopathy? *Pain.* 2013;154(suppl 1):S10–S28.

68. Mapplebeck JC, Beggs S, Salter MW. Sex differences in pain: A tale of two immune cells. *Pain.* 2016;157(suppl 1):S2–S6.

69. Gao YJ, Zhang L, Ji RR. Spinal injection of TNF-alpha-activated astrocytes produces persistent pain symptom mechanical allodynia by releasing monocyte chemoattractant protein-1. *Glia*. 2010;58(15):1871–1880.
70. McKelvey R, Berta T, Old E, Ji RR, Fitzgerald M. Neuropathic pain is constitutively suppressed in early life by anti-inflammatory neuroimmune regulation. *J Neurosci*. 2015;35(2):457–466.
71. Petho G, Reeh PW. Sensory and signaling mechanisms of bradykinin, eicosanoids, platelet-activating factor, and nitric oxide in peripheral nociceptors. *Physiol Rev*. 2012;92(4):1699–1775.
72. Schaible HG. Nociceptive neurons detect cytokines in arthritis. *Arthritis Res Ther*. 2014;16(5):470.
73. Stemkowski PL, Smith PA. Sensory neurons, ion channels, inflammation and the onset of neuropathic pain. *Can J Neurol Sci*. 2012;39(4):416–435.
74. Moalem G, Tracey DJ. Immune and inflammatory mechanisms in neuropathic pain. *Brain Res Brain Res Rev*. 2006;51(2):240–264.
75. Xie W, Strong JA, Zhang JM. Early blockade of injured primary sensory afferents reduces glial cell activation in two rat neuropathic pain models. *Neuroscience*. 2009;160(4):847–857.
76. Strong JA, Xie W, Bataille FJ, Zhang JM. Preclinical studies of low back pain. *Mol Pain*. 2013;9:17.
77. Hanani M. Role of satellite glial cells in gastrointestinal pain. *Front Cell Neurosci*. 2015;9:412.
78. Huang LY, Gu Y, Chen Y. Communication between neuronal somata and satellite glial cells in sensory ganglia. *Glia*. 2013;61(10):1571–1581.
79. Zhang X, Chen Y, Wang C, Huang LY. Neuronal somatic ATP release triggers neuron-satellite glial cell communication in dorsal root ganglia. *Proc Natl Acad Sci U S A*. 2007;104(23):9864–9869.
80. Harden RN, Oaklander AL, Burton AW, et al. Complex regional pain syndrome: Practical diagnostic and treatment guidelines, 4th edition. *Pain Med*. 2013;14(2):180–229.
81. Straub RH, Wiest R, Strauch UG, Harle P, Scholmerich J. The role of the sympathetic nervous system in intestinal inflammation. *Gut*. 2006;55(11):1640–1649.
82. Koopman FA, Stoof SP, Straub RH, Van Maanen MA, Vervoordeldonk MJ, Tak PP. Restoring the balance of the autonomic nervous system as an innovative approach to the treatment of rheumatoid arthritis. *Mol Med*. 2011;17(9–10):937–948.
83. Padro CJ, Sanders VM. Neuroendocrine regulation of inflammation. *Semin Immunol*. 2014;26(5):357–368.
84. Elenkov IJ. Neurohormonal-cytokine interactions: Implications for inflammation, common human diseases and well-being. *Neurochem Int*. 2008;52(1–2):40–51.
85. Xie W, Chen S, Strong JA, Li A-L, Lewkowich IP, Zhang J-M. Localized sympathectomy reduces mechanical hypersensitivity by restoring normal immune homeostasis in rat models of inflammatory pain. *J Neurosci*. 2016;36(33):8712–8725.
86. Rodriguez-Pinto I, Agmon-Levin N, Howard A, Shoenfeld Y. Fibromyalgia and cytokines. *Immunol Lett*. 2014;161(2):200–203.

87. Alexander GM, Peterlin BL, Perreault MJ, Grothusen JR, Schwartzman RJ. Changes in plasma cytokines and their soluble receptors in complex regional pain syndrome. *J Pain*. 2012;13(1):10–20.

88. Bjurstrom MF, Giron SE, Griffis CA. Cerebrospinal fluid cytokines and neurotrophic factors in human chronic pain populations: A comprehensive review. *Pain Pract*. 2016;16(2):183–203.

89. Wang JG, Strong JA, Xie W, et al. The chemokine CXCL1/growth related oncogene increases sodium currents and neuronal excitability in small diameter sensory neurons. *Mol Pain*. 2008;4:38.

90. Xie WR, Deng H, Li H, Bowen TL, Strong JA, Zhang J-M. Robust increase of cutaneous sensitivity, cytokine production and sympathetic sprouting in rats with localized inflammatory irritation of the spinal ganglia. *Neuroscience*. 2006;142(3):809–822.

91. Johnson ZI, Schoepflin ZR, Choi H, Shapiro IM, Risbud MV. Disc in flames: Roles of TNF-alpha and IL-1beta in intervertebral disc degeneration. *Eur Cell Mater*. 2015;30:104–116; discussion 116–107.

92. Hess A, Axmann R, Rech J, et al. Blockade of TNF-alpha rapidly inhibits pain responses in the central nervous system. *Proc Natl Acad Sci U S A*. 2011;108(9):3731–3736.

93. Hooten WM. Chronic pain and mental health disorders: Shared neural mechanisms, epidemiology, and treatment. *Mayo Clin Proc*. 2016;91(7):955–970.

94. Leonard BE. Pain, depression and inflammation: Are interconnected causative factors involved? *Mod Trends Pharmacopsychiatry*. 2015;30:22–35.

4

Shared Brain Synaptic Mechanisms of Pain and Anxiety

Insight From Preclinical Studies

IPEK YALCIN AND MIN ZHUO ■

INTRODUCTION

Pain is defined as an unpleasant sensory and emotional experience associated with actual or potential tissue damage or described in terms of such damage (International Association for the Study of Pain). It is thus a multidimensional and subjective experience. Pain experience is composed of three dimensions: the **sensory-discriminative** dimension, which identifies the location, timing, and physical characteristics of the noxious stimulus and leads to withdrawal reflexes to prevent or limit tissue damage; the **affective-motivational dimension**, linked with emotion, which underlies the unpleasantness associated with exposure to a noxious stimulus and activates behaviors enabling the individual to cope with the noxious stimulus; and the **cognitive dimension**, which influences the appraisal of the meanings and consequences of pain. Our understanding of basic pain mechanisms at cortical levels is highly limited, especially at affective aspects of suffering.

AFFECTIVE ASPECTS OF PAIN

The affective dimension of pain is primarily due to the feelings of unpleasantness and secondary to the long-term impact of having pain. The unpleasantness[1,2] reflects aversive and motivational aspect of pain, providing a teaching signal that shapes subsequent behavior. For instance, the immediate unpleasant aspect of pain motivates behaviors such as escape or fight to reduce this feeling state; in contrast, after an injury, pain could diminish movement as a protective measure. The persistence of pain enhances unpleasantness over time and leads to a secondary affect such as anxiety and depression. These psychiatric comorbidities that progressively emerge in the context of chronic pain tightly determine clinical outcomes, with more frequent pain complaints and greater disability.

Role of Cortex in Unpleasantness

Cortical areas such as the somatosensory I (SI) and II (SII), the anterior cingulate, and the insular cortices are involved in mediating and modulating the pain experience.[3] Among these areas, the somatosensory cortices are primarily thought to play a role in discriminating the location and intensity of painful stimuli,[4] while other cortical areas, including the cingulate cortex and the insula, were proposed to support the affective, motivational, and cognitive aspects of pain. While most of the data focus on the possible role of the anterior cingulate and insular cortices in the emotional component of pain, it is important to note that the other cortical regions, such as the somatosensory cortex, may exert indirect influence. Indeed, a rapid rewiring of SI induced by peripheral nerve injury causes SI hyperexcitability.[5] This synaptic remodeling, including an increased synaptogenesis and synapse elimination and an enhanced strength of persisting synapses, causes SI hyperexcitability in response to peripheral stimulation and might also affect the anterior cingulate cortex (ACC) or other pain-related cortical areas.[6]

Clinical imaging and lesion studies have largely supported the recruitment of the ACC[7,8] and insula[9] for the unpleasantness of pain, and preclinical studies have more precisely associated the activation of the ACC with pain-like aversive behavior, while the inhibition of these neurons blocks such behavior.[1,10] Besides, ACC also contributes to the anticipation of pain,[11] empathy for pain,[12] and avoidance learning observed as a secondary reaction to pain.[13]

Both clinical and preclinical studies also highlighted cortical segregation between different components of pain, reporting that SI and posterior insular cortex are necessary for the somatosensory component while ACC and anterior portion of the insula (AI) are essential for the pain affect.[7,14] This dichotomy is also observed during witnessing others' pain, which also recruits AI and medial ACC (mACC).[15] It has been proposed that neural signals in AI/mACC might not code for specific experiences (e.g., pain, disgust, unfairness), but instead mediate a broader function across different region. It has been recently shown that there exists both shared and independent coding in AI/mACC. Left AI and mACC disclose activity patterns that are shared between different modalities (pain, disgust, and unfairness) but also between first-hand and vicarious aversive experiences, pointing to common coding of affective unpleasantness. Instead, right AI discloses activity patterns that are specific for the events' sensory properties and the target of the experience.[16]

Interestingly, neural representation of pain unpleasantness is shown to be sex dependent. Indeed, results revealed that subjective pain unpleasantness is strongly associated with increased perigenual ACC activity in women and decreased ventromedial prefrontal cortex (PFC) activity in men.[17]

Role of Cortex in Secondary Affect: Insight From Anxiety and Depression

When pain becomes chronic, the emotional aspect of pain can become pathological. For instance, mood disorders such as depression and anxiety are frequently observed, with prevalence rates ranging from 30% in neuropathic pain patients[18] to close to 80% in patients with fibromyalgia.[19] For implementing research on this question, it is difficult to assess, in patients, whether the mood disorders are a consequence of the chronic pain or were preexisting and favored the development of chronic pain.[20] In this regard, clinical research has recently tried to identify factors that may increase or predict the risk for pain chronification[21,22] and risk for developing mood disorders. While preclinical research offers a unique opportunity to test cellular and molecular hypotheses, human clinical investigations provide critical neuroanatomical insights, particularly through functional imaging studies. Indeed, recent human studies in chronic pain point out morphological and functional changes as well as reorganization in cortical regions associated with affective and cognitive disorders, such as the medial PFC (mPFC)[23,24] and the ACC.[4]

NEUROANATOMICAL ALTERATIONS AND NEUROPLASTICITY

In the past two decades, several authors have considered the possibility that plasticity of brain structures and cellular remodeling are involved in the pathophysiology and treatment of mood disorders.[25,26] This hypothesis may also apply to pain-induced mood disorders because cortical and subcortical functional and structural neuroplastic alterations have been observed in chronic pain. Imaging studies showed that the increased functional connectivity between nucleus accumbens (NAc) and the PFC is predictive for the pain chronification.[22] Preclinical imaging and molecular evidence are also supportive of a time-dependent reorganization of functional connectivity of the NAc to the insula, and the SI/SII cortices demonstrated significant decreases at postneuropathy day 28 but not at early-phase (days 2–5).[27] A study using functional magnetic resonance imaging (fMRI) showed that the depressed mood increases the pain unpleasantness associated with greater inferior frontal gyrus and amygdala activation and that responses to noxious thermal stimuli in these patients were characterized by increased activity in a broad network, including prefrontal areas, subgenual ACC, and hippocampus.[28]

The recent development of preclinical models also allowed exploring the anxiodepressive consequences of chronic pain and started to provide mechanistic insights. Again, the ACC, an integration center that interconnects neurons from the frontal cortex, the thalamus, and the amygdala and processes cognitive, emotional, and autonomic functions[29,30] seems to be implicated in the secondary pain affect such as anxiety and depression. By using an MRI approach, the longitudinal cortical changes associated with pain-like and anxiety-like behaviors were determined in the rat model of neuropathic pain.[31] The volume of the ACC as well as of the retrosplenial, entorhinal, and insular cortices bilaterally decreased in a time-dependent manner, and the changes in the prefrontal and retrosplenial cortices were correlated with anxiety-related behaviors. Preclinical studies on the mPFC, comprising the ACC, reported significant morphological alterations with neuropathic pain, such as increased arborization and length of basal but not apical dendrites of pyramidal cells and increased spine density in the early phase of spinal nerve injury.[32] While these results may seem to differ from MRI data[31] and from the report showing no changes in dendritic length of amygdala neurons in neuropathic animals,[33] it is important to point out that the alterations are likely region and time dependent and may also depend on whether the chronic pain is accompanied by anxiodepressive behaviors. In particular, the time-dependent morphological alterations may be critical. Indeed, the decreased frontal cortex volume after sciatic nerve injury only appeared after a long delay, coincident with the onset of anxiety-like behaviors.[31] Such time dependency could rely on long-term molecular and neural plasticity, which could, for example, imply epigenetic and gene expression changes, neurotrophins recruitment, and stimulation of dendritic arborization as well as changes in neurogenesis, as observed in the depression field.[34,35]

Transcriptional Mechanisms

Recent studies reported that chronic pain promotes adaptive changes in gene expression in brain networks involved in stress and depression. These studies point out the existence of different transcriptome profiles across brain regions such as ACC, mPFC, NAc, and periaqueductal gray (PAG) and identify a substantial number of similar and distinct signaling pathway–associated gene alterations between chronic pain– and chronic stress–induced depression.[36,37] For instance, one of the main negative regulators of the MAPK signaling cascade, MAPK phosphatase 1 (MKP-1), also known as dual-specificity phosphatase 1, is overexpressed in the ACC in chronic pain– and chronic stress–induced depression, suggesting that this pattern is consistent regardless of the cause of depression.[36] Besides, multiple other genes, including histone deacetylases (HDAC) such as HDAC5, brain-derived neurotrophic factor, 5-hydroxytryptamine, Btg2, Cyr61, Tph2, Ccl3, Fos, and Slc17a that have been previously implicated in anxiodepressive and nociceptive states, were altered in the mPFC of animals displaying anxiodepressive behavior following sciatic nerve surgery.[37]

Monoamine Hypothesis

The monoamine hypothesis, despite its limitations, remains one of the most studied hypotheses of depression.[38,39] It proposes that depression results from decreased cerebral monoamine function since antidepressant drugs increase monoamine transmission by inhibiting monoamine oxydase or by inhibiting the reuptake of serotonin and/or noradrenaline. This hypothesis is also supported by biochemical studies reporting alterations in the receptor density and the metabolites of noradrenaline and serotonin in cortical and limbic structures. Imaging studies show decreased dopamine receptor binding, and genetic studies provide evidence for polymorphisms of catechol-O-methyl-transferase[40] or serotonin transporter[41] in depressed patients.

The monoaminergic systems are also implicated in pain control as the serotonergic and noradrenergic brainstem regions provide descending pain modulating pathways. Antidepressants acting on noradrenergic, but not on serotonergic, uptakeonly are first-line treatments against neuropathic pain.[42,43] Recent studies also evidenced that neuropathic pain–induced anxiodepressive behaviors coincided with marked modifications in noradrenergic locus coeruleus neurons, such as increased tyrosine hydroxylase and noradrenaline transporter expression and α_2-adrenoceptor hypersensitivity, influencing locus coeruleus firing and noradrenaline release in the PFC terminal areas.[44] Similar changes in tyrosine hydroxylase, noradrenaline transporter, and

α_2-adrenoceptor levels in the locus coeruleus have also been described in animal models of depression and in the postmortem brain tissue of depressed individuals.[45]

Neuroimmune Hypothesis

Neuroimmune alterations are increasingly recognized to play important roles in the pathophysiology of depression[46] and chronic pain.[47] During the course of an immune challenge, the release of pro-inflammatory cytokines is usually transient and highly regulated by anti-inflammatory mechanisms, but clinical[48] and preclinical studies[47,49] have presented evidence for a sustained imbalance between pro-inflammatory and anti-inflammatory cytokines in chronic pain. Pro-inflammatory cytokines also cause sickness behaviors, including emotional dysregulation such as sadness, anxiety, decreased social interaction, and low energy.[50] While primarily studied with the peripheral nervous system and the spinal cord, the recruitment of neuroimmune mechanisms in chronic pain also affects the brain. For instance, at an early phase of the neuropathic pain, an increase in microglial staining is observed in the PAG and the hypothalamus,[51] and an astroglial activation is detected in the PAG[52]; while at a later phase, when an anxiety-like behavior is present, astrogliosis is observed in the cingulate cortex.[50] Moreover, the upregulation of IL-1β, a pro-inflammatory cytokine implicated in the induction and maintenance of neuropathic pain, has been reported in the prefrontal cortex during the early phase of a peripheral neuropathic pain.[53] Unfortunately, these studies do not directly address the potential link between cytokines and the emotional consequences of chronic pain. Another important drawback is that most research focuses on early changes, from 1 hour to 7 days after nerve injury, rather than on long-term changes, whereas emotional consequences of neuropathic pain develop over time.

Cellular and Molecular Insights

ACC Post-LTP: NMDA Receptor–Dependent Postsynaptic Form of LTP

Long-term potentiation (LTP) and long-term depression (LTD) are enduring increase and decrease, respectively, in synaptic strength induced by specific patterns of synaptic activity. Excitatory synapses in the ACC of adult animals can undergo LTP, which can be induced by different stimulation protocols, including theta-burst stimulation (TBS), paired training, and spike-excitatory postsynaptic potential (EPSP) pairing.[54,55] Activation of postsynaptic glutamate N-methyl-D-aspartate (NMDA) receptors as well as L-type voltage-gated calcium channels is important for the induction of ACC LTP.[54] For instance, bath application of the NMDA receptor antagonist AP-5 blocks the induction of LTP through TBS,[54] while NMDA receptor subtype 2A (NR2A)- or NR2B-selective antagonists separately only reduce LTP but completely eliminate it when they are combined.[54]

Postsynaptic increases in intracellular Ca^{2+} are critical for the induction of ACC LTP. Intracellular Ca^{2+} binds to calmodulin (CaM), leading to the activation of various calcium-stimulated signaling pathways.[56] Postsynaptic application of the polyamino carboxylic acid BAPTA, which blocks Ca^{2+}-activated currents, has been shown to completely abolish LTP induction within the ACC.[55,57] In addition, selective expression within the ACC of a CaM mutant with two impaired Ca^{2+}-binding sites on the N-terminal lobe resulted in a complete block of LTP induction within ACC slices.[58] Additional intracellular signaling proteins such as Ca^{2+}-CaM stimulated adenylyl cyclases (ACs), including AC1 and Ca^{2+}-CaM–dependent protein kinase subtype IV (CaMKIV), have also been implicated in the induction of ACC LTP. For instance, genetic deletion of AC1 completely abolishes ACC LTP induction through TBS.[59] The requirement of AC1 is further confirmed by the use of the selective AC1 inhibitor NB001.[60] A recent study using both genetic and pharmacological approaches found that AC1 is required for late-phase LTP in the ACC.[61] The role of CaMKIV in ACC LTP has also been confirmed using brain slices of CaMKIV knockout mice because TBS stimulation failed to induce ACC LTP, whereas wild-type mice displayed a robust level of LTP under this protocol.[62] In addition, activation of AC1 and AC8 leads to the activation of cyclic adenosine monophosphate (cAMP)-dependent protein kinase A (PKA). In turn, cAMP response element–binding protein (CREB) and other immediate early genes such as c-Fos and Egr1 activate targets that are thought to lead to structural changes.[56] Interestingly, genetic deletion of Egr1 significantly attenuates ACC LTP, implicating that intracellular protein synthesis may play a role in LTP.

A critical feature of ACC LTP expression is the functional recruitment of postsynaptic AMPA receptors. Both pharmacological and genetic studies have found that the involvement of AMPA receptors in ACC LTP is subtype selective and that the AMPA receptor subtype 1 is critical for the expression of ACC LTP. Indeed, genetic deletion of GluA1 completely abolishes ACC LTP, while deletion of AMPA GluA2 has no significant effect.[63] This is further supported by pharmacological studies using peptide inhibitors. For example, the AMPA receptor subunit GRIA1 appears to play a critical role in ACC LTP expression because postsynaptic, preapplication of the GRIA1-inhibiting peptide Pep1-TGL completely blocks LTP induction by paired training.[64] The involvement of the GRIA1 subunit appears to be time dependent as the LTP-blocking effect of Pep1-TGL did not occur if the antagonist was introduced 5 minutes after the pairing protocol commenced, suggesting that the functional recruitment of AMPA receptor GRIA1 subunits is complete within 5 to 10 minutes.

Phosphorylation of postsynaptic AMPA receptors by PKA-dependent phosphorylation is important for ACC LTP since ACC LTP was significantly impaired in mice with a GluA1 knock-in mutation at the PKA phosphorylation site serine 845 (s845A).[65] In addition, PKMζ is required for the expression of ACC LTP.[66] Application of the PKMζ inhibitor ζ-pseudosubstrate inhibitory peptide (ZIP) erases late-phase LTP in the ACC.[66]

ACC Pre-LTP: NMDA Receptor–Independent Presynaptic Form of LTP
Recent studies reported the existence of pre-LTP in ACC brain slices from adult mice.[67–69] The induction of pre-LTP is NMDA receptor independent, a key feature differentiating pre-LTP from post-LTP in the ACC. Furthermore, pre-LTP and post-LTP have been observed in the same neurons, presumably at the same excitatory synapses.[68]

Glutamate kainite (GluK1), but not GluK2, receptor is important for the induction of pre-LTP. This was nicely demonstrated by the use of GluK1 knockout mice as well as a selective GluK1 inhibitor.[68] By contrast, NMDA receptors and postsynaptic Ca^{2+} signaling pathways are not required for pre-LTP. A PKMζ inhibitor, ZIP, which erases post-LTP in ACC, did not affect pre-LTP.

Using both pharmacological and genetic approaches, it has been shown that AC1 and PKA are required for pre-LTP. For instance, genetic deletion of AC1 or inhibition of AC1 by NB001 completely prevents the induction of ACC LTP. The expression of pre-LTP is through different protein channels. Indeed, pre-LTP requires a mechanism involving hyperpolarization-activated cyclic nucleotide-gated (HCN) channels. A role of Fragile X Mental Retardation Protein in pre-LTP in ACC has also been reported recently.[67] Future studies are clearly needed to map out the molecular pathways for pre-LTP in ACC.

Pre-LTP: A New Mechanism for the Connection Between Pain and Anxiety
In the ACC, previous studies suggested that both presynaptic and postsynaptic transmission are upregulated in chronic pain conditions.[70,71] Behavioral studies indicate that pre-LTP is related to the anxiety induced by chronic pain.[57] Inhibiting the expression of pre-LTP by HCN channel inhibitors in the ACC reduced enhanced anxiety-like behaviors in animals with chronic pain. Post-LTP, which is important for behavioral sensitization, was not affected by HCN channel inhibition. Pre-exposure to a stimulus that causes anxiety can reduce the probability that synapses undergo pre-LTP in brain slices, further suggesting that pre-LTP is involved in anxiety.[68] These results also suggest that

pre-LTP may serve as one of the general mechanisms for anxiety, especially the one caused by chronic pain.

CONCLUSION AND FUTURE DIRECTIONS

Besides the somatosensory component, there is an unmet need to take charge of the affective consequences of chronic pain. Advances in our understanding of synaptic and molecular mechanisms would provide new opportunities to develop medicines to treat chronic pain and its comorbidity. For instance, the linkage of pre-LTP with chronic pain–induced anxiety provides new insight for identifying drug targets and helps us to understand why chronic anxiety is long-lasting and resistant to drugs targeting neurotransmission and modulation. Thus, manipulating pre-LTP may provide a unique opportunity to reverse or even erase this often debilitating condition. Future studies on basic molecular and signaling pathways that trigger and maintain pathological changes of central synapses are important. At the network and systemic levels, it is critical to understand how neuronal processing takes place among different brain regions.

REFERENCES

1. Johansen JP, Fields HL, Manning BH. The affective component of pain in rodents: Direct evidence for a contribution of the anterior cingulate cortex. *Proc Natl Acad Sci U S A*. 2001;98(14):8077–8082.
2. Vierck CJ, Hansson PT, Yezierski RP. Clinical and pre-clinical pain assessment: Are we measuring the same thing? *Pain*. 2008;135(1–2):7–10.
3. Garcia-Larrea L, Peyron R. Pain matrices and neuropathic pain matrices: A review. *Pain*. 2013;154(suppl 1):S29–S43.
4. Peyron R, Laurent B, Garcia-Larrea L. Functional imaging of brain responses to pain: A review and meta-analysis. *Neurophysiol Clin*. 2000;30(5):263–288.
5. Kim SK, Nabekura J. Rapid synaptic remodeling in the adult somatosensory cortex following peripheral nerve injury and its association with neuropathic pain. *J Neurosci*. 2011;31(14):5477–5482.
6. Kim SK, Eto K, Nabekura J. Synaptic structure and function in the mouse somatosensory cortex during chronic pain: In vivo two-photon imaging. *Neural Plast*. 2012;2012:640259.
7. Rainville P, Duncan GH, Price DD, Carrier B, Bushnell MC. Pain affect encoded in human anterior cingulate but not somatosensory cortex. *Science*. 1997;277(5328):968–971.
8. Tolle TR, Kaufmann T, Siessmeier T, et al. Region-specific encoding of sensory and affective components of pain in the human brain: A positron emission tomography correlation analysis. *Ann Neurol*. 1999;45(1):40–47.

9. Ostrowsky K, Magnin M, Ryvlin P, Isnard J, Guenot M, Mauguiere F. Representation of pain and somatic sensation in the human insula: A study of responses to direct electrical cortical stimulation. *Cereb Cortex.* 2002;12(4):376–385.

10. Qu C, King T, Okun A, Lai J, Fields HL, Porreca F. Lesion of the rostral anterior cingulate cortex eliminates the aversiveness of spontaneous neuropathic pain following partial or complete axotomy. *Pain.* 2011;152(7):1641–1648.

11. Porro CA, Baraldi P, Pagnoni G, et al. Does anticipation of pain affect cortical nociceptive systems? *J Neurosci.* 2002;22(8):3206–3214.

12. Lamm C, Decety J, Singer T. Meta-analytic evidence for common and distinct neural networks associated with directly experienced pain and empathy for pain. *Neuroimage.* 2011;54(3):2492–2502.

13. LaGraize SC, Fuchs PN. GABAA but not GABAB receptors in the rostral anterior cingulate cortex selectively modulate pain-induced escape/avoidance behavior. *Exp Neurol.* 2007;204(1):182–194.

14. Barthas F, Sellmeijer J, Hugel S, Waltisperger E, Barrot M, Yalcin I. The anterior cingulate cortex is a critical hub for pain-induced depression. *Biol Psychiatry.* 2015;77(3):236–245.

15. Singer T, Seymour B, O'Doherty J, Kaube H, Dolan RJ, Frith CD. Empathy for pain involves the affective but not sensory components of pain. *Science.* 2004;303(5661):1157–1162.

16. Corradi-Dell'Acqua C, Tusche A, Vuilleumier P, Singer T. Cross-modal representations of first-hand and vicarious pain, disgust and fairness in insular and cingulate cortex. *Nat Commun.* 2016;7:10904.

17. Girard-Tremblay L, Auclair V, Daigle K, Leonard G, Whittingstall K, Goffaux P. Sex differences in the neural representation of pain unpleasantness. *J Pain.* 2014;15(8):867–877.

18. Bair MJ, Robinson RL, Katon W, Kroenke K. Depression and pain comorbidity: A literature review. *Arch Intern Med.* 2003;163(20):2433–2445.

19. Fietta P, Manganelli P. Fibromyalgia and psychiatric disorders. *Acta Biomed.* 2007;78(2):88–95.

20. Blackburn-Munro G, Blackburn-Munro RE. Chronic pain, chronic stress and depression: Coincidence or consequence? *J Neuroendocrinol.* 2001;13(12):1009–1023.

21. Attal N, Masselin-Dubois A, Martinez V, et al. Does cognitive functioning predict chronic pain? Results from a prospective surgical cohort. *Brain.* 2014;137(part 3):904–917.

22. Baliki MN, Petre B, Torbey S, et al. Corticostriatal functional connectivity predicts transition to chronic back pain. *Nat Neurosci.* 2012;15(8):1117–1119.

23. Baliki MN, Chialvo DR, Geha PY, et al. Chronic pain and the emotional brain: Specific brain activity associated with spontaneous fluctuations of intensity of chronic back pain. *J Neurosci.* 2006;26(47):12165–12173.

24. Baliki MN, Geha PY, Apkarian AV, Chialvo DR. Beyond feeling: Chronic pain hurts the brain, disrupting the default-mode network dynamics. *J Neurosci.* 2008;28(6):1398–1403.

25. Ota KT, Duman RS. Environmental and pharmacological modulations of cellular plasticity: Role in the pathophysiology and treatment of depression. *Neurobiol Dis.* 2013;57:28–37.

26. Pittenger C, Duman RS. Stress, depression, and neuroplasticity: A convergence of mechanisms. *Neuropsychopharmacology.* 2008;33(1):88–109.

27. Chang PC, Pollema-Mays SL, Centeno MV, et al. Role of nucleus accumbens in neuropathic pain: Linked multi-scale evidence in the rat transitioning to neuropathic pain. *Pain.* 2014;155(6):1128–1139.

28. Berna C, Leknes S, Holmes EA, Edwards RR, Goodwin GM, Tracey I. Induction of depressed mood disrupts emotion regulation neurocircuitry and enhances pain unpleasantness. *Biol Psychiatry.* 2010;67(11):1083–1090.

29. Shackman AJ, Salomons TV, Slagter HA, Fox AS, Winter JJ, Davidson RJ. The integration of negative affect, pain and cognitive control in the cingulate cortex. *Nat Rev Neurosci.* 2011;12(3):154–167.

30. Vogt BA. Pain and emotion interactions in subregions of the cingulate gyrus. *Nat Rev Neurosci.* 2005;6(7):533–544.

31. Seminowicz DA, Laferriere AL, Millecamps M, Yu JS, Coderre TJ, Bushnell MC. MRI structural brain changes associated with sensory and emotional function in a rat model of long-term neuropathic pain. *Neuroimage.* 2009;47(3):1007–1014.

32. Metz AE, Yau HJ, Centeno MV, Apkarian AV, Martina M. Morphological and functional reorganization of rat medial prefrontal cortex in neuropathic pain. *Proc Natl Acad Sci U S A.* 2009;106(7):2423–2428.

33. Goncalves L, Silva R, Pinto-Ribeiro F, et al. Neuropathic pain is associated with depressive behaviour and induces neuroplasticity in the amygdala of the rat. *Exp Neurol.* 2008;213(1):48–56.

34. Coyle JT, Duman RS. Finding the intracellular signaling pathways affected by mood disorder treatments. *Neuron.* 2003;38(2):157–160.

35. Tsankova NM, Berton O, Renthal W, Kumar A, Neve RL, Nestler EJ. Sustained hippocampal chromatin regulation in a mouse model of depression and antidepressant action. *Nat Neurosci.* 2006;9(4):519–525.

36. Barthas F, Humo M, Gilsbach R, et al. Cingulate overexpression of mitogen-activated protein kinase phosphatase-1 as a key factor for depression. *Biol Psychiatry.* 2017;82(5):370–379.

37. Descalzi G, Mitsi V, Purushothaman I, et al. Neuropathic pain promotes adaptive changes in gene expression in brain networks involved in stress and depression. *Sci Signal.* 2017;10(471).

38. Goldberg JS, Bell CE Jr, Pollard DA. Revisiting the monoamine hypothesis of depression: A new perspective. *Perspect Med Chem.* 2014;6:1–8.

39. Krishnan V, Nestler EJ. The molecular neurobiology of depression. *Nature.* 2008;455(7215):894–902.

40. Antypa N, Drago A, Serretti A. The role of COMT gene variants in depression: Bridging neuropsychological, behavioral and clinical phenotypes. *Neurosci Biobehav Rev.* 2013;37(8):1597–1610.

41. Kenna GA, Roder-Hanna N, Leggio L, et al. Association of the 5-HTT gene-linked promoter region (5-HTTLPR) polymorphism with psychiatric disorders: Review of psychopathology and pharmacotherapy. *Pharmgenomics Pers Med.* 2012;5:19–35.

42. Attal N. [Pharmacological treatment of neuropathic pain in primary care]. *Rev Prat.* 2013;63(6):795–802.

43. Finnerup NB, Sindrup SH, Jensen TS. Recent advances in pharmacological treatment of neuropathic pain. *F1000 Med Rep.* 2010;2:52.

44. Alba-Delgado C, Llorca-Torralba M, Horrillo I, et al. Chronic pain leads to concomitant noradrenergic impairment and mood disorders. *Biol Psychiatry.* 2013;73(1):54–62.

45. Zhu MY, Klimek V, Dilley GE, et al. Elevated levels of tyrosine hydroxylase in the locus coeruleus in major depression. *Biol Psychiatry.* 1999;46(9):1275–1286.

46. Dantzer R, O'Connor JC, Freund GG, Johnson RW, Kelley KW. From inflammation to sickness and depression: When the immune system subjugates the brain. *Nat Rev Neurosci.* 2008;9(1):46–56.

47. Clark AK, Old EA, Malcangio M. Neuropathic pain and cytokines: Current perspectives. *J Pain Res.* 2013;6:803–814.

48. Backonja MM, Coe CL, Muller DA, Schell K. Altered cytokine levels in the blood and cerebrospinal fluid of chronic pain patients. *J Neuroimmunol.* 2008;195(1–2):157–163.

49. Calvo M, Dawes JM, Bennett DL. The role of the immune system in the generation of neuropathic pain. *Lancet Neurol.* 2012;11(7):629–642.

50. Narita M, Kuzumaki N, Kaneko C, et al. Chronic pain-induced emotional dysfunction is associated with astrogliosis due to cortical delta-opioid receptor dysfunction. *J Neurochem.* 2006;97(5):1369–1378.

51. Takeda K, Muramatsu M, Chikuma T, Kato T. Effect of memantine on the levels of neuropeptides and microglial cells in the brain regions of rats with neuropathic pain. *J Mol Neurosci.* 2009;39(3):380–390.

52. Mor D, Bembrick AL, Austin PJ, et al. Anatomically specific patterns of glial activation in the periaqueductal gray of the sub-population of rats showing pain and disability following chronic constriction injury of the sciatic nerve. *Neuroscience.* 2010;166(4):1167–1184.

53. Apkarian AV, Lavarello S, Randolf A, et al. Expression of IL-1beta in supraspinal brain regions in rats with neuropathic pain. *Neurosci Lett.* 2006;407(2):176–181.

54. Zhao M-G, Toyoda H, Lee Y-S, et al. Roles of NMDA NR2B subtype receptor in prefrontal long-term potentiation and contextual fear memory. *Neuron.* 2005;47(6):859–872.

55. Zhuo M. Cortical excitation and chronic pain. *Trends Neurosci.* 2008;31(4):199–207.

56. Bliss TVP, Collingridge GL, Kaang B-K, Zhuo M. Synaptic plasticity in the anterior cingulate cortex in acute and chronic pain. *Nat Rev Neurosci.* 2016;17(8):485–496.

57. Zhuo M. Neural mechanisms underlying anxiety-chronic pain interactions. *Trends Neurosci.* 2016;39(3):136–145.

58. Wei F, Xia X-M, Tang J, et al. Calmodulin regulates synaptic plasticity in the anterior cingulate cortex and behavioral responses: A microelectroporation study in adult rodents. *J Neurosci.* 2003;23(23):8402–8409.

59. Liauw J, Wu L-J, Zhuo M. Calcium-stimulated adenylyl cyclases required for long-term potentiation in the anterior cingulate cortex. *J Neurophysiol.* 2005;94(1):878–882.

60. Wang H, Xu H, Wu L-J, et al. Identification of an adenylyl cyclase inhibitor for treating neuropathic and inflammatory pain. *Science Transl Med.* 2011;3(65):65ra63–65ra63.

61. Chen T, O'Den G, Song Q, Koga K, Zhang M-M, Zhuo M. Adenylyl cyclase subtype 1 is essential for late-phase long term potentiation and spatial propagation of synaptic responses in the anterior cingulate cortex of adult mice. *Mol Pain.* 2014;10:65.

62. Wei F, Qiu C-S, Liauw J, et al. Calcium-calmodulin-dependent protein kinase IV is required for fear memory. *Nat Neurosci.* 2002;5(6):573–579.

63. Toyoda H, Zhao M-G, Ulzhöfer B, et al. Roles of the AMPA receptor subunit GluA1 but not GluA2 in synaptic potentiation and activation of ERK in the anterior cingulate cortex. *Mol Pain.* 2009;5:46.

64. Toyoda H, Wu L-J, Zhao M-G, Xu H, Zhuo M. Time-dependent postsynaptic AMPA GluR1 receptor recruitment in the cingulate synaptic potentiation. *Dev Neurobiol.* 2007;67(4):498–509.

65. Song Q, Zheng H-W, Li X-H, et al. Selective phosphorylation of AMPA receptor contributes to the network of long-term potentiation in the anterior cingulate cortex. *J Neurosci.* 2017;37(35):8534–8548.

66. Li X-Y, Ko H-G, Chen T, et al. Alleviating neuropathic pain hypersensitivity by inhibiting PKMζ in the anterior cingulate cortex. *Science.* 2010;330(6009):1400–1404.

67. Koga K, Descalzi G, Chen T, et al. Coexistence of two forms of LTP in ACC provides a synaptic mechanism for the interactions between anxiety and chronic pain. *Neuron.* 2015;85(2):377–389.

68. Koga K, Liu M-G, Qiu S, et al. Impaired presynaptic long-term potentiation in the anterior cingulate cortex of Fmr1 knock-out mice. *J Neurosci.* 2015;35(5):2033–2043.

69. Koga K, Yao I, Setou M, Zhuo M. SCRAPPER selectively contributes to spontaneous release and presynaptic long-term potentiation in the anterior cingulate cortex. *J Neurosci.* 2017;37(14):3887–3895.

70. Xu H, Wu LJ, Wang H, et al. Presynaptic and postsynaptic amplifications of neuropathic pain in the anterior cingulate cortex. *J Neurosci.* 2008;28(29):7445–7453.

71. Zhao M-G, Ko SW, Wu L-J, et al. Enhanced presynaptic neurotransmitter release in the anterior cingulate cortex of mice with chronic pain. *J Neurosci.* 2006;26(35):8923–8930.

5

The Epigenetic Bridge Between Stress, Chronic Pain, and Psychiatric Disorders

SIOUI MALDONADO-BOUCHARD AND MARIO INCAYAWAR ■

CLINICAL CASE

Mrs. X, 46 years old, comes into the clinic with a refractory chronic pain complaint: For the past year, she has had lower back pain that comes and goes. Radiographs and magnetic resonance imaging (MRI) are negative, as are blood tests. Mrs. X has consulted various primary care physicians and specialists, with no apparent success. Common pain medicines have had no effect.

On further investigation, it is found that the patient also presents with mild depressive and anxiety symptoms and that she is currently experiencing several life stressors: divorce, loss of employment, and a recent home burglary. Furthermore, when Mrs. X. was 8 years old, she escaped her country at war with her mother and lived precariously before entering the United States as a refugee. She sometimes has dreams related to these experiences, even today.

It would be reasonable, in such a case, after having discarded other potential diagnoses (e.g., disk herniations, cancers, fractures), to consider the possibility of chronic stress (including early-life stress) causing and/or maintaining the chronic back pain. Such an approach will lead to a different list of possible treatments, such as antidepressants and anti-inflammatory drugs to control the pain and referral to a psychologist or psychiatrist to address the depression and anxiety.

The link between early-life stress and chronic stress, depression-anxiety, and current chronic pain is explained through epigenetic mechanisms and chronic inflammation, as we will discuss in this chapter. To understand the relationship between stress, epigenetics, pain, and psychopathology, one must first review the physiology of stress. The stress response is an adaptive mechanism that has allowed us to survive dangers. However, chronic stress is becoming more and more common and unfortunately underlies the causation of many ailments and diseases.

PHYSIOLOGY OF STRESS

When people sense danger, the brain first reacts through the neural route. It activates the sympathetic nervous system, which induces the adrenal glands to release catecholamines, namely epinephrine and norepinephrine. The endocrine route (the hypothalamic-pituitary-adrenal [HPA] axis) also activates, but more slowly. The hypothalamus secretes corticotropin-releasing hormone (CRH) into the pituitary portal circulation. This, in turn, stimulates the pituitary gland to release the adrenocorticotropic hormone (ACTH), which triggers glucocorticoid release by the adrenal glands.[1] Circulating glucocorticoids exert negative neuroendocrine feedback; high plasma levels signal the hypothalamus to stop producing CRH and signal the anterior pituitary to stop producing ACTH, completing a feedback loop (Figure 5.1). This sequence of events describes the overall functioning of the stress response.

In response to acute stress, glucocorticoids and their receptors enhance cellular resiliency and plasticity through the inhibition of inflammation and apoptosis. Ninety percent of glucocorticoid molecules are bound to glucocorticoid-binding globulin, and only unbound glucocorticoids can cross the blood–brain barrier and body cell membranes. The small percentage of molecules that do cross the membrane of cells and reach the cytoplasm can bind to two types of receptors: mineralocorticoid receptors and glucocorticoid receptors. Mineralocorticoid receptors have an affinity to glucocorticoids 10 times greater than that of glucocorticoid receptors. This means that of the small percentage of glucocorticoid molecules that are able to cross cell membranes, only a fraction actually bind to glucocorticoid receptors.[1] Glucocorticoid receptors are found in virtually all cells of the body. In normal, acute stress circumstances, glucocorticoids have an anti-inflammatory effect. At the cellular and molecular levels, glucocorticoid molecules in the cytoplasm can bind

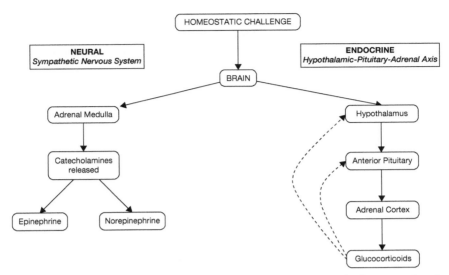

Figure 5.1. Schematic diagram of the psychological stress response, both its neural and endocrine route. *Dotted lines* represent inhibitory feedback loops.

to glucocorticoid receptors and trigger conformational changes that allow the glucocorticoid receptors to translocate to the cell nucleus through microtubular highways.[2] When in the nucleus, the glucocorticoid receptors can act as ligand-binding transcription factors that inhibit the expression of inflammatory genes.[3]

Conversely, in chronic stress, glucocorticoid receptors have the opposite effect; they can aggravate inflammation and apoptosis. Chronic exposure to elevated levels of glucocorticoids that ensues to early-life trauma,[4,5] chronic psychological stress[6,7] such as social isolation, bullying, marital conflict, physical abuse, exposure to racist attacks, and discrimination can lead to the development of glucocorticoid resistance. Indeed, stressful environments can lead to the chronic activation of the HPA axis and the autonomic nervous system, resulting in a high level of glucocorticoids and a decrease in glucocorticoid receptor sensitivity and function, which, by hindering the inhibitory effect of glucocorticoids, increases inflammation. The signaling pathways of pro-inflammatory cytokines, such as NF-κB, mitogen-activated protein kinases, and cyclooxygenase, can affect the travel of glucocorticoid receptors from the cytoplasm of the cell to the nucleus, or the ability of the glucocorticoid receptor to function as a transcription factor to inhibit the expression of pro-inflammatory genes by transcription factors such as NF-κB and activator protein 1 (AP-1).[8,9] The result is the increased production of pro-inflammatory agents. In turn, chronic elevated pro-inflammatory cytokine levels can contribute to the development of chronic pain.[10,11] The immune cells, including lymphocytes and macrophages, will lose sensitivity to glucocorticoids as well.[12]

The extended exposure of the body to the glucocorticoid hormones[13] and epinephrine and norepinephrine hormones[14] results in a diminished expression and function of the glucocorticoid receptor[6] through epigenetic mechanisms, detailed next.

EPIGENETIC CHANGES, PAIN, AND PSYCHOPATHOLOGY

Epigenetic modifications are potentially heritable and reversible changes in gene expression that do not alter the DNA sequence.[15,16] Epigenetic changes are exceptional because they can be triggered by the outside environment, can be stable, can be heritable, but can also be reversible, giving them a powerful potential for drug discoveries and the development of treatment strategies for diseases and mental illness. Regulation of gene expression occurs in various ways. In genetics, regulation is observed during transcription,[17] post-transcription,[18-20] and translation.[21] Three main levels of regulation are recognized today: direct regulation, in which a controlling factor directly alters a gene; indirect regulation, where a controlling factor affects the transcriptional machinery; and epigenetic regulation, which involves modifications to the DNA that do not change the DNA sequence.

Chromatin is a crucial element in epigenetics because its structure determines whether genes on the DNA are transcribed.[22-24] Chromatin is the combination of the DNA and the proteins found in the cell nucleus. The chromatin is referred to as *heterochromatin* or *euchromatin*, depending on its conformation.[16] When it is tightly wound, it is referred to as heterochromatin. The transcriptional machinery cannot access the DNA sequence, and genes are silenced, or inactivated. When the chromatin is loose or unwound, it is referred to as euchromatin. In this state, the transcriptional machinery can access the DNA, and genes can be expressed, or activated.[25] The chromatin is shaped by nucleosomes. A DNA segment containing 147 base pairs wraps around a histone octamer, forming a nucleosome.[26] These histone proteins contain a large number of arginine and lysine amino acids, which allow them to interact with the DNA.[27] There are five main types of histones: H1, H2A, H2B, H3, and H4. H1 is considered a linking histone, binding the DNA strand to the nucleosome and preventing it from moving by anchoring its entry and exit sites to the nucleosome. The H2, H3, and H4 histones are the core histones; they are the building blocks of the nucleosome. The nucleosome is composed of an H3-H4 tetramer, which is flanked on either side by an H2A-H2B dimer.[25,26] The chromatin can be remodeled through various mechanisms, but we summarize here three main types of epigenetic modifications. These include the addition of a methyl group to certain nucleotides of the DNA (DNA methylation), histone modifications,* and the changes induced by small regulatory noncoding RNA such as microRNAs. Research in the past decade has revealed the role of these epigenetic mechanisms in physical diseases, including cancer,[29] cardiovascular diseases,[30] neurodegenerative diseases,[31] chronic pain,[32] and various psychiatric conditions, such as depression and anxiety.[33]

Poverty, abuse, rape, bullying, war, or other psychosocial stressors at an early age can induce powerful epigenetic changes. Recent research shows that even prenatal maternal and paternal psychosocial stress could affect their offspring's brain development and psychopathology.[34-36] A stressful environment can affect the sensitivity of glucocorticoid receptors.[7] It can also alter its expression, and therefore concentration,[4,5,37] through epigenetic mechanisms. For example, epigenetic modifications to the glucocorticoid receptor have been found in individuals having suffered childhood abuse, and these modifications dramatically increased their risk for suicide later on.[4] Stressful environments lead to a decrease in glucocorticoid receptor expression: The promoter of the glucocorticoid receptor gene is not demethylated.[38,39] This epigenetic alteration remains until adulthood and can be transmitted to the next generation. The resulting downregulation of the glucocorticoid receptor leads to chronically increased levels of circulating glucocorticoids, reduced glucocorticoid feedback sensitivity, and no dampening of HPA responsivity to stress in adulthood; in other words, less resilience to stressors in adulthood.[5,40,41] Chronic stress also affects the sympathetic autonomic system. For example, chronic psychological stress is associated with the development of essential hypertension. This type of hypertension is associated with silencing of the norepinephrine transporter gene. The silencing of this transporter seems to occur in individuals exposed to chronic stress.[42,43]

These epigenetic changes to the glucocorticoid receptors cause chronically stressed individuals to be at higher susceptibility to stress-related health problems, such as autoimmune diseases, cardiovascular diseases, chronic pain, metabolic syndrome, diabetes, obesity, cardiovascular disease,[42,44] development of chronic pain, neurological disorders (e.g., Alzheimer disease),[45] and psychiatric conditions such as depression,[46] anxiety, and schizophrenia through changes to the epigenome.[47]

These are the most clearly understood mechanisms associated with stress, but there are likely more to discover. A recent wave of studies indicates that

---

*There is a significant body of literature on the heritability of epigenetic modifications due to DNA methylation, but less is known about histone modifications. For this reason, some do not consider histone modifications to be an example of epigenetic modification, but the definition of epigenetics we adopt here does recognize them.[28]

the microbiota can influence the regulation of the HPA axis and, more broadly speaking, inflammation and pain.[48] Short-chain fatty acids (SCFAs), signaling molecules produced by microorganisms in the gut, inhibit histone deacetylase and activate certain G-protein–coupled receptors in the brain. When the microbiota changes, the gut epithelium can become more permeable and let a greater number of these SCFAs into the bloodstream; these molecules then modulate the HPA axis.[49] Unexpectedly for many, osteocalcin has also been recently found to play an important role in the stress response. According to the Karsenty study,[50] circulating osteocalcin that is produced in bones increases after the experience of stress. Osteoblasts have been found to increase in glutamate uptake as a result of stress exposure, thereby preventing osteocalcin inactivation. Increased osteocalcin activation then appears to inhibit the postsynaptic parasympathetic neurons (which inhibit fear or the fight or flight response), thus allowing the full development of the stress response. This recent discovery of the role of osteocalcin in the neuropharmacology of stress could also have a significant impact on the understanding and management of stress-related diseases, chronic pain, and mental illness. Skeletal health could be a factor to consider for the management of the stress response as it relates to physical and mental illness.

CLINICAL EXAMPLES

Perceived Loneliness

Increasing evidence suggests that epigenetic changes can also occur in adulthood. Individuals with elevated cortisol levels are at high risk for inflammation-related diseases, such as cardiovascular diseases, arthritis, irritable bowel syndrome, and mental illness, among others. In a study by Cole et al., individuals who consistently *perceived* themselves as lonely (throughout a 3-year period) as adults based on the validated University of California, Los Angeles (UCLA) Perceived Loneliness Scale showed decreased transcription of the anti-inflammatory glucocorticoid target genes and an increase in transcription of the pro-inflammatory NF-κB target genes.[51,52] The promoters of overexpressed genes in lonely individuals had a nearly three-fold greater presence of NF-κB motifs compared with the promoters of overexpressed genes in nonlonely individuals.[52] This confirms the role of the NF-κB signaling pathway in adult lonely individuals and suggests epigenetic mechanisms at play in adulthood.

In addition, Cole[52] found that in lonely individuals, transcription factors involved in cell growth and differentiation were upregulated, as were certain chromatin structure regulators such as histone acetyltransferases. Genes involved in cytoskeleton remodeling and cell cycle progression, as well as a number of genes involved directly in inflammation, such as cytokines, chemokines, and, importantly, cyclooxygenase-2, the regulator of prostaglandin synthesis,[52] were upregulated. Other genes were also markedly downregulated, specifically, certain genes involved in B-lymphocyte function and antiviral responses.[52] This suggests that loneliness leads to epigenetic changes that decrease the adaptive immune response and increase inflammation.

Overall, this reflects the observed condition of lonely individuals: high-risk for inflammatory-related diseases and weakened defense against viral infection as well as humoral immune response. This evidence supports the role of both early-life events and adult-life stressful social environment in triggering epigenetic changes to the glucocorticoid receptor gene. On a positive note, an essential property of epigenetic mechanisms is that they are, in theory, reversible, giving them powerful potential in the development of treatment strategies (psychotherapy and pharmacotherapy) for various physical diseases and mental illnesses.

Irritable Bowel Syndrome

Epigenetics also explains the association of chronic stress and some forms of chronic pain. Tran et al.[53] found that in rats, repeated acute stress in the form of a water-avoidance task caused visceral pain resembling that of irritable bowel syndrome. More specifically, this repeated stress caused epigenetics changes to the glucocorticoid receptor and to the corticotropin-releasing factor. In the amygdala, this stress caused decreased methylation of the corticotropin-releasing factor promoter and increased methylation of the glucocorticoid receptor gene. Consequently, it caused increased expression of the corticotropin-releasing factor and decreased expression of the glucocorticoid receptor. This means higher levels of unbound glucocorticoids, some of which reached the central nucleus of the amygdala, a crucial site for the development of visceral pain.

Not only was epigenetics found as the mediator between chronic stress and pain, but also this relationship was shown to be reversible in rodents. Tran et al.[54] found that in rats, repeated psychological stress induced chronic pain through histone deacetylation. In a follow-up experiment, they were able to reverse cortisol-induced pain and anxiety by administering trichostatin A (TSA), a histone deacetylase inhibitor at H3K9 on the glucocorticoid receptor promoter. These new studies are beginning to uncover the link between chronic psychological stress, epigenetics, and the development of chronic pain. Intriguingly, the disproportionally frequent, severe, and disabling chronic pain experienced by African Americans has been linked to epigenetic changes. It is proposed that psychosocial stresses affecting this group, such as poverty, child-hood stress, low socioeconomic status, and racial discrimination, could affect DNA methylation and explain their vulnerability and the disparities.[55]

Although it is very early to make any conclusions, such findings help us to better understand the role of stress in the development of chronic pain and mental illness, as well as how psychotherapeutic interventions and pharmacotherapy targeting the reversal of epigenetic changes can contribute to controlling chronic pain and certain mental disorders at a molecular level.

CHRONIC STRESS, MICROGLIA, AND MICROBIOTA IN PAIN AND SUFFERING

Twenty years ago, Professor Linda R. Watkins delivered a seminal lecture at the University of California, Irvine, on the role of microglia in pain and the sickness response. She revealed that when activated by infection, trauma, or stress, microglia released pro-inflammatory cytokines that created or maintained enhanced pain states and what she called the sickness response, which included fever, prostration, appetite and sleep disturbances, and decreased social interactions. Today, it is recognized that glial cells (microglia and astrocytes), which are located in the brain and spinal cord, not only accomplish their function as neural resident macrophages but also have important functions in the development of chronic pain, mental disorders, and neurodegenerative diseases. Their function is critical for the homeostasis of the central nervous system in both neural health and disease

Role of Stress and Glial Cells

Glial cells, including microglia and astrocytes, interact with pain-related neurons to process pain.[56,57] Although glial cells can be activated and induce a pro-inflammatory effect by a range of factors and conditions, such as stress, hypoxia, infection, tissue damage, overfeeding, nicotine, cocaine, morphine exposure, lipopolysaccharide stimulus, hormones, exercise, and aging, the effect of psychosocial stress on glial cells is particularly relevant for understanding the pain response and its effects on mental health. Physiologically, glial cells are activated either by the sympathetic adrenergic activity[58] that follows the experience of stress or by peripheral nerve fibers (vagal afferents) that have been stimulated by peripherally produced pro-inflammatory cytokines. Microglia and astrocytes stimulated by central and peripheral input seem to sensitize neurons (neuroinflammation) and explain allodynia, hyperalgesia, spontaneous and chronic pain, and ultimately the illness response.[59,60] This unexpected bidirectional and long-distance brain–immune system communication occurs throughout the glial cells and leukocytes capable of receiving brain input through their adrenergic receptors.[61] In fact, this brain–immune system makes evolutionary sense because microglia embryologically originate from immune cells.

The diathesis-stress model is a theory that assumes individual vulnerabilities to stress and subsequent mental illness. This theory could be extended to pain. Early psychosocial stress (e.g., physical and sexual abuse, bullying, maternal separation) and repeated social defeat (e.g., low socioeconomic status, racial discrimination) could potentially affect immunity and produce inflammation by increasing glial cells reactivity.[62–64] In fact, the experience of such stressful events is associated with the development of chronic pain later in life and psychopathology. Indeed, in this book alone, the reader can consult the many chapters on pain conditions that are associated with stress and mental disorders. The complex mechanism underlying clinical chronic pain is likely related to glial cell activation, inflammation, and epigenetic changes. Interestingly, a recent study of integrated positron emission tomography–MRI demonstrated glial activation in chronic low back pain.[65]

Similarly, glial activation, the release of pro-inflammatory cytokines, and subsequent inflammation have been found in many psychiatric conditions. The most revealing evidence of brain inflammation and microglial activation exists for major depressive episodes.[66] This highlights the possible use of repurposed minocycline (a tetracycline antibiotic that inhibits microglial activation) and other anti-inflammatory drugs as a potential treatment for depression and other psychiatric disorders, when underlying neuroinflammation is suspected.[67] The innate immune system activation, including microglia, has been found to play a role in schizophrenia as well,[68–70] opening new and promising ways to develop new treatments. The immune system appears also to be involved in the pathogenesis of bipolar disorder. The pro-inflammatory cytokine interleukin-10 (IL-10) was found to be elevated in bipolar patients with psychotic features,[71] and other proinflammatory cytokines were involved in panic disorder, although there are discrepant findings in the literature.[72] Undoubtedly, inflammatory processes will be found in other psychiatric disorders in the near future.

The Microbiota and Glial Cells Link

Another intertwined relationship appears to exist between stress, epigenetics, microglia, and microbiota. As briefly mentioned earlier, the microbiome seems to exert a modulatory influence over the microglia.[73] The eradication of gut microbiota in lab rats severely changed microglia characteristics, and its reintroduction by transplant partially restored microglia function. SCFAs (gut microbiota bacterial fermentation products) regulate microglia maturation and activation thought epigenetic mechanisms and other biological processes.[49] It is worth noting that microglia behavior can also be subjected to epigenetic changes[74] and that genes related to epigenetic modifications have been found to be dysregulated in microglia, making the microglia function highly adaptable to changes in the physical and psychosocial environment. It is thought that DNA methylation, histone modification, and noncoding RNAs, as main epigenetic processes, have important roles in modulating neuroinflammation, which is considered one of the critical underlying mechanisms at the origin of chronic pain and mental illness.

CONCLUSION

For many years, researchers and clinicians have suspected psychosocial stress to play a role in mental health and pain, or at least noticed a certain association between the two. It is only recently that mechanisms explaining this association have been uncovered. Epigenetics, microglia, the microbiome, and now even skeletal molecules are demonstrating a role in this complex tableau of stress, mental health, and pain. Recent research developments on microglia, microbiome, and epigenetic changes in pain medicine and psychiatry are paving the way for future exciting discoveries. It will allow a multilayered evaluation of pain and psychiatric patients that takes into account their complex individual biological characteristics. The new knowledge on psychosocial stress, epigenetics, glial cells, and microbiome is contributing to the goal of developing person-centered or individualized pain medicine and psychiatry.

REFERENCES

1. Sorrells SF, Caso JR, Munhoz CD, Sapolsky RM. The stressed CNS: When glucocorticoids aggravate inflammation. *Neuron*. 2009;64(1):33–39.
2. Pratt W, Galigniana M, Morishima Y, Murphy P. Role of molecular chaperones in steroid receptor action. *Essays Biochem*. 2004;40(41–58).
3. Lu NZ, Cidlowski JA. Translational regulatory mechanisms generate N-terminal glucocorticoid receptor isoforms with unique transcriptional target genes. *Mol Cell*. 2005;18(3):331–342.
4. McGowan PO, Sasaki A, D'Alessio AC, et al. Epigenetic regulation of the glucocorticoid receptor in human brain associates with childhood abuse. *Nat Neurosci*. 2009;12(3):342–348.

5. Liu D, Diorio J, Tannenbaum B, et al. Maternal care, hippocampal glucocorticoid receptors, and hypothalamic-pituitary-adrenal responses to stress. *Science.* 1997;277(5332):1659–1662.

6. Miller GE, Cohen S, Ritchey AK. Chronic psychological stress and the regulation of pro-inflammatory cytokines: A glucocorticoid-resistance model. *Health Psychol.* 2002;21(6):531–541.

7. Cohen S, Janicki-Deverts D, Doyle WJ, et al. Chronic stress, glucocorticoid receptor resistance, inflammation, and disease risk. *Proc Natl Acad Sci U S A.* 2012;109(16):5995–5999.

8. Pace TWW, Hu F, Miller AH. Cytokine-effects on glucocorticoid receptor function: Relevance to glucocorticoid resistance and the pathophysiology and treatment of major depression. *Brain Behav Immun.* 2007;21(1):9–19.

9. Rebeyrol C, Saint-Criq V, Guillot L, et al. Glucocorticoids reduce inflammation in cystic fibrosis bronchial epithelial cells. *Cell Signal.* 2012;24(5):1093–1099.

10. Alexander JK, Popovich PG. Neuroinflammation in spinal cord injury: Therapeutic targets for neuroprotection and regeneration. *Prog Brain Res.* 2009;175:125–137.

11. Stemkowski PL, Smith PA. Sensory neurons, ion channels, inflammation and the onset of neuropathic pain. *Can J Neurol Sci.* 2012;39(4):416–435.

12. Stark JL, Avitsur R, Padgett DA, Campbell KA, Beck FM, Sheridan JF. Social stress induces glucocorticoid resistance in macrophages. *Am J Physiol.* 2001;280(6):R1799–R1805.

13. DeRijk R, Michelson D, Karp B, et al. Exercise and circadian rhythm-induced variations in plasma cortisol differentially regulate interleukin-1β (IL-1β), IL-6, and tumor necrosis factor-α (TNFα) production in humans: High sensitivity of TNFα and resistance of IL-6. *J Clin Endocrinol Metab.* 1997;82(7):2182–2191.

14. DeRijk RH, Petrides J, Deuster P, Gold PW, Sternberg EM. Changes in corticosteroid sensitivity of peripheral blood lymphocytes after strenuous exercise in humans. *J Clin Endocrinol Metab.* 1996;81(1):228–235.

15. Szyf M. Epigenetic therapeutics in autoimmune disease. *Clin Rev Allergy Immunol.* 2010;39(1):62–77.

16. Szyf M, Meaney M. Epigenetics, behaviour, and health. *Allergy Asthma Clin Immunol.* 2008;4(1):37–49.

17. Cramer P. Multisubunit RNA polymerases. *Curr Opin Struct Biol.* 2002;12(1):89–97.

18. Yap K, Makeyev EV. Regulation of gene expression in mammalian nervous system through alternative pre-mRNA splicing coupled with RNA quality control mechanisms. *Mol Cell Neurosci.* 2013;56:420–428.

19. Kloc M, Zearfoss NR, Etkin LD. Mechanisms of subcellular mRNA localization. *Cell.* 2002;108(4):533–544.

20. Maquat LE, Carmichael GG. Quality control of mRNA function. *Cell.* 2001;104(2):173–176.

21. Mendez R, Richter JD. Translational control by CPEB: A means to the end. *Nat Rev Mol Cell Biol.* 2001;2(7):521–529.

22. Groudine M, Eisenman R, Gelinas R, Weintraub H. Developmental aspects of chromatin structure and gene expression. *Prog Clin Biol Res.* 1983;134:159–182.

23. Szyf M, McGowan P, Meaney MJ. The social environment and the epigenome. *Environ Mol Mutag.* 2008;49(1):46–60.

24. Ramain P, Bourouis M, Dretzen G, Richards G, Sobkowiak A, Bellard M. Changes in the chromatin structure of *Drosophila* glue genes accompany developmental cessation of transcription in wild type and transformed strains. *Cell.* 1986;45(4):545–553.

25. Horn PJ, Peterson CL. Chromatin higher order folding: Wrapping up transcription. *Science.* 2002;297(5588):1824–1827.

26. Luger K, Mader AW, Richmond RK, Sargent DF, Richmond TJ. Crystal structure of the nucleosome core particle at 2.8 A resolution. *Nature.* 1997;389(6648):251–260.

27. Bhasin M, Reinherz EL, Reche PA. Recognition and classification of histones using support vector machine. *J Comput Biol.* 2006;13(1):102–112.

28. Bird A. Perceptions of epigenetics. *Nature.* 2007;447(7143):396–398.

29. Feinberg AP. Epigenetic stochasticity, nuclear structure and cancer: The implications for medicine. *J Intern Med.* 2014;276(1):5–11.

30. Baccarelli A, Rienstra M, Benjamin EJ. Cardiovascular epigenetics: Basic concepts and results from animal and human studies. *Circ Cardiovasc Genet.* 2010;3(6):567–573.

31. Fernandez-Santiago R, Ezquerra M. Epigenetic research of neurodegenerative disorders using patient iPSC-based models. *Stem Cells Int.* 2016;2016:9464591.

32. Descalzi G, Ikegami D, Ushijima T, Nestler EJ, Zachariou V, Narita M. Epigenetic mechanisms of chronic pain. *Trends Neurosci.* 2015;38(4):237–246.

33. Hoffmann A, Sportelli V, Ziller M, Spengler D. Epigenomics of major depressive disorders and schizophrenia: Early life decides. *Int J Mol Sci.* 2017;18(8).

34. Graham AM, Rasmussen JM, Entringer S, et al. Maternal cortisol concentrations during pregnancy and sex-specific associations with neonatal amygdala connectivity and emerging internalizing behaviors. *Biol Psychiatry.* 2019;85(2):172–181.

35. Palma-Gudiel H, Córdova-Palomera A, Eixarch E, Deuschle M, Fañanás L. Maternal psychosocial stress during pregnancy alters the epigenetic signature of the glucocorticoid receptor gene promoter in their offspring: A meta-analysis. *Epigenetics.* 2015;10(10):893–902.

36. Dietz DM, Laplant Q, Watts EL, et al. Paternal transmission of stress-induced pathologies. *Biol Psychiatry.* 2011;70(5):408–414.

37. Szyf M. The early life environment and the epigenome. *Biochim Biophys Acta.* 2009;1790(9):878–885.

38. Weaver ICG, D'Alessio AC, Brown SE, et al. The transcription factor nerve growth factor-inducible protein a mediates epigenetic programming: Altering epigenetic marks by immediate-early genes. *J Neurosci.* 2007;27(7):1756–1768.

39. Hellstrom IC, Dhir SK, Diorio JC, Meaney MJ. Maternal licking regulates hippocampal glucocorticoid receptor transcription through a thyroid hormone–serotonin–NGFI-A signalling cascade. *Philos Trans R Soc Lond B.* 2012;367(1601):2495–2510.

40. Feder A, Nestler EJ, Charney DS. Psychobiology and molecular genetics of resilience. *Nat Rev Neurosci.* 2009;10(6):446–457.

41. Weaver ICG, Cervoni N, Champagne FA, et al. Epigenetic programming by maternal behavior. *Nat Neurosci.* 2004;7(8):847–854.

42. Esler M, Eikelis N, Schlaich M, et al. Human sympathetic nerve biology: Parallel influences of stress and epigenetics in essential hypertension and panic disorder. *Ann N Y Acad Sci.* 2008;1148:338–348.

43. Esler M, Eikelis N, Schlaich M, et al. Chronic mental stress is a cause of essential hypertension: Presence of biological markers of stress. *Clin Exp Pharmacol Physiol.* 2008;35(4):498–502.
44. Ahn SY, Gupta C. Genetic programming of hypertension. *Front Pediatr.* 2017;5:285.
45. Bisht K, Sharma K, Tremblay M-È. Chronic stress as a risk factor for Alzheimer's disease: Roles of microglia-mediated synaptic remodeling, inflammation, and oxidative stress. *Neurobiol Stress.* 2018;9:9–21.
46. Story Jovanova O, Nedeljkovic I, Derek S, et al. DNA methylation signatures of depressive symptoms in middle-aged and elderly persons: Meta-analysis of multiethnic epigenome-wide studies. *JAMA Psychiatry.* 2018;75(9):949–959.
47. Kramer NE, Cosgrove VE, Dunlap K, Subramaniapillai M, McIntyre RS, Suppes T. A clinical model for identifying an inflammatory phenotype in mood disorders. *J Psychiatr Res.* 2019;113:148–158.
48. Ho P, Ross DA. More than a gut feeling: The implications of the gut microbiota in psychiatry. *Biol Psychiatry.* 2017;81(5):e35–e37.
49. Pearson-Leary J, Zhao C, Bittinger K, et al. The gut microbiome regulates the increases in depressive-type behaviors and in inflammatory processes in the ventral hippocampus of stress vulnerable rats. *Mol Psychiatry.* 2019; Mar 4 [Epub ahead of print].
50. Berger JM, Singh P, Khrimian L, et al. Mediation of the acute stress response by the skeleton. *Cell Metab.* 2019;30(5):890–902.
51. Hughes ME, Waite LJ, Hawkley LC, Cacioppo JT. A short scale for measuring loneliness in large surveys. *Res Aging.* 2004;26(6):655–672.
52. Cole SW, Hawkley LC, Arevalo JM, Sung CY, Rose RM, Cacioppo JT. Social regulation of gene expression in human leukocytes. *Genome Biol.* 2007;8:R189.181–R189.113.
53. Tran L, Chaloner A, Sawalha AH, Greenwood Van-Meerveld B. Importance of epigenetic mechanisms in visceral pain induced by chronic water avoidance stress. *Psychoneuroendocrinology.* 2013;38(6):898–906.
54. Tran L, Schulkin J, Ligon CO, Greenwood-Van Meerveld B. Epigenetic modulation of chronic anxiety and pain by histone deacetylation. *Mol Psychiatry.* 2015;20(10):1219–1231.
55. Aroke EN, Joseph PV, Roy A, et al. Could epigenetics help explain racial disparities in chronic pain? *J Pain Res.* 2019;12:701–710.
56. Watkins LR, Maier SF. *Cytokines and Pain.* Basel: Birkhauser Verlag; 1999.
57. Chiang CY, Sessle BJ, Dostrovsky JO. Role of astrocytes in pain. *Neurochem Res.* 2012;37(11):2419–2431.
58. Norris JG, Benveniste EN. Interleukin-6 production by astrocytes: Induction by the neurotransmitter norepinephrine. *J Neuroimmunol.* 1993;45(1–2):137–145.
59. Old EA, Clark AK, Malcangio M. The role of glia in the spinal cord in neuropathic and inflammatory pain. *Handb Exp Pharmacol.* 2015;227:145–170.
60. Watkins LR, Maier SF. Beyond neurons: Evidence that immune and glial cells contribute to pathological pain states. *Physiol Rev.* 2002;82(4):981–1011.
61. Beis D, von Kanel R, Heimgartner N, et al. The role of norepinephrine and alpha-adrenergic receptors in acute stress-induced changes in granulocytes and monocytes. *Psychosom Med.* 2018;80(7):649–658.
62. Roque A, Ochoa-Zarzosa A, Torner L. Maternal separation activates microglial cells and induces an inflammatory response in the hippocampus of male rat

pups, independently of hypothalamic and peripheral cytokine levels. *Brain Behav Immunity.* 2016;55:39–48.

63. Wohleb ES, Hanke ML, Corona AW, et al. beta-Adrenergic receptor antagonism prevents anxiety-like behavior and microglial reactivity induced by repeated social defeat. *J Neurosci.* 2011;31(17):6277–6288.

64. Thames AD, Irwin MR, Breen EC, Cole SW. Experienced discrimination and racial differences in leukocyte gene expression. *Psychoneuroendocrinology.* 2019;106:277–283.

65. Loggia ML, Chonde DB, Akeju O, et al. Evidence for brain glial activation in chronic pain patients. *Brain.* 2015;138(part 3):604–615.

66. Setiawan E, Wilson AA, Mizrahi R, et al. Role of translocator protein density, a marker of neuroinflammation, in the brain during major depressive episodes. *JAMA Psychiatry.* 2015;72(3):268–275.

67. Berk M, Walker AJ, Nierenberg AA. Biomarker-guided anti-inflammatory therapies: From promise to reality check. *JAMA Psychiatry.* 2019;76(8):779–780.

68. Mongan D, Ramesar M, Focking M, Cannon M, Cotter D. Role of inflammation in the pathogenesis of schizophrenia: A review of the evidence, proposed mechanisms and implications for treatment. *Early Interv Psychiatry.* 2019; Jul 31 [Epub ahead of print].

69. Zhang L, Zheng H, Wu R, Kosten TR, Zhang XY, Zhao J. The effect of minocycline on amelioration of cognitive deficits and pro-inflammatory cytokines levels in patients with schizophrenia. *Schizophr Res.* 2019;212:92–98.

70. Canetta S, Sourander A, Surcel HM, et al. Elevated maternal C-reactive protein and increased risk of schizophrenia in a national birth cohort. *Am J Psychiatry.* 2014;171(9):960–968.

71. Lesh TA, Careaga M, Rose DR, et al. Cytokine alterations in first-episode schizophrenia and bipolar disorder: Relationships to brain structure and symptoms. *J Neuroinflammation.* 2018;15(1):165.

72. Quagliato LA, Nardi AE. Cytokine alterations in panic disorder: A systematic review. *J Affect Disord.* 2018;228:91–96.

73. Erny D, Hrabe de Angelis AL, Jaitin D, et al. Host microbiota constantly control maturation and function of microglia in the CNS. *Nat Neurosci.* 2015;18(7):965–977.

74. Garden GA. Epigenetics and the modulation of neuroinflammation. *Neurotherapeutics.* 2013;10(4):782–788.

PART II

Diagnostic Issues

6

Identifying and Assessing Overlapping Chronic Pain and Mental Illness

GLENN J. TREISMAN ■

INTRODUCTION

Patients presenting with chronic pain of uncertain etiology have frustrated clinicians since the dawn of medicine. Physicians have long observed that identical clinical problems present with varying degrees of pain and suffering. Even in conditions with a known etiology, patients vary widely in the course of illnesses with similar pathology. Some patients are completely disabled, while others experience minimal impact on their function and life course. Psychiatric disorders play a very large role in determining the expression, course, and degree of impairment caused by chronic pain conditions.

The identification of psychiatric comorbidities in patients with chronic pain is essential. The global message for this chapter is that patients who fail to respond in the expected manner to treatment need further evaluation. The current fad of simply giving more of a treatment that has failed has distorted our practice. Limited time for each patient, a focus on short lengths of stay in hospital, emphasis on conserving resources, incentives for good patient satisfaction scores, and a consumerist view of medicine as a commodity have incentivized clinicians to give "pain medicines" for pain and to treat patients with procedures rather than use an interdisciplinary rehabilitative approach. For example, the resulting opiate epidemic is taking the lives of more people in the United States than motor vehicle crashes, despite cell phones and texting while driving.

Better evaluation of patients is time-consuming and requires expert observation across repeated follow-up interactions. This chapter is divided into different types of psychiatric conditions and ways they can be identified and incorporated into the diagnostic formulation of a patient with chronic pain.

CHRONIC PAIN IS COMPLICATED BY THE CIRCUMSTANCES OF THE PATIENT'S LIFE

Patients with chronic pain have often been led to believe that their pain should be eliminated. The "pain is a vital sign" campaign and the constant rating of pain in offices and in hospitals are partially responsible for this belief. Patients may be hostile to efforts to help them when the efforts do not fit their concept of what they "should" receive. These elements add to the "comorbidity" that arises from a variety of sources, including the culture, the medical system, the family, and the individual.

The life circumstances of a patient are often overlooked. The patient lives in a system that rewards illness rather recovery. An example is a patient who had been injured and was able to go back to work at about 70 % of his previous level. His boss urged him to go out on disability until he could come back at 100% because he could hire someone else after our patient had "moved over" to getting disability income. He cooperated and "went out on disability." His family became financially vulnerable, and his wife was concerned about him returning to work part-time because they might lose his disability income. He became focused on the idea that he could not return to work unless his pain was "completely better." His physical therapy benefits "ran out," and he kept reinjuring himself in the process of trying to achieve 100% function, while his dose of opiates was continually increased.

Elements that complicate the experience of pain include a sense of helplessness, poor coping skills, limited family support, limited expectations of self, and a sense of victimization and misuse by others or the system. Elements at the family level include the idea that pain is "holding everyone together," including difficult marriages and difficult family relationships, and an identified ill person on whom to focus all of the family distress. Infantilized and overprotected ill children often are the anchors holding families together. They are unable to mature and develop independence because of their chronic pain condition, which seems inadequate to explain their degree of dependence.

Families are sometimes held together by dysfunctional efforts to take care of the identified sick member suffering from intractable pain.

Economic elements also play a role in the circumstances of the patient. The medical system is set up to take care of common acute problems, many of which can be diagnosed using checklists and can be solved by following guidelines for treatment. More complex, chronically ill patients with interlocking problems are repeatedly run through these algorithms without success. The "problem-focused visit" does not serve the needs of these patients, and they are shunted from doctor to doctor. Emergency departments are rewarded for providing brief pain interventions, usually in the form of opioids and sometimes accompanied by brief admissions. Doctors are told to conserve costs and are rewarded for doing less workup as well as providing inexpensive and acute solutions to chronic problems. The medical system is reluctant to pay for integrated care, including psychotherapy, family therapy, cognitive behavioral therapy, and specialty rehabilitative programs, and for the physicians who provide coherent integrated rehabilitative individualized treatment.

The culture is also a part of the patient's world. Our consumerist culture believes that medical personnel are "providers" and that patients are customers. Patients in pain are victims and need their pain relieved. The media suggests that poor outcomes are the fault of malicious doctors, evil drug companies, and profit-driven hospitals and, at the same time, promotes that there are quick and cheap fixes for all problems. The current "patient satisfaction" craze is so politically driven that findings of increased patient satisfaction correlating with increased mortality[1] are ignored.

These factors amplify both the suffering and the behaviors associated with pain that motivate doctors to prescribe opiates.[2] Patients are not faking nor consciously exaggerating their pain. Pain is intensified as it becomes a central focus, and it distracts patients from rehabilitation and drives toward disability.

The evaluation of the life circumstances of the patient should include the support system that the patient has (including spouse, romantic partners, children and parents, and any other significant elements such as employer, social worker, or parole officer) as well as factors that maintain disability. Identification of family systems that sustain pain-related problems is essential to successful treatment of chronic pain.

Patients should be evaluated for their ideas about the meaning of their pain, the medical field, their predicament, and their legal situation. What are their goals, what would they like their treatment to achieve, what is their view of themselves after treatment, and most important, what do they hope to get from their health care practitioners? This history sets up the "role induction," in which the patient is told a diagnostic formulation and the role of the practitioner is defined, and their role in the upcoming treatment is proposed. The role induction is a neglected art in current medical practice but is fundamental in the rehabilitative treatment of chronic pain.

Patients should be encouraged to question anything about the diagnosis and treatment, but it is not a debate, it is informational. Patients may disagree, but by disagreeing, they are declining treatment, and again, it is not a negotiation, it is a recommendation. By disagreeing with their diagnostic formulation or the proposed treatment, they are declining treatment with you. This is not to say that practitioners will not discuss the plan. As practitioners, we are happy to discuss and even bargain about how fast we taper opiates, when we stop stimulants, or how slowly we discontinue benzodiazepines, but we must agree on the goals of care, including discontinuation of medications that play no useful role or make things worse. If we do not have the same goals, we cannot work together. Most important, we point out to patients that if they disagree with the diagnosis or treatment plan, they probably do want to work with us.

BEHAVIOR AND CHRONIC PAIN

Maladaptive behavior arises in most patients who are disordered by chronic pain. These behaviors must be identified and changed for patients to get better. The concept of using a behavioral approach for patients owes much credit to Wilbert (Bill) Fordyce at the University of Washington in Seattle after he discovered the work of B. F. Skinner. Fordyce was a psychologist in the Department of Physical Medicine and Rehabilitation. In the early 1960s, he began working with patients with chronic pain using a behavioral approach adapted from Skinner's work on behavior modification.[3] He researched the reinforcers of pain behaviors, ways that patients had been "conditioned" to behave in response to pain, and how to change the behavior. Surprisingly, changing the behavior improved health and decreased pain. Table 6.1 shows the essential elements of operant or "Skinnerian" conditioning.

As part of patient evaluation, a careful behavioral assessment of patients must be included in the formulation and can be used to help patients develop a plan to overcome the patterns of maladaptive behavior. Analysis of the positive reinforcers of pain behavior, such as opiates, attention, and support, as well as the negative reinforcers of pain behavior, such as relief from distress, relief from expectations and demands, and relief from criticism, are just a few of the ways pain behavior is increased by conditioning. Analysis of this kind allows clinicians to develop treatment programs that address these reinforcers and help counter-condition patients into healthier behavioral patterns.

Table 6.1 ESSENTIAL ELEMENTS OF OPERANT OR "SKINNERIAN" CONDITIONING

		Stimulus quality	
		Positive	**Negative**
Stimulus when	Deliver	Positive reinforcement	Punishment
behavior occurs		Privileges	Discharge
		Attention and praise	Additional requirements
		(behavior increases)	(behavior decreases)
	Withdraw	Extinction	Negative reinforcement
		Decreasing attention	Relief from distress
		Loss of privileges	Relief from responsibilities
		(behavior decreases)	(behavior increases)

OPIATES AND ADDICTION

A more severe behavioral disturbance involves addiction to opioids, sedative-hypnotics, alcohol, and stimulants. This may originate with efforts to treat pain but can develop into formal addiction. Although the area is contentious, we define dependence as a state in which physical withdrawal occurs in the absence of drug use, while addiction is the state in which the patient increases the use of the drug despite increasing negative consequences from using it in a way that disrupts function in all spheres of life. Often, patients taking high doses of opiates have lost everything of importance in their life, continue to rate their pain as 10 out of 10 despite increasing doses of the opiates, and continue to request increases their opiate doses. These patients need a rehabilitative approach that includes treatment of addiction as part of the program.

Many patients with chronic pain are dependent on opiates, benzodiazepines, and stimulants and are vulnerable to addiction. The concept of pseudoaddiction is not a useful construct, and no research has shown that it is distinct in any valid way from addiction.[4] Evaluating patients for addiction includes taking a careful history for use of illicit drugs, use of addictive drugs for pain and distress, and a correlation between escalating use of the drug and increasing dysfunction, loss of psychosocial support, estrangement from family and friends, loss of outside interests, loss of romantic connections, and deterioration of intimate relationships. This requires obtaining information from an outside informant because the very nature of addiction makes denial a central mechanism of the condition. Most patients with chronic pain will have varying degrees of overcommitment to the reinforcing medications they are taking, making it hard to see how much addiction plays a role in the problems.

Addiction also causes "out of character" behavior as the addiction worsens. Behaviors such as lying, deceiving, hiding medication, taking more than prescribed doses, and manipulating people in their life in ways that were not present before the medications are hallmarks of addiction. Others may excuse these behaviors, underreport them, and even hide them because they believe, as the addicted patient does, that these medications are "needed" and that the medical community just does not understand those needs. We have seen parents, children, and friends "sneak" drugs into an inpatient unit despite knowing that the person is there to get off those drugs.

A discussion of the treatment of addiction in patients with chronic pain is beyond the scope of this chapter, but the careful evaluation of behavioral elements of every case (including both conditioned behaviors and addiction) sets the stage for a discussion with patients about this part of the formulation and treatment plan. The lack of compelling evidence for long-term benefit from opiates in patients with chronic pain allows a discussion of discontinuation of the drugs as part of the treatment plan. In addition, it shifts the conversation to emphasizing the need for a behaviorally based rehabilitative program for improving function to treat their pain syndrome.

PERSONALITY AND CHRONIC PAIN

All personality traits have survival value in the right circumstances, and these traits become maladaptive in circumstances in which the natural response of patients to their condition makes them worse rather than better. Traits adaptive in a particular environment are maladaptive in the opposite environment. We tend to see personality vulnerabilities in our patients, such as impulsivity, emotional excess, and insensitivity to consequences, as negative traits, but they are positive traits in many settings outside the clinic. Clinicians fear patients with personality disorder more than any other psychiatric diagnosis, but treatment of these disorders is a necessary part of caring for our patients.

Many authors have described relationships between chronic pain and personality. In the five-factor model of Costa and McCrae,[5] neuroticism and extraversion are associated with vulnerability to maladaptation to chronic pain. Patients with personality disorders, particularly those associated with extraversion and neuroticism, have also been shown to have a vulnerability to disordering chronic pain syndromes.[6]

A simplified model of personality can be used to discuss the elements of personality in patients with chronic pain.[7] Patients who focus on the present rather than the future, on feelings rather than function, and on rewards rather than avoidance of consequences (Figure 6.1) are described as extraverted. They are more likely to seek symptom relief than to look for a long-term therapeutic solution to a problem and are vulnerable to having their behavior directed by the need to modify discomfort at the cost of future function. They may seek

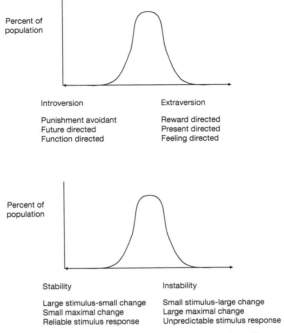

Figure 6.1. Simplified diagrams of the introversion–extraversion dimension and the stability–instability dimension.

"painkillers" to overcome their pain (even at excessive doses), when doctors have recommended the slower process of rehabilitative exercises. Patients with emotions that are highly reactive to stimuli have been referred to as neurotic (i.e., emotional instability) and are likely to develop disordered behaviors in response to pain.

Extraverted patients focus on feelings and the present. The experience of pain is a problem they may approach by trying to "feel better" immediately rather than work to improve function and avoid problems in the future. In medical settings, they often seek out medical solutions that blunt pain at the cost of function and future capacity because of their nature. Unstable (neurotic) patients respond to unpleasant sensations with a large surge in emotions. This may lead them to develop catastrophic reactions to the helpless feelings they develop when they are overwhelmed by pain. They place an intense emotional pressure on the clinician because they "need" to feel better. In the setting of chronic pain, this style of response is frequently ineffective and even destructive. They are inclined to pressure doctors to give them opioids and benzodiazepines. They may also pressure clinicians to help them apply for disability, while declining rehabilitative interventions and long-term solutions that require patience and effort.

Disordering traits of personality in patients with chronic pain are usually easy for experienced clinicians to recognize. The patient continues to try to solve their problems using the same maladaptive style despite repeated failures. They arrive on high doses of opiates with a pain rating of 10 out of 10 and want more narcotics even when we point out that the opiates are not helping their pain. The emotional pressure patients apply to obtain what they feel they need can identify these patients. Clinicians feel manipulated or like they are having their "arm twisted." Their history is distorted by their misperceptions and emotional responses to events. They describe events as happening to them and see themselves as victims, and they are difficult to redirect. In the words of Thomas Sydenham, "All is caprice. They love without measure those whom they will soon hate without reason. Now they will do this, now that; ever receding from their purpose."[8]

These patients are among the most disabled patients and are often on the highest doses of medications. Their vulnerabilities in terms of temperament are magnified by the current cultural problems in medicine described previously. Unfortunately, clinicians often have the mistaken belief that they cannot be helped and that personality disorders cannot be treated. This is not true, and they respond to interventions for chronic pain, but they are harder to treat and require more time and patience. Helping patients to see that the same traits that have helped them in many situations are working against them now allows an opportunity to guide patients in styles that are more effective in dealing with their pain.

The social response to the epidemic of opiate overprescribing is to "clamp down" on overprescribing, with no plan to deal with patients dependent on high-dose narcotics, no real plan to educate the public, and no provision of resources for alternative and more effective treatment has been particularly problematic for these patients. They are at high risk of using illicit opiates such as heroin and moving to alternative methods of getting what they think they "need."

PSYCHIATRIC DISEASE STATES AND CHRONIC PAIN

These conditions are presumed to have an etiology based in brain pathology. The most common conditions to complicate chronic pain are the disorders that affect mood, reward, energy, well-being, cognition, and sleep. We will focus on major depression and bipolar disorder. Major depression has a prevalence of about 5% of the population, depending a great deal on definition and ascertainment method. Bipolar disorder, including bipolar type 2 and other variants, has a prevalence of 1 to 2% of the population, meaning that the general population has at least a 7 to 8% prevalence of one of these disorders of affective function.

Major depression is much more common in patients with chronic illness and has its highest prevalence in conditions that distort immune function and the stress axis. Conditions associated with central nervous system (CNS) inflammation such as transverse myelitis, multiple sclerosis, HIV, and other diseases, are associated with a very high prevalence of major depression (4–10 times that of the general population). Patients with other devastating illnesses that have minimal effects on immune regulation and CNS inflammation, such as amyotrophic lateral sclerosis, have rates of major depression only modestly higher than the general population.[9] Major depression is a common comorbid condition in chronic pain syndromes and makes pain much more difficult to treat.[10]

Depressive Disorders and Pain Management

Patients with major depression have been shown to be less responsive to treatments for pain, particularly opiates. Because they have diminished rewards from other activities, the pleasurable response and rewarding elements of opiate medications (or alcohol and other sedative hypnotic drugs) make patients with depression particularly susceptible to overuse and addiction to these drugs. Additionally, because of disrupted reward sensitivity, patients with depression are less likely to engage in rehabilitative treatments. The sense of hopelessness drives escapist coping, less personal investment in getting better (and often a sense that getting better is unattainable), and a reliance on immediate relief rather than sacrifice of comfort in favor of function. To further complicate matters, depressed patients are less able to use distraction and self-hypnotic techniques of pain management that are often used in rehabilitative settings. Depression has even been hypothesized to have a role in the development of some pain amplification syndromes.

The treatment of major depression is noteworthy because many of the antidepressants, particularly those that have noradrenergic reuptake blockade as part of their mechanism, are useful in treating chronic pain syndromes. Also useful for chronic pain are several other medications that may enhance the antidepressant action of antidepressants, such as the anticonvulsants (e.g., lamotrigine, valproic acid, and carbamazepine). This "double action" is useful in treatment of neuropathic pain but can also help patients identify the presence of a depressive disorder. It is often difficult to convince patients that their depression may be more than a simple reaction to their pain.

Major depression in classic cases occurs with clear episodes of decreased mood, feeling bad about oneself (low self-attitude), and decreased sense of wellness (low vital sense), with recovery to baseline after an episode that may last for a few weeks to a few months. The diagnosis of major depression may be much more difficult to appreciate in patients with chronic illness and chronic pain. The loss of rewards or pleasure from appetite-driven behaviors like eating, sleeping, and sex and from productivity-related behaviors like work, hobbies, and exercise may have more validity in the setting of illness or pain. Other features include increased anxiety, increased hopelessness, a sense of dependency, an amplification of negative thinking and poor coping, and early morning awakening with difficulty returning to sleep. All elements of depression are often mistakenly attributed to the pain and to the drugs used to treat chronic pain.

A family history of depression should be carefully sought out in the evaluation of patients with chronic pain. Alcohol or other drug use disorders in family members (particularly female family members) are often indications of a mood disorder. Episodic difficulties in adolescence and young adult life that disrupt function are often indicators of major depression. Disruptions of important relationships may also be indicators of depressive episodes. Patients with disproportionate dependency on others, disproportionate distress or resignation over prognosis, and unexplained diminished function should raise clinician's suspicion of a depressive illness in addition to the chronic pain issues. Sleep disturbance, particularly with early morning awakening, may be a symptom of depression. Weight loss or weight gain, often accompanied by a change in appetite or food preference, excessive food cravings, day–night sleep cycle reversal, and other "neurovegetative" markers of depression are often confused with the effects of pain or opiate withdrawal and should raise suspicion for occult depression. Patterned mood changes through the day (usually worse it the morning, better in the afternoon, and worse again in the evening) are a common feature of depression, although mood may also be destabilized by opiate blood level variations.

Patients may reject the diagnosis of depression, and this may be an issue for treatment. They usually believe that a diagnosis of depression implies that their pain is not real. The information that depression can make real pain even worse is often reassuring for patients. Family members might also believe that the diagnosis of depression implies that the pain is not real, and they may respond with rejecting the diagnosis or alternatively thinking that the patient is lying or exaggerating their pain. Family meetings are essential to manage potential misunderstandings regarding the diagnosis of depression.

While other psychiatric disease states such as obsessive-compulsive disorder, schizophrenia, and panic disorder may complicate chronic pain syndromes, these conditions are usually easier to diagnose and separate from the pain condition and associated behavioral issues. Bipolar disorder is also a complicating feature in many patients but is in need of better research and is beyond the scope of this discussion.

INTEGRATED CARE OF CHRONIC PAIN

Solutions to straightforward medical problems lend themselves to operationalized criteria and treatment protocols and algorithms. This does not diminish the technical need to identify and treat these problems, but they are generally well served by the current medical specialization approach in which clinicians develop great technical skill in a single area of medical care. Medical miracles occur on a daily basis, unappreciated by critics of the US medical system. The unique evolution of the US system has also placed enormous pressures on practitioners to provide care more efficiently, maximize profits, concentrate on "problem-focused visits," and shorten lengths of stay. It is a system that limits reimbursement for "cognitive specialties" in medicine and wants problems cured with time-limited, predictable, low-cost treatments. Patients with complex problems that cut across specialties, particularly psychiatric disorders, are expensive, so they have been "carved out," excluded, and under-reimbursed to the point at which, for example, Cedars-Sinai Hospital closed their psychiatric services in 2012.[11] This loss of coordinated care passed nearly unnoticed in the medical community. The gradual elimination of comprehensive care programs for patients with chronic pain (shown to have successful outcomes) throughout the United States went similarly unnoticed. These comprehensive pain rehabilitation programs were unable to secure adequate reimbursement and were financially untenable in the current reimbursement scheme. These programs spent extensive time simultaneously detoxifying patients from short-term symptomatic treatments, doing trials of neuromodulators that would have long-term efficacy, treating comorbidity, and engaging patients in rehabilitation. The Johns Hopkins program is one of a handful of those still operating. They were replaced by "pain clinics," which, in the absence of a quick-fix intervention or short-term rehabilitation, became opiate-prescribing clinics and fueled the current opiate epidemic. Most patients with injuries recover function with support and treatment. Those who do not recover need intensive multidisciplinary evaluation to understand why they are not responding and to develop plans for comprehensive treatment, including identifying and treating the psychiatric comorbidities described.

Many clinicians have discussed the need for integrated care, a model in which psychiatry, psychology, physical medicine, neurology, anesthesiology, orthopedics, and the other related specialties have clinics with integrated evaluation and treatment. Identification and treatment of the kinds of problems we have described in this chapter require expertise in both pain and psychiatry. These comorbidities are common and are a common reason for treatment failure, unnecessary tests and procedures, disability, decreased function, and poor outcomes. While integrated care is expensive, treatment failure is more expensive. If society does not pay for effective care, all of us pay for disability, loss of productivity, and loss of infrastructure.

CONCLUSION

Psychiatric comorbidity profoundly affects the outcomes for patients with chronic pain. Unfortunately, many patients suffer from several of these complications that all further exacerbate each other. Problems of poor coping, limited life skills, poor social and behavioral modeling, limited resources, and poor self-efficacy all are problems from the narrative of a patient's life that can complicate and exacerbate chronic pain disorders. Operant conditioning of behavior with rewards for chronic pain behavior, punishment for getting better, and negative reinforcement that increases reliance on addictive medication all worsen pain, decrease recovery, and cause patients to be disengaged from rehabilitative care. Also in the realm of behavior, iatrogenic addiction and preexisting addiction make it much more difficult for patients to engage in rehabilitative approaches to care. Features of temperament, including extraversion and instability, lead to maladaptive responses to managing pain and difficulty engaging with physicians. Lastly, diseases of mood, such as major depression and bipolar disorder, decrease reward responses to healthy behavior and shunt patients toward avoidance coping, nihilistic views of recovery, and disengagement from support systems and medical care.

REFERENCES

1. Fenton JJ, Jerant AF, Bertakis KD, Franks P. The cost of satisfaction: A national study of patient satisfaction, health care utilization, expenditures, and mortality. *Arch Intern Med.* 2012;172(5):405–411.
2. Turk DC, Okifuji A. What factors affect physicians' decisions to prescribe opioids for chronic noncancer pain patients? *Clin J Pain.* 1997;13(4):330–336.
3. Fordyce WE, Fowler RS, DeLateur B. An application of behavior modification technique to a problem of chronic pain. *Behav Res Ther.* 1968;6(1):105–107.
4. Greene MS, Chambers RA. Pseudoaddiction: Fact or fiction? An investigation of the medical literature. *Curr Addict Rep.* 2015;2(4):310–317.

5. Wade JB, Dougherty LM, Hart RP, Rafii A, Price DD. A canonical correlation analysis of the influence of neuroticism and extraversion on chronic pain, suffering, and pain behavior. *Pain*. 1992;51(1):67–73.

6. Reynolds CJ, Carpenter RW, Tragesser SL. Accounting for the association between BPD features and chronic pain complaints in a pain patient sample: The role of emotion dysregulation factors. *Personal Disord*. 2018;9(3):284–289.

7. McHugh PR, Slavney PR. *Perspectives of psychiatry*. 2nd ed. Baltimore, MD: Johns Hopkins University Press; 1998.

8. Sydenham T. *The Works of Thomas Sydenham M.D.* Translated from the Latin edition of Dr. Greenhill. London: Printed for the Sydenham Society; 1850.

9. Rabkin JG, Wagner GJ, Del Bene M. Resilience and distress among amyotrophic lateral sclerosis patients and caregivers. *Psychosom Med*. 2000;62:271–279.

10. Clark MR, Treisman GJ. Perspectives on pain and depression. *Adv Psychosom Med*. 2004;25:1–27.

11. Gorman A. Cedars-Sinai to cut most psychiatric services: The closing of the inpatient and outpatient programs is prompted by changes in the healthcare system. *Los Angeles Times*. 2011; Dec 1.

7

Assessment and Monitoring of Patients With Chronic Pain and Co-occurring Substance Use and Abuse

JON STRELTZER ■

INTRODUCTION

A pain patient can be considered to fall within three categories of potential comorbidity with substance abuse disorders: (a) substance abuse that preexisted a pain state without any etiological connection between the two; (b) substance use that predisposes to the experience of pain; or (c) substance use disorders that are, at least in part, presumed to be caused or exacerbated by the pain state. The latter is likely to be of most concern to the physician because of its greater prevalence in clinical practice. All of these comorbidities complicate pain management, and pain, particularly chronic pain, may interfere with the treatment of any substance use disorder. The pain patient with substance abuse may continually seek narcotic analgesics, feigning or exaggerating pain, making the physician uncomfortable and the actual pain state very difficult to assess. Many consider substance abuse or "addiction" to be the major comorbid condition of concern related to chronic pain.

The comorbidity of substance abuse and pain is particularly problematic in the United States and Canada. Most countries with advanced health care systems do not have significant issues in this regard. This is because the medical culture of most countries is that pain is treated with opioids only briefly if at all, and primarily for severe, acute painful conditions. Treatment of pain with long-term opioids, particularly in high doses, is known to be associated with substantial medical comorbidity, including trauma, infections, occupational dysfunction, interpersonal and family problems, psychiatric disorders,[1] and, in the United States, unintentional overdoses and death. It is also being increasingly realized that it is associated with the enhancement and persistence of chronic pain.

CHRONIC PAIN WITH OPIOID DEPENDENCE

Estimates of the percentage of chronic pain patients in the United States who have a substance use disorder vary widely. Not long ago, it was suggested that the prevalence of addiction resulting from prescription of opioid analgesics for pain was quite low, and was even advertised as less than 1% in a drug company–sponsored video used for marketing purposes (see http://www.youtube.com/watch?v=hwtSvHb_PRk). There is now broad realization that this belief was mistaken and contributed to the vast increase in opioid prescribing and concurrent addiction problems seen in chronic pain patients today. Recent estimates suggest that the prevalence of substance use disorders in the chronic pain population in the United States is between 20 and 40%.[2,3]

A case example is a 60-year-old man who has used daily opioids for back and leg pain for 12 years, with doses reaching very high levels. He has had several hospitalizations in recent years. There was no premorbid history of substance abuse. The absence of such a history appears to be approximately equally as likely as among opioid-dependent chronic pain patients.[4] Patients taking megadoses of opioids often have medical admissions to rule out various medical conditions when they may be actually having complications from their opioid use. The complications can include abdominal pain from severe constipation or even bowel obstruction, withdrawal symptoms from using up their pain pills too quickly, and altered mental status. The problem must be recognized to devise a treatment plan, which necessarily requires coordination among the treating physicians.

In a study of veterans receiving opioids for chronic back pain compared with those only receiving nonsteroidal anti-inflammatory drugs (NSAIDs) but with identical pain ratings, depression, personality disorders, and history of substance abuse were more common in the veterans receiving opioids. Comparing the opioid-treated group to the nonopioid treated group, depression was found in 65% versus 20%, substance use disorder was present in 43% versus 13%, and a personality disorder was found in 14% versus 1%, all significant at $P < .001$. There was no difference in the two groups in anxiety disorders or psychosis.

In this sample, the average daily morphine equivalent dose was only 46 mg, a low dose in today's clinical population.[5] Similar findings are present in recent studies from several countries.[6,7] It is reasonable to consider that the comorbidity in opioid-using chronic pain patients would be even greater in a population using larger doses.

CONSULTATION WITH THE OPIOID-DEPENDENT CHRONIC PAIN PATIENT

The treatment of chronic pain has changed significantly in the United States in recent years. It is far more complex than it used to be. A pain specialist is now more likely to be referred patients who are being maintained on opioids. This was a relatively rare in 1980 and has now become commonplace.[8,9] In the 1980s, literature began to appear that suggested that some chronic nonmalignant pain patients would benefit from treatment with long-term opioids.[10] Anecdotal cases were minimally described, opioid doses were low, and improvement in functioning could not be documented. The American Pain Society and the American Academy of Pain Management issued guidelines published in a joint statement in 1997 that actively promoted chronic opioid therapy for chronic pain.[11] In the 1990s, pharmaceutical marketing of opioids became increasingly aggressive. Patients who previously had been described as "pain-prone"[12] or hypochondriacal, with the treatment being primarily psychological, were subsequently prescribed opioids and in ever higher doses.[13] As the prescription of opioids skyrocketed in the United States and Canada, morbidity, including addiction and mortality from unintended overdoses, grew exponentially.[14]

In recent years, a movement opposing this trend has been gaining momentum. Both the scientific literature and the lay press are increasingly describing the lack of safety and effectiveness of chronic opioid therapy.[15,16] Organizations concerned with the treatment of chronic pain are issuing guidelines increasingly restrictive of chronic opioid therapy. In a joint publication in 2009, the American pain societies retreated a great deal from their enthusiasm for liberal opioid prescribing.[17] They concluded that evidence of efficacy was weak, as was evidence for almost all the previously suggested procedures to ensure safety that had been based on "expert opinion."

Editorials are now frequently seen in prominent journals calling attention to problems associated with excessive prescription of opioid pain medications.[18–20] One school of thought has promoted the use of risk management strategies to solve the problem. Recommendations involve screening for past substance abuse behaviors and only prescribing opioids for chronic pain when alternative treatment methods have been tried first, because of the risk for addiction. This school of thought recommends close monitoring of the patient after the decision to prescribe opioids on a long-term basis has been made. Treatment contracts are often recommended. These may make the prescribing physician more comfortable, but evidence is lacking for their effectiveness as an adjunct to managing pain.[21] The use of treatment contracts and frequent urine drug screens makes this type of management similar to what is used in drug treatment programs. Most prescribing practitioners do not have the training, resources, or experience to provide such management, however. While such management is legal under the guise of pain management, this may often be more accurately described as office-based treatment of opioid dependence. Office-based treatment of opioid dependence (not associated with pain management) with controlled substances is legally allowed in the United States only to practitioners who obtain a special license to use buprenorphine for such treatment.

With regard to risk management, it appears that the major risk factor in the development of opioid dependence (or an opioid use disorder) is *exposure*.[22] Risk management strategies that focus on patient characteristics to predict risk have failed to influence mortality and morbidity associated with opioid prescribing, nor is there any evidence that such strategies produce increased effectiveness of chronic pain management.

Many patients who are seen in consultation for pain management have no significant past history of substance abuse but have become dependent on opioids following a medical and surgical condition that was treated overzealously and overlong with opioids. This dependence is usually associated with adverse consequences, including anxiety about taking the drug frequently enough to avoid withdrawal discomfort, irritability, sleep disturbance, and impairment in social and occupational activities.

A typical case involves a middle-aged man or woman with chronic musculoskeletal pain who had been prescribed opioid drugs, such as morphine, hydrocodone, or oxycodone, and whose dose escalated over time from a few tablets per day to higher and higher doses, eventually reaching a relatively stable plateau. Such a patient is likely to receive a prescription for a fixed daily dose of an opioid, usually with the availability of additional "breakthrough" opioids, as needed for pain not controlled by the fixed dose. The patient will report that this additional medication is taken only as needed, but careful history usually reveals that roughly the same amount is taken each day, and the amount prescribed remains the same from month to month.

The pain complaints tend to be continuous all day long, and they often have increased in subjective intensity and spread beyond their original location. The patient reports that narcotic pain medications are the only effective method of temporary relief because other modalities such as physical therapy do not affect the overall course of the chronic pain.

Case Vignette

A 43-year-old man had been treated for chronic back pain for 5 years following an acute onset of severe low back pain after lifting heavy boxes at work. He had been initially treated with physical therapy and oxycodone. He improved, and after 2 months he returned to work where he was valued because of his skills and experience. He continued to use oxycodone, however, feeling uncomfortable after each dose wore off. His dose steadily escalated in an attempt to match the comfortable feeling the original dose provided, and the patient expressed great appreciation for the increased doses, reporting that the pain medication allowed him to keep working and caring for his 8-year-old son as a single father. Over the next 3 years, the dose escalated further despite opioid rotation, reaching 540 mg of morphine daily. The patient agreed to a consultation with a pain specialist at the urging of a nurse associated with the insurance company covering his work injury.

The consultant noted that there were no abnormal neurological findings, and several lumbar magnetic resonance imaging (MRI) studies revealed only degenerative changes commonly found in normal populations. The consultant diagnosed an opioid dependency associated with enhanced pain sensitivity. He recommended treating the opioid dependency with buprenorphine and pain flareups with non-narcotics, such as acetaminophen as needed. Three years later, the patient was doing very well.

The treating physician and the patient originally believed that prescriptions of high-dose daily opioids were necessary and effective for pain and allowed the patient to keep his job and continue functioning. The physician had assumed that opioids were continuing to provide effective analgesia even while tolerance had developed. After his opioid dependence was treated, however, the patient realized that opioids had actually been a significant burden to him, causing a significant struggle to maintain his employment and his role as a father. There is no good evidence that opioids taken chronically retain the efficacy seen in acute treatment. In contrast, there is substantial evidence that opioids taken daily over the long-term induce changes in the central nervous system that cause enhanced sensitivity to pain by numerous mechanisms.

Evidence for the Lack of Analgesic Efficacy of Chronic Opioid Intake on Pain

The pain consultant should also know the evidence of the lack of analgesic efficacy of chronic opioid intake on pain. The evidence, cited here, is compelling at the cellular, physiological, experimental, epidemiological, and clinical levels.

Nerve cells involved in pain pathways adapt to chronic opioid intake through a number of chemical mechanisms.[23] These processes seem to overlap in a redundant fashion. For example, administration of chronic opioids suppresses the function of intracellular cyclic adenosine monophosphate (AMP). This leads to an adaptive response, an upregulation of adenylyl cyclase and the system responsible for synthesizing cyclic AMP. This upregulation of the cyclic AMP system leads to increase in cyclic AMP response element–binding protein, an intracellular peptide that stimulates RNA to make dynorphin in those cells capable of responding, including the pain-transmitting cells of the dorsal horn of the spinal cord.[24] Dynorphin is associated with abnormal pain sensitivity (hyperalgesia).[25]

Hyperalgesia is also induced by other neuropeptides elicited under the influence of chronic opioid intake, including substance P,[26] cholecystokinin,[27] orphanin/FQ,[28] and inflammatory cytokines.[29] Thus, cellular responses to stimulation by long-term exogenous opioids are multiple and overlapping, and they counteract and ultimately reverse the acute analgesic effects.

Several studies have confirmed that methadone maintenance patients are more sensitive to experimental pain than controls who do not take daily opioids.[30] Clinically, methadone maintenance patients on very high doses of the powerful analgesic are not protected from pain at all. If they need surgery, or have an acute painful condition, they do not need less pain medication, they need more than opioid-naïve individuals to effectively combat acute pain.[31] Studies of non–substance-abusing chronic pain patients reveal the same enhanced pain sensitivity to chronic opioid therapy.[32]

There is also evidence that patients with somatic symptom disorders are more likely to become dependent on daily opioids. Somatic symptom disorders are emotional or behavioral reactions characterized by preoccupation with somatic concerns not necessarily associated with physiological or organic lesions. Patients with serious objectively verifiable injuries rarely take daily opioids in the long-term after the acute condition heals or stabilizes. Patients with a somatoform pain disorder, however, are more likely to have pain that spreads to new sites from the original injury, to have more diagnostic tests, to have nonphysiological findings on exam, and to have received more treatments, such as physical therapy, than those with more serious injuries.[33] Thus, when a consultation is called for a chronic pain patient, careful consideration must be given to the possibility of a somatic symptom disorder explaining the degree and persistence of the pain.

As summed up by Ballantyne and Mao,[34] and recently confirmed in a report from the Centers for Disease Control and Prevention,[35] the use of chronic high doses of opioids for the management of pain is neither safe nor effective. It is likely to contribute to morbidity and mortality in a vicious cycle of pain leading to prescription of higher doses of opioid analgesics, which will induce greater pain sensitivity. Doses that appear to be stable over months, or even a few years, are likely to escalate when viewed from a long-term perspective, unless something happens to disrupt this process.[36] Disruptions tend to occur because of medical complications or loss of the prescribing doctor.

MONITORING TOOLS

Physician Drug Monitoring Programs

Most states now have prescription drug monitoring programs online. Consulting these websites will usually reveal complete and up-to-date information on what prescriptions for controlled substances the patient has filled. For new patients, this can be a good check to see if the patient is actually receiving the medication that is claimed. For patients who are being followed, this provides information with regard to how frequently the patient is refilling prescriptions and also whether other doctors are providing controlled substances.

Toxicology

If there is any suspicion that the patient is using illicit or licit substances of abuse, urine or blood maybe screened for their presence. This is particularly valuable in assessing new patients and monitoring compliance during ongoing treatment.

TREATMENT

Treatment of opioid dependence for chronic pain can be effective not just for the opioid dependence but also for chronic pain.[37]

A case example is a 36-year-old man who was hospitalized because of an excruciating headache unrelieved by extended release oxycodone, 240 mg, three to four times per day. The headache partially improved on intravenous morphine, given through a patient-controlled analgesia pump, with the total dose averaging an astonishing 95 mg/hour. At that dose, he could sleep and converse without apparent cognitive impairment. The referring physician had consulted various specialists in the past and tried many different treatments in a vain effort to control the pain and reduce the huge opioid intake. He was at a loss at this point, and just wanted help. The patient gave a history of suffering migraine headaches since age 22 years. His sister and mother had similar headaches. Originally, his headaches had been only occasional and were well-controlled with medication. The headaches got progressively worse in severity, however, and by the time he was 29 years old, he was using opioid analgesics daily. His opioid doses gradually rose, with temporary benefit whenever he raised the dose, but then the headaches would become worse again. He had been hospitalized with increasing frequency because of intractable pain or complications from high-dose opioids.

The pain consultant recognized that the patient's headaches were probably due to a combination of rebound headaches associated with opioids and the enhanced pain sensitivity produced by them. He discussed this assessment with the patient, who became intrigued by the potential of not living with constant pain yet was fearful of changing his habits, and he preferred to go back to his oxycodone, but at a higher dose.

The consultant pointed out that the patient had been through this many times before, and the recommendation was going to have to be what the consultant thought was best. Moreover, he was sure that the referring physician would agree with the recommendation because he had discussed it with him already. The consultant assured the patient that he would visit him every day and monitor his comfort closely.

The patient-controlled morphine was changed to a fixed continuous dose of intravenous morphine, initially at 70 mg per hour. Each day this was reduced by 10 mg, until it reached 40 mg per hour, when the hourly dose was reduced by 5 mg per day. The patient was assured that should he feel severe pain coming on, he could ask for something. He wanted to know what, and was told it would be haloperidol, a major tranquilizer with analgesic effects that would not interfere with his other medications or the changes in narcotic dose. It would be given intramuscularly for more rapid effect. If it did not help, it would be changed. This satisfied his long-developed habit of having "something strong" under his control.

The patient asked for the injection several times the next day, and once or twice each day for the remainder of his hospitalization. The dose was 0.5 mg, low enough to minimize the possibility of side effects. More important, he was visited daily. The pain consultant carefully listened to his concerns. Minor adjustments were made to his treatment as a result, but the narcotic dose consistently came down. He was praised for how well he was doing, and after a few days, he would greet the consultant with a smile.

When his dose was down to 25 mg/hour, there was pressure to discharge him because he looked so comfortable. He was then switched to oral methadone 15 mg three times a day for the first day, being reduced to 10 mg three times a day after that. In 3 more days, he was discharged. He was then placed on an outpatient tapering schedule that concluded in 2 weeks. He was seen twice as an outpatient. He was put on an anticonvulsant by a neurology consultant for headache prophylaxis. Otherwise, he was taking only acetaminophen and a rare haloperidol tablet. He gratefully stated that his life had been restored to him. Three months later, he phoned the consultant, reported he was doing well, and talked about his sister who had migraine headaches also and was dependent on prescription narcotics.

This case example is consistent with the rapidly accumulating evidence that daily opioids, at least in high doses, enhance pain sensitivity in general and, clinically, that dependency issues are a major problem. It was necessary for the patient's primary physician to allow the detoxification. Perhaps most important, the patient had to see that the consultant had his best interests in mind and would stick with him through the psychologically stressful change in habits. The detoxification went surprisingly smoothly considering the huge dose of opioid to which the patient was tolerant. Reducing a continuous intravenous dose is not difficult in the hospital because the dose is constant without the fluctuations that occur with oral dosing or when the patient controls the dose. Reducing or, even better, eliminating opioid analgesics in the opioid-dependent chronic pain patient has consistently been found to be beneficial.[38]

A Treatment Model

A six-step treatment model,[39] for which there is evidence of effectiveness, has proved successful in these patients. The first step involves explaining the role of opioids in maintaining chronic pain and enhancing pain sensitivity.

The patient should be told of the changes to the pain regimen and given a rationale for doing this. An appropriate message might be, "It is only natural that you are seeking to relieve your pain. You have been unsuccessful, however, despite very high doses of pain medications. In fact, these medications (opioids) have contributed to your chronic painful condition. Your body needs to recover from the changes induced by the constant intake of opioids, and it is likely that you will become stronger and feel better as a result." Despite the anxiety engendered by modifying habitual ways of medicating pain, this approach, when given confidently, often inspires hope. For many patients, this makes sense because they have suspected that the medication is a problem and that they have become dependent on it.

Other patients are convinced that they need opioids and cannot live without them. This is similar to the cigarette smoker who believes smoking is something he or she cannot stop, despite all the warnings about the health consequences. Such patients may argue that opioids are not the problem but the solution. The patient may still do well if the physician is supportive but strict in eliminating opioids. The physician does best by not focusing on addiction as an issue, but rather insisting that the best long-term solution for the pain is not the use of (high-dose) opioids that will enhance pain sensitivity.

The second step is detoxification. After the level of opioid dependence is determined, the dose can be fixed and steadily reduced. If the patient is on high doses to start with, detoxification with the rapidly metabolized drug that the patient is usually dependent on, such as oxycodone, hydrocodone, or morphine, is exquisitely difficult because of the feared withdrawal pain that occurs toward the end of each dosing interval. Opioid substitution with oral methadone or sublingual buprenorphine, however, works particularly well with minimal discomfort because of their reliable absorption and long duration of action. Methadone is remarkably powerful in a patient naïve to this drug, so care must be taken not to start with too high a dose.

Detoxification using sublingual buprenorphine, a partial mu opioid receptor agonist, is the easiest, safest, and most comfortable, but the patient must have a base average of only 30 mg or less of methadone or its equivalent. Because buprenorphine binds so tightly to the receptor, it displaces other opioids. Since the other opioids will be full agonists stimulating the receptor more than buprenorphine, their displacement at high doses will cause a relative withdrawal. A useful technique is to detoxify with methadone down to 30 mg or less, and then switch to sublingual buprenorphine after 24 to 48 hours of abstinence from methadone.

The third step is to manage pain with nonopioid medications simultaneously with detoxification. Most of the time, the psychiatric consultant will be dealing with patients whose chronic pain is related to a stable medical condition. The objective medical findings will be similar to those for most patients who are not dependent on opioid pain medications. The primary need of the patient for opioid medications, then, is psychological, related to conditioning factors and the opioid dependence itself. The patient should be told that the opioids used for detoxification are not actually treating his or her pain but are counteracting the enhanced pain sensitivity caused by the opioids. Pain treatment will be with other medications. Most often, acetaminophen is satisfactory. The next choice would be NSAIDs.

The long-term opioid dependent patient will often reject these choices saying that they don't work. The patient can be told that, of course, they don't work while he or she is dependent on high-dose opioids, but as the pain sensitivity improves, they may once again work as they should.

A crucial element in treating the opioid-dependent chronic pain patient is the provision of psychological support to the patient. The patient must be supported through that critical stage when long-established drug-taking habits are changing. The patient may be quite anxious and often dubious of this new approach. Frequent visits to inpatients and frequent appointments for outpatients, listening to their concerns, and providing confident explanations, often repeatedly, go a long way. When the patient realizes that the consultant is genuinely interested in his or her well-being and not simply leaving orders that will induce suffering and then disappearing, the patient will begin to develop some trust in the consultant.

The fifth step involves coordinating care with other providers and with key family members. Coordinating care with the staff (for inpatients) and the referring physician is critical so that they understand the treatment and do not inadvertently sabotage it. A house officer covering at night, unfamiliar with the pain management plan, may order opioids when the patient complains of pain, rather than utilizing the as-needed medications available. For outpatients, the physician who had been prescribing the opioids must be contacted to prevent a return to the former medications that created the problem.

Spouses or other family members can be extremely helpful unless they are opioid dependent themselves, or are abusing and diverting the drugs. Family members frequently recognize opioid-related problems that the patient denies. They can help the patient comply with his or her new, alternative medications, and they can encourage increased functionality. The encouragement and appreciation of family members can help solidify and sustain the patient's improvement.

The final step is to reinforce healthy behaviors in general. Many, if not most, of these patients smoke tobacco. This should be discussed and consideration of quitting encouraged. The patient can be given advice about how to stop smoking if any interest is expressed. Some patients will indicate that with a medication dependency and all their other problems, smoking is the last thing they want to worry about. It is still useful to recommend stopping smoking simultaneously with the detoxification process because it is part of health behaviors in general, and you are concerned with the patient's overall health status. Even if the patient does not show interest in stopping smoking, the underlying message to the patient is not that he or she is being considered addicted to medications but that his or her health is the primary consideration. This helps with rapport and trust over the whole process.

Similarly to discussing smoking, other health behaviors should be brought up. There should be attention to diet and exercise, framed as important to the whole process. Finally, it is helpful to encourage a positive attitude about the patient's willingness to go through this process and to develop a healthier lifestyle. In fact, he or she can be told that the most difficult part of all of this is the psychological part, breaking old habits. Many patients want to see themselves as psychologically strong, and this approach may spur them on to have a more positive attitude.

CONCLUSION

Substance abuse complicates pain management in general. Treatment of opioid dependence in the chronic pain patient is necessary for effective pain management, whether or not the patient uses drugs illicitly. Opioids, particularly in high doses, produce central nervous system neuroadaptations that reduce or eliminate analgesic effectiveness and enhance sensitivity to pain in general. The neuroadaptations often result in opioid dependency and, in the long-term, craving. Excessive morbidity and mortality occur. Weaning patients from chronic opioids can be exquisitely difficult if simple dose reduction is attempted. The process can be quite successful and gratifying, however, if certain principles are followed. These include education; comfortable detoxification using long-acting opioids, usually methadone or buprenorphine; nonopioid pain management; psychological support; and coordinated care.

REFERENCES

1. Streltzer J. Assessment of pain and psychiatric comorbidities. In: Ebert M, Kerns R, eds. *Behavioral and Psychopharmacologic Pain Management*. Cambridge, UK: Cambridge University Press; 2011:82–93.
2. Cheatle MD. Prescription opioid misuse, abuse, morbidity, and mortality: Balancing effective pain management and safety. *Pain Med*. 2015;16:S3–S8.
3. Chou R, Turner JA, Devine EB, et al. The effectiveness and risks of long-term opioid therapy for chronic pain: A systematic review for a National Institutes of Health Pathways to Prevention Workshop. *Ann Intern Med*. 2015;162:276–286.
4. Streltzer J, Davidson, R, Goebert, D. An observational study of buprenorphine treatment of the prescription opioid dependent pain patient. *Am J Addict*. 2015;24;357–361.
5. Breckenridge J, Clark JD. Patient characteristics associated with opioid versus nonsteroidal anti-inflammatory drug management of chronic low back pain. *J Pain*. 2003;4:344–350.
6. Azevedo LF, Costa-Pereira A, Mendonça L, Dias CC, Castro-Lopes JM. A population-based study on chronic pain and the use of opioids in Portugal. *Pain*. 2013;154:2844–2852.
7. Fredheim OM, Mahic M, Skurtveit S, Dale O, Romundstad P, Borchgrevink PC. Chronic pain and use of opioids: A population-based pharmacoepidemiological study from the Norwegian prescription database and the Nord-Trøndelag health study. *Pain*. 2014;155:1213–1221.
8. Streltzer J. Chronic pain and addiction. In: Leigh H, ed. *Consultation-Liaison Psychiatry: 1990 and Beyond*. New York, NY: Plenum Press; 1994:43–51.
9. Von Korff M, Deyo RA. Potent opioids for chronic musculoskeletal pain: Flying blind? *Pain*. 2004;109:207–209.

10. Portenoy RK, Foley KM. Chronic use of opioid analgesics in non-malignant pain: Report of 38 cases. *Pain.* 1986;25:171–186.

11. American Academy of Pain Medicine, American Pain Society. The use of opioids for the treatment of chronic pain: A consensus statement from the American Academy of Pain Medicine and the American Pain Society. *Clin J Pain.* 1997;13:6–8.

12. Engel GL. Psychogenic pain and pain-prone patient. *Am J Med.* 1959;26:899–918.

13. Martin BI, Deyo RA, Mirza SK, Turner JA, Comstock BA, Hollingworth W, Sullivan SD. Expenditures and health status among adults with back and neck problems. *JAMA.* 2008;299:656–664.

14. Paulozzi LJ, Ryan GW. Opioid analgesics and rates of fatal drug poisoning in the United States. *Am J Prev Med.* 2006;31:506–511.

15. Katz M. Long-term opioid treatment on nonmalignant pain: A believer loses his faith. *Arch Intern Med.* 2010;170:1422–1423.

16. Juurlink DN, Dhalla IA, Nelson LS. Improving opioid prescribing: The New York City recommendations. *JAMA.* 2013;309:879–80.

17. Chou R, Fanciullo GJ, Fine PG, et al. (2009). American Pain Society–American Academy of Pain Medicine Opioids Guidelines Panel. Clinical guidelines for the use of chronic opioid therapy in chronic noncancer pain. *J Pain.* 2009;10:113–130.

18. Sullivan MD, Von Korff M, Banta-Green C, Merrill JA, Saunders K. Problems and concerns of patients receiving chronic opioid therapy for chronic non-cancer pain. *Pain.* 2010;149:345–353.

19. Kelly MA. Current postoperative pain management protocols contribute to the opioid epidemic in the United States. *Am J Orthop (Belle Mead NJ).* 2015;44(10 suppl):S5–S8.

20. Grady D, Berkowitz SA, Katz MH. Opioids for chronic pain. *Arch Intern Med.* 2011;(12)171:1426–1427.

21. Arnold RM, Han PK, Seltzer D. Opioid contracts in chronic nonmalignant pain management: Objectives and uncertainties. *Am J Med.* 2006;119:292–296.

22. Rossow I, Bramness JG. The total sale of prescription drugs with an abuse potential predicts the number of excessive users: A national prescription database study. *BMC Public Health.* 2015;15:288.

23. White J. Pleasure into pain: The consequences of long-term opioid use. *Addict Behav.* 2004;29:1311–1324.

24. Nestler EJ. Molecular neurobiology of addiction. *Am J Addict.* 2001;10:201–217.

25. Vanderah TW, Gardell LR, Burgess SE, et al. Dynorphin promotes abnormal pain and spinal opioid antinociceptive tolerance. *J Neurosci.* 2000;20:7074–7079.

26. King T, Gardell LR, Wang R, et al. Role of NK-1 neurotransmission in opioid-induced hyperalgesia. *Pain.* 2005;116:276–288.

27. Xie J, Herman D, Stiller C, et al. Cholecystokinin in the rostral ventromedial medulla mediates opioid-induced hyperalgesia and antinociceptive tolerance. *J Neurosci.* 2005;25:409–416.

28. Stinus L, Allard M, Gold L, Simmonet G. Changes in CNS neuropeptide FF-like material, pain sensitivity, and opiate dependence following chronic morphine treatment. *Peptides.* 1995;16:1235–1241.

29. Hutchinson MR, Shavit Y, Grace PM, Rice KC, Maier SF, Watkins LR. Exploring the neuroimmunopharmacology of opioids: An integrative review of mechanisms

of central immune signaling and their implications for opioid analgesia. *Pharmacol Rev.* 2011;63:772–810.

30. Doverty M, White JM, Somogyi AA, Bochner F, Ali R, Ling W. Hyperalgesic responses in methadone maintenance patients *Pain*. 2001;90:91–96.

31. Compton P, Charuvastra VC, Kintaudi K, Ling W. Pain responses in methadone-maintained opioid abusers. *J Pain Symptom Manage*. 2000;20:237–245.

32. Hay JL, White JM, Bochner F, Somogyi AA, Semple TJ, Rounsefell B. Hyperalgesia in opioid-managed chronic pain and opioid-dependent patients. *J Pain*. 2009;10:316–322.

33. Streltzer J, Eliashof BA, Kline AE, Goebert D. Chronic pain disorder following physical injury. *Psychosomatics*. 2000;41:227–234.

34. Ballantyne J, Mao J. Opioid therapy for chronic pain. *NEJM*. 2003;349:1943–1953.

35. Dowell D, Haegerich TM, Chou R. CDC guideline for prescribing opioids for chronic pain—United States, 2016. *MMWR Recomm Rep.* 2016;65:1–49.

36. Streltzer J, Johansen L. Prescription drug dependence and evolving beliefs about pain management. *Am J Psychiatry*. 2006;163:594–598.

37. Miller NS, Swiney T, Barkin RL. Effects of opioid prescription medication dependence and detoxification on pain perceptions and self-reports. *Am J Ther*. 2006;13:436–444.

38. Harden P, Ahmed S, Ang K, Wiedemer N. Clinical implications of tapering chronic opioids in a veteran population. *Pain Med*. 2015;16:1975–1981.

39. Streltzer J. Pain management in the opioid-dependent patient. *Curr Psychiatry Rep*. 2001;3:489–496.

8

Psychometrics for Detecting Pain-Related Malingering

BLAKE H. TEARNAN ■

INTRODUCTION

Pain is ubiquitous. It is a part of the human experience. It is protective because it promotes healing by encouraging rest, and it motivates us to seek help. As the body heals, pain subsides, returning the body to homeostasis. In a minority of individuals, the universal experience of short-lived pain persists beyond the normal time for healing, leading to sometimes severe activity limitation, mood disturbance, loss of work productivity, relationship strain, dependency on narcotics, and a whole host of other problems. The impact of chronic pain on the individual and society is tremendous, and despite remarkable advances in medicine and psychology over the past decades, the material, emotional, and economic costs of chronic pain have steadily increased year-in and year-out.[1] Causes related to the persistence of pain are believed to be multifactorial, with learning playing a critical role in the development of disabling chronic pain.[2]

When pain does not subside as expected, avoidance behaviors and the threat attached to pain increase. This in turn can lead to greater pain sensitivity and body awareness, in which pain sensations are amplified and normal sensations are misinterpreted as harmful. This phenomenon is related to a complex interplay of emotional, cognitive, and neurophysiological changes, which are driven by the need to protect the individual from further physical and psychological harm. Within a relatively short span of time, muscle atrophy occurs from disuse, leading to increased pain and strengthening the avoidance response and the threat associated with pain.[2]

The longer pain persists, the more psychological factors begin to affect the expression of pain, disability, and suffering. Fears of pain deepen and avoidance strategies strengthen with short-term relief of pain from diminished activity. Patients desperate to find a cure for pain pursue treatments that often result in more pain and debility. Levels of stress increase because patients are unable to meet the obligations of work and family. Mood and sleep begin to deteriorate, and social and family relationships become strained.

Pain, disability, and suffering are also shaped by incentives. Family members, friends, and health care providers often inadvertently reinforce illness behavior by directing attention to an individual's complaints of pain and disability. They can also discourage wellness activities, worried the pain might worsen. Moreover, family members frequently encourage more health care in a futile effort to eliminate pain. Evidence also shows that when there are significantly powerful incentives to appear disabled, people will engage in behaviors to maximize the appearance of more disability.[3-5] Work-related injuries, Social Security disability benefits, and personal injury lawsuits expose individuals to financial incentives that can influence reported levels of disability. One well-designed meta-analytical study examined the pain ratings and treatment response of patients receiving compensation for their injuries. They found greater levels of pain intensity and poorer treatment outcomes in patients receiving compensation compared with chronic pain patients receiving no incentives.[6] Compensation benefits also prolonged recovery. Social and financial incentives can increase the likelihood of claims, intensify the level of pain-related disability, and delay or prevent recovery from injury.[7]

DEFINING MALINGERING

Increasingly, it is recognized that a significant minority of patients also feign their pain and the extent to which pain has affected their lives. The *Diagnostic and Statistical Manual of Mental Disorders*, fourth edition (DSM-IV)[8] and fifth edition (DSM-5)[9] define malingering as the "intentional production of false or grossly exaggerated physical or psychological symptoms, motivated by external incentives such as avoiding military duty or work, obtaining financial compensation, evading criminal prosecution, or obtaining drugs."[9(p. 726)] Malingering should be considered when there is concurrent litigation, the individual has a diagnosis of antisocial personality disorder, there are significant discrepancies between objective findings and subjective reports of distress or disability, or the person is uncooperative or medically noncompliant.

Although widely used, the DSM-IV and DSM-5 criteria have been criticized for failing to adequately conceptualize malingering and for ineffectively discriminating malingerers from nonmalingerers.[10] In one investigation,[11] the DSM-IV criteria produced an unacceptably high rate of false positives, leading to a misclassification rate of more than 80%. Some have advised against using the DSM criteria to classify malingerers.[10] Instead, Rogers[5] recommends the definition of malingering be restricted to the gross exaggeration of physical or psychological symptoms (i.e., feigning), motivated by external incentives. He argues that the presence of minor exaggeration or isolated symptoms does not meet the criteria for malingering and that the co-occurrence of internal incentives (e.g., avoidance of a loss of self-esteem) does not rule out malingering. However, the behavior of patients whose primary motivation is to gratify an internal need to assume the sick role is considered factitious and not malingering.

The construct of malingering is built around the idea that individuals motivated to deceive will manifest behaviors, thoughts, and emotions that are inconsistent or at odds with patients experiencing genuine symptoms.[12] This includes the magnitude and intensity of symptoms, complaints, discrepancies between observed behaviors and reported symptoms, and disagreements between claims of disability and evidence on medical records and collateral observations.[7] Inconsistency also refers to the unreliability of reported and observed symptoms across time, situations, and domains of functioning (e.g., cognitive, physical/medical, and psychological). The greater the inconsistencies, the more likely individuals reporting pain-related disability are thought to be deliberately misrepresenting their true capabilities.

It is important in the discussion of malingering to distinguish simple exaggeration from gross or severe exaggeration because the recognition of deception depends on the clinician distinguishing the two. Exaggeration is common, especially in patients with chronic pain. Patients exaggerate for many reasons, including fear of being minimized or dismissed by their health care providers or family members and efforts to influence the relationship with health care providers and to demonstrate the extent of their suffering. The clinician must decide whether patients are reporting their symptoms accurately and honestly or engaging in simple, major, or gross exaggeration in which symptom severity exceeds what the majority of chronic pain patients normally report.[13]

Malingering is not considered a stable state or related to any character flaw.[5] The individual's decision to deceive fluctuates depending on the situation; relations with medical or legal professionals; the perceived costs and benefits of feigning, such as the amount of monetary gain expected versus the cost of being discovered; and the behaviors and energy required to achieve a successful deception.[7] Results from all studies show that compensation is the key factor in explaining malingered pain.[14]

INCIDENCE OF MALINGERING

Malingering until recently was dismissed as a serious but infrequent problem assigned to less than 5 to 10% of patients reporting chronic pain.[15] However, with the advent of new technologies, especially in the neuropsychological arena, and a better understanding of the construct of malingering and feigning, several investigations have determined that the base rate of malingering in chronic pain is considerably higher. In one of the more comprehensive studies, it was found that 39% of patients with fibromyalgia who were seeking benefits related to their pain exaggerated symptoms of pain.[16] Another investigation reported a 36% base rate of malingering in chronic pain claimants.[17] Clearly, the rate of exaggerated response bias and malingering is higher than originally thought.

SOCIETAL IMPACT OF MALINGERING

The cost of malingered chronic pain is substantial. One study estimated that the annual cost related to malingered mental illness of Social Security disability payments far exceeds $20 billion.[18] This does not include payments for malingered chronic pain or various other medical conditions that often overlap with chronic pain, such as traumatic brain injury. There is an obvious societal need to identify patients who malinger pain-related disability. Advances in assessment methodology over the past two decades in the detection of malingering have substantially increased the accuracy and reliability of detecting malingered pain complaints.[19] The remaining part of this chapter will be devoted to these assessment methods.

DETECTING DECEPTION

Most clinicians cannot reliably detect deception through observation or the application of widely used diagnostic criteria (e.g., DSM-V).[19] This is especially true in the assessment of chronic pain. Patients often report symptoms that are disproportionate to objective medical findings. This is partly the case because it is estimated that the underlying cause of low back pain in nearly 85% of patients is poorly understood.[7] Relying solely on objective medical findings to determine the legitimacy of symptoms reported by patients is wholly inadequate. It will cause the clinician in the vast majority of cases to overestimate malingering.

The assessment of malingered chronic pain must reflect the diversity of problems reported by patients and as such should be as complex and multifactorial. To this end, clinicians should paint with a broad brush and include methods to examine all three functional domains: cognitive, psychological, and physical/medical. This is the case because patients with debilitating chronic pain report deficits in thinking, general health, and psychological well-being.[4]

DETECTION STRATEGIES

Detecting feigning is markedly improved when the clinician employs various detection strategies, ideally encompassing all three functional domains. According to Rogers,[5] a detection strategy is "conceptually based and empirically validated for systematically differentiating a specific response style." In the assessment of malingering, the goal of the clinician is to be able to reliably and accurately differentiate feigning from honest responders. Without the use of well-defined and empirically sound detection strategies, the clinician is prone to make inferential leaps based on an array of ill-defined, complex, and sometimes conflicting data sets. For example, some authors suggest that the presence of evasiveness should alert the clinician to the possibility of symptom exaggeration.[7] The obvious problem for the clinician is operationalizing what evasiveness means in the context of the clinical interview and how can it be quantified and reliably measured. Another example is noncompliance with treatment. How much compliance should be expected before a suspicion of feigning is dismissed? Empirically sound detection strategies should ideally demonstrate, for instance, that scores on a particular health inventory exceeding X will correctly classify 85% of malingered patients and only incorrectly classify 5%. This level of methodological sophistication gives the clinician the confidence that malingering is correctly identified.

Finally, of paramount importance in the development of empirically validated deception strategies is the inclusion of target symptoms relevant to chronic pain. This involves querying about musculoskeletal pain, pain-related disability, and treatment-related variables.[20] In most investigations of malingered chronic pain, these symptoms have been ignored, particularly by narrowly defined questionnaires.[21]

TYPES OF DETECTION STRATEGIES

Investigations of malingering have relied largely on knowledge-based strategies. According to Lanyon,[22] most patients who misrepresent health problems tend to lack knowledge of the target symptoms; therefore, procedures that capitalize on this "knowledge gap" are more effective in revealing an exaggerated response style. One of the more widely used knowledge-deficient strategies relies on a lack of normative information.[23] Most patients who feign pain complaints are unaware of the frequency and intensity of various symptoms in the general population of patients reporting chronic pain and will tend to overstate their reported symptoms. For example, patients motivated to feign are more likely to admit to experiencing very rare symptoms (e.g., coughing up blood) than the general population of chronic pain patients.

Rogers[5] proposed various strategies that align with Lanyon's[23] model of knowledge deficiency, including the indiscriminate endorsement of symptoms. This approach capitalizes on the tendency of simulators to endorse a broad array of physical (e.g., musculoskeletal, gastrointestinal, and neurological) and psychological symptoms (e.g., sleep disturbance, mood disturbance, social avoidance, diminished energy, poor appetite, and little confidence for coping with daily stressors). Related to indiscriminate endorsement of symptoms is the strategy of intensity of medical complaints. This strategy relies on the tendency of malingerers to overstate the frequency, duration, and intensity of pain-related symptoms.[5] The endorsement of unusual symptoms is a third strategy that also exploits simulators' tendencies to broadly endorse physical and psychological symptoms, including those that are infrequent, rare, or nonsensical, or that contain unusual symptom combinations. Another strategy is *reported versus observed*, which examines the dissimilarities between the patient's personal accounts of their symptoms versus what is observed clinically. Finally, there are two additional strategies, termed *projected disability* and *projected virtue*,[20] in which patients motivated to malinger exploit opportunities to complain of excessive pain-related disability (e.g., activity interference) and portray themselves as high in moral standing to obfuscate their tendencies to malinger (e.g., "I always tell the truth").

EMPIRICAL SUPPORT FOR DETECTION STRATEGIES

The detection strategy with the greatest empirical support in malingered health complaints is the indiscriminate endorsement of symptoms. In one of the earliest reports, Furnham and Henderson[24] showed that patients feigning medical illness reported a broad array of physical and psychological symptoms.

More recently, McGuire and Shores,[25] employing the Symptom Checklist-90-Revised,[26] discriminated between a clinical sample of patients reporting pain and a group of pain simulators. In a similar investigation, Larrabee[27] used the 13-item Modified Somatic Perception Questionnaire[28] to demonstrate that patients reporting chronic pain who were classified with definite or probable malingering of neurocognitive dysfunction endorsed a significantly higher number of symptoms than a sample of clinical patients reporting chronic pain.

The use of unusual symptoms as a detection strategy has received far less attention in investigations of malingered health complaints.[5] In one of the few reported studies, Wygant et al.[29] examined the use of rare symptoms. They studied more than 50,000 Minnesota Multiphasic Personality Inventory-2 (MMPI-2)[30] profiles of patients with medical concerns and chronic pain for uncommon symptoms, resulting in the development of the Infrequent Somatic Complaints Scale (Fs), which included items that were endorsed by less than 25% of the sample. The Fs demonstrated large to very large effect sizes in its ability to discriminate patients who are feigning. Tearnan and Ross[20] also found that rare and even nonsensical symptom complaints effectively classified patients instructed to simulate pain complaints from normal controls in their investigation of the Life Assessment Questionnaire (LAQ).[20]

Investigations of projected disability and virtue are limited. Although heuristically appealing, our own studies[20] showed very little discrimination between clinical controls and chronic pain patients instructed to malinger pain-related disability and various aspects of personal virtue. We found that both groups endorsed relevant responses to excess.

ASSESSMENT METHODS FOR MALINGERED PAIN

Various assessment methods have been used to examine malingered pain complaints, including clinical interview, physical examination, review of medical records, diagnostic testing, collateral interviews, physical performance capability (e.g., Functional Capacity Evaluation), and psychometric testing.[7] Although they all have their merits, the most effective means of understanding malingered pain complaints is psychometric testing. The reasons are primarily four-fold. First, the psychometric method is objective. The results are achieved independent of the clinician's beliefs or biases using standard test administration and scoring procedures. The drawbacks to most other methods of assessment are a reliance on subjective ratings or significant clinician input, which can potentially corrupt the information-gathering process.

Second, the psychometric method is more efficient for assessing a wide array of cognitive, physical/medical, and psychological symptoms. It requires considerably less time for the patient to respond to hundreds of true and false questions on a self-report questionnaire than it would take for a clinician to ask the same amount of questions in a face-to-face interview. In a related vein, the standardized nature of the psychometric method reduces the errors inherent in assessing complex data sets by a priori selection of information to be targeted for assessment.

Third, many psychometric tests, especially multiscale inventories, employ multiple detection strategies. For example, both the LAQ[20] and MMPI-2 use numerous detection strategies for assessing response bias. Studies have shown the need to employ multiple strategies to capture the varied approaches patients use when feigning.[5]

Fourth, psychometric tests can assist the clinician in decisions about malingering. Rules for deciding if a patient has feigned are very unclear in most other methods of assessment. If a patient, for example, has a positive straight-leg raise in the supine but not sitting position, does this meet criteria for a feigned pain response? If the patient is observed ambulating with significantly less pain behavior when walking outside the exam room, does this finding suggest feigning? In well-validated psychometric tests with empirically derived detection strategies, criteria for determining a moderate to high level of suspicion of feigning are usually made clear. For example, most studies recommend a cut score of 29 on the Symptom Validity Test[31,32] for determining a feigned response style; and on the LAQ, a raw score on the Feigning Index (FI) scale exceeding 144.5 is highly suggestive of feigning.

Although psychometric tests have distinct advantages, they should not be the exclusive method of assessment for detecting malingering. A review of records, for example, is invaluable for determining the patient's level of functioning before developing chronic pain. Prior records may also shed a light on the mechanisms of injury. Furthermore, the medical records might also reveal problems with noncompliance, past history of legal problems, and unstable employment.[7] Information from neuropsychological testing can also be an invaluable supplement to knowledge gleaned from psychometric testing, especially in chronic pain. Most patients with chronic pain report cognitive deficits (e.g., impaired concentration and memory). Multiple studies have shown individuals who are malingering pain-related symptoms perform poorly on many neuropsychological tests.[33,34]

SELECTION OF A PSYCHOMETRIC TEST

The selection of a psychometric test should be guided by the primary intended use of the test. A psychometric test for use in detecting feigning in a chronic pain population should be validated with chronic pain patients and should include symptoms germane to chronic pain.

Psychometric tests should ideally include multiple detection strategies including indiscriminate endorsement of symptoms, intensity of medical complaints, and unusual symptoms. Unfortunately, there are few validated tests, with the exception of the LAQ[20] and the MMPI-2, that meet these criteria. However, some singularly focused tests, such as the Modified Somatic Perception Questionnaire,[28] have demonstrated moderate to high levels of discrimination in classifying malingerers from normal controls. The argument for including multiple detection strategies relates to the increased sensitivity for detecting feigning because patients often adopt numerous strategies when feigning their symptoms.[5]

The classification accuracy of a psychometric test is measured by sensitivity and specificity. The sensitivity (true positive) of a test refers to the test's ability to correctly detect feigning. Highly sensitive tests are more likely to classify patients as potential malingerers. Specificity (false positive), on the other hand, measures the proportion of patients who are not feigning that are correctly identified. The goal of an optimal test is to maximize both sensitivity and specificity. However, there is usually a tradeoff between measures. The level of the cut score used for classifying patients depends on the purpose of the test. In most medical screenings, the goal is high sensitivity, casting the widest net possible to detect disease. This is at the expense of classifying some patients as disease carriers because the cost of a missed discovery could be catastrophic. However, in the detection of malingering, misclassifying patients as malingerers could have disastrous consequences for the patient. Since the cost of committing a type I error is high when making decisions about whether a patient was truthful or not, detection strategies for use in feigning tend to forgo the likeliness for discovery, or type II error, by lowering the sensitivity of the test. Rogers[5] recommends the minimum sensitivity of the test be as low as .50 while striving to achieve high levels of specificity.

Two complementary measures to sensitivity and specificity are useful when evaluating psychometric tests, positive predictive power (PPP) and negative predictive power (NPP). PPP is the probability of correct classification of a particular cut score.[3] Both PPP and the level of sensitivity need to be considered when evaluating the accuracy of cut scores. As Rogers[5] points out, high sensitivity levels can be reached, but often at the expense of low PPP values. If a particular cut score identifies 30 of 35 feigning patients, but misclassifies 85 actual patients, the PPP is only .25 (30/115). Rogers[5] recommends a minimum PPP value of a test to be .75. NPP reflects the type II error rate where the probability that an individual is not feigning when negative test results are achieved. PPP and NPP values are very useful when evaluating the utility of a test. Unfortunately, many, if not most, psychometric tests do not include these utility estimates.[5]

Finally, the selection of a psychometric test for use in malingering detection must be guided by the degree of scientific validity of the test. There is no perfect measure. The validation of any psychometric test is an evolving process that is reached in degrees over sometimes multiple investigations, demonstrating the test's ability to reliably and accurately measure what it was designed to measure. However, since the opinions of clinicians rendering judgments about the patient's truthfulness will sometimes come under the close scrutiny of the legal system, the scientific basis for the use of certain psychometric tests will be challenged. It will be the burden of the clinician to demonstrate that the test has sufficient validation to warrant the opinions reached and whether the test meets federal standards for the admissibility of scientific evidence.[35]

DETERMINING THE LIKELIHOOD OF FEIGNING

The first step when examining the results of a psychometric test is determining whether the patient's responses were reliable. If the patient was disengaged from the testing process or careless in his or her responses to items on the test, the results will be uninterpretable. The tests employed for use in malingering detection should include measures of reliability. Scores that are deemed unreliable cannot be used to make judgments about honest versus feigned response styles. After the test results are determined to be reliable, the clinician must decide whether the patient's scores exceeded recommended cut score values. Scale scores exceeding the recommended cut score should alert the clinician that there is a likelihood the patient feigned his responses. Tests will vary in a number of detection strategies (i.e., scales) used to reach conclusions about feigning. For example, the MMPI-2 uses multiple detection strategies or validity scales for determining whether patients have engaged in an honest versus feigned response style.

Making a determination of feigning should rest on the PPP and NPP values associated with each scale. To reiterate, PPP is the probability of correct classification at a particular cut score. For example, the FI scale on the LAQ has a PPP of 86% at the cut score of 144.5. This means there is an 86% likelihood that a patient scoring above 144.5 on the FI scale is feigning. NPP reflects the probability that an individual is not feigning when negative results are achieved. The NPP reflects the type II error rate.

Finally, the clinician needs to also turn to other sources of evidence to support the impression that the patient is feigning.[4,7] The more varied the sources of information, the greater the confidence the clinician will have in reaching the conclusion that the patient deceived. It was argued earlier that the psychometric method is the best method of assessing a variety of information, and it is an efficient way of collecting large bits of information about patients. All three domains of functional disability can be assessed with the psychometric method, especially if multiscale inventories are used. The limitation is that other methods of assessment can retrieve additional information the psychometric method cannot. The caveat is that most nonpsychometric data are based on detection strategies that are not empirically derived, but rely instead on observation or conclusions reached from record review or physical exam. Some also recommend using occurrences of feigning behavior that are rare or very impractical to implement (e.g., filming patients). That being said, reaching conclusions about feigning is strengthened when various sources of evidence using different methods of assessment across different domains of functioning are utilized.

The following schematic can be useful in assisting the clinician in determining the likelihood that the patient engaged in a feigned response style. The degree of feigning is rated from insignificant to high:

Insignificant: No evidence of feigning. Patient's responses indicate an honest response style.

Minimal: Honest reporting of symptoms with some exaggeration of symptoms, but no scale exceeds recommended cut score values. There is also no strong evidence of intention, such as failure on cognitive SVT or exceeding cut scores on unusual symptom scales (e.g., LAQ Nonsensical Scale).

Mild: Gross exaggeration of several symptoms with at least one scale exceeding recommended cut score values. There is no strong evidence of intention, such as failure on cognitive SVT or exceeding cut scores on unusual symptom scales (e.g., LAQ Nonsensical Scale).

Moderate: Gross exaggeration of numerous symptoms and more than one scale exceeding recommended cut score values. Also, the significantly elevated scales examine more than one functional domain. Additional information from other sources (e.g., physical exam or medical records) also supports the impression the patient feigned. There is no evidence of intention, such as failure on cognitive SVT or exceeding cut scores on unusual symptom scales (e.g., LAQ Nonsensical Scale).

High: Gross exaggeration of numerous symptoms and two or more detection strategy scales exceeding recommended cut score values. Also, the significantly elevated scales examine more than one functional domain. Additional information from other sources (e.g., physical exam or medical records) also supports the impression the patient feigned. There is also evidence of intention, such as failure on cognitive SVT or exceeding cut scores on unusual symptom scales (e.g., LAQ Nonsensical Scale).

DIAGNOSING MALINGERING

If the clinician concludes the evidence for feigning is moderate to high, the next step in the process is to determine the primary motivation that best explains the patient's feigned response style. If the patient was presumed motivated by an internal need to assume the sick role, the behavior is deemed factitious and not malingering. If the primary motivation is considered external, such as receiving monetary gain, avoiding work responsibilities, obtaining drugs, avoiding prosecution, or influencing sentencing, the feigning is considered malingering. The matter is complex because most patients who feign are motivated by a multitude of incentives, and these will change with circumstances, opportunity, and psychological need.[5] The clinician must decide what the primary motivation is that best explains the patient's behavior at the time of the evaluation.

The clinician also needs to rule out somatic symptom disorder[9] when reaching decisions about malingering. Somatic symptom disorder is defined as a preoccupation with physical symptoms, such as pain, or associated health concerns. The symptoms produce significant distress and impairment. The distinction between somatic symptom disorder, factitious disorder, and malingering is difficult to make because individuals belonging to each group report numerous symptoms at high intensity, significant distress, and impairment in daily functioning. However, the degree of difference is important. Patients exceeding cut point scores on more than one valid detection strategy are likely feigning. Another important distinction between a feigned response style and somatic symptom disorder is how individuals score on less somatically charged detection strategies. In essence, patients with somatic symptom disorder will endorse items that reflect excessive somatic concerns, but they will not fail more traditional validity scales unless they are engaged in feigning (e.g., F and Fb on the MMPI-2), and their scores will usually not be so extreme to exceed recommended cut point scores for detecting feigning.[4] Also, information from additional sources other than testing is also helpful in reaching conclusions about somatic symptom disorder, such as gender, history of sexual abuse, and concurrent chronic physical illness.

Additionally, the clinician must exclude any alternative explanations that might account for why the patient feigned, other than to gain monetarily or otherwise.[4,13] Was there some medical or psychological condition, for instance, that rendered the patient incapable of appreciating the consequences of feigning, legally and morally?

CHOICE OF PSYCHOMETRIC INSTRUMENT

There are numerous pain instruments, several widely used health inventories, and multiscale personality inventories used in chronic pain assessment.[2]

However, few have scales sensitive to response bias, and those that do have not demonstrated adequate sensitivity and specificity to recommend their use in malingering detection with patients purporting chronic pain.[3,5] Psychometric instruments should contain one or more empirically derived detection strategies. They should be validated with chronic pain patients and present levels of sensitivity and specificity.[20] They should also contain utility measures (e.g., PPP and NPP). Two instruments that meet these criteria are the MMPI-2[17] and the LAQ.[20] Both questionnaires are multiscale inventories that have been validated with chronic pain patients, and they have been shown to be very useful in uncovering response bias.

ETHICAL ISSUES

The use of psychometric tests should be guided by ethical principles. Clinicians need to be thoroughly familiar with whatever psychometric instrument is used when assessing chronic pain. This should include the strengths and weaknesses of each test, particularly as they relate to the PPP and NPP values of the tests. When reaching decisions about malingering, clinicians should never base their conclusions on one or even two tests. Multiple sources of information need to be considered, including data from medical records, other psychometric testing, neuropsychological testing, interview, and physical exam if available.

ACKNOWLEDGMENTS

I would like to thank Jesel Garcia for her tremendous help in the literature searches.

REFERENCES

1. Freburger JK, Holmes GM, Agans RP, et al. The rising prevalence of chronic low back pain. *Arch Intern Med.* 2009;169(3):251–258.
2. Gatchel RJ. *Clinical Essentials of Pain Management.* Washington, DC: American Psychological Association; 2005.
3. Young G. *Malingering, Feigning, and Response Bias in Psychiatric/Psychological Injury: Implication for Practice and Court.* New York, NY: Springer; 2014.
4. Etherton JL. Diagnosing malingering in chronic pain. *Psychol Inj and Law.* 2014;7:362–369.

5. Rogers R. Detection strategies for malingering and defensiveness. In: Rogers R, ed. *Clinical Assessment of Malingering and Deception*. New York, NY: The Guilford Press; 2008:14–35.

6. Rohling ML, Binder LM, Langhinrichsen-Rohling, J. Money matters: A meta-analytic review of the association between financial compensation and the experience and treatment of chronic pain. *Health Psychol*. 1995;14(6):537–547.

7. Aronoff, GM, Mandel S, Genovese E, et al. Evaluating malingering in contested injury or illness. *Pain Pract*. 2007;7(2):178–204.

8. American Psychiatric Association. *Diagnostic and Statistical Manual of Mental Disorders*. 4th ed. Washington, DC: Author; 2000.

9. American Psychiatric Association. *Diagnostic and Statistical Manual of Mental Disorders: DSM-5*. 5th ed. Washington, DC: Author; 2013:726.

10. Vitacco MJ. Syndromes associated with deception. In: Rogers R, ed. *Clinical Assessment of Malingering and Deception*. New York, NY: Guilford Press; 2008:39–50.

11. Rogers R, Vitacco MJ. Forensic assessment of malingering and related response styles. In: Van Dorsten B, ed. *Forensic Psychology: From Classroom to Courtroom*. New York, NY: Kluwer Academic; 2002:83–104.

12. Bianchini KJ, Greve KW, Glynn G. On the diagnosis of malingered pain-related disability: Lessons from cognitive malingering research. *Spine J*. 2005;5:404–417.

13. Iverson G. Identifying exaggeration and malingering. *Pain Pract*. 2007;7(2):94–102.

14. McDermott BE, Feldman MD. Malingering in the medical setting. *Psychiatr Clin N Am*. 2007;30:645–662.

15. Fishbain DA, Cutler R, Rosomoff HL, Rosomoff RS. Chronic pain disability exaggeration/malingering and submaximal effort research. *Clin J Pain*. 1999;15:244–274.

16. Mittenberg W, Patton C, Canyock EM, Condit DC. Base rates of malingering and symptom exaggeration. *J Clin Exp Neuropsychol*. 2002;24(8):1094–1102.

17. Meyers JE, Millis SR, Volkert K. A validity index for the MMPI-2. *Arch Clin Neuropsychol*. 2002;17(2):157–69.

18. Chafetz M, Underhill J. Estimated costs of malingered disability. *Arch Clin Neuropsychol*. 2013;28:633–639.

19. Bass C, Halligan P. Factitious disorders and malingering: Challenges for clinical assessment and management. *Lancet*. 2014;383:1422–1432.

20. Tearnan BH, Ross SA. The development and classification accuracy of the Life Assessment Questionnaire in the detection of pain-related malingering. *Behav Sci Law*. 2012;30(4):516–536.

21. Arbisi PA, Butcher JN. Psychometric perspectives on detection of malingering of pain: Use of the Minnesota Multiphasic Personality Inventory-2. *Clin J Pain*. 2004;20(6):383–391.

22. Lanyon RI. Detecting deception: Current models and directions. *Clin Psychol Sci Prac*. 1997;4(4):377–387.

23. Lanyon RI. Assessing the misrepresentation of health problems. *J Pers Assess*. 2003;81(1):1–10.

24. Furnham A, Henderson M. Response bias in self-report measures of general health. *Pers Indiv Differ*. 1983;4(5):519–525.

25. McGuire BE, Shores EA. Simulated pain on the symptom checklist 90—revised. *J Clin Psychol.* 2001;57(12):1589–1596.
26. Derogatis LR. *SCL-90-R: Symptom Checklist—90-R.* Bloomington, MN: Pearson; 1994.
27. Larrabee, GJ. Exaggerated pain report in litigants with malingered neurocognitive dysfunction. *Clin Neuropsychol.* 2003;17(3):395–401.
28. Main CJ. The modified somatic perception questionnaire. *J Psychosom Res.* 1983;27:503–514.
29. Wygant DB, Ben-Porath YS, Berry DTR, Arbisi PA. An MMPI-2 validity scale designed to detect somatic overreporting in civil forensic settings. Paper presented at: Annual meeting of the American Psychology–Law Society Conference; 2006; St. Petersburg Beach, FL.
30. Butcher JN, Dahlstrom WG, Graham JR, Tellegen AM, Kreammer B. *MMPI-2: Manual for Administration and Scoring.* Minneapolis, MN: University of Minnesota Press; 1989.
31. Ben-Porath YS, Tellegen A. *MMPI-2 Fake Bad Scale (FBS).* 2007. http://www.upress.umn.edu/tests/mmpi2_fbs.html. Accessed December 4, 2007.
32. Ben-Porath YS, Tellegen A. *MMPI-2 FBS (Symptom Validity Scale).* 2007. http://www.pearsonassessments.com/resources/fbs.html. Accessed December 4, 2007.
33. Meyers JE, Diep A. Assessment of malingering in chronic pain patients using neuropsychological tests. *Appl Neuropsychol.* 2000;7(3):133–139.
34. Greve KW, Ord J, Curtis KL, Bianchini KJ, Brennan A. Detecting malingering in traumatic brain injury and chronic pain: A comparison of three forced-choice symptom validity tests. *Clin Neuropsychol.* 2008;22:896–918.
35. *Daubert v. Merrell Dow Pharmaceuticals, Inc.,* 113 S. Ct. 2786; 1983.

9

Neuroimaging Correlates for Psychological and Chronic Pain Experiences

JOHN A. STURGEON AND KATHERINE T. MARTUCCI ∎

OVERVIEW OF THE RELATIONSHIP BETWEEN PAIN AND PSYCHOLOGY

In its acute form, pain is a useful biological signal that protects the organism by signaling tissue damage, injury, or other threats. However, pain can progress to a chronic stage whereby pain loses its value as a protective signal and instead complicates effective functioning. Individuals with chronic pain are vulnerable to greater levels of physical, occupational, and psychosocial impairment,[1] poorer sleep,[2] and increased psychiatric disorders.[3] The presence of a chronic pain condition is a risk factor for several mood disorders, including major depressive disorder; several anxiety disorders, including generalized anxiety disorder and panic disorder; and post-traumatic stress disorder.[4] Individuals with chronic pain also tend to show vulnerabilities in other areas, including problems in interpersonal relationships[5] and substance use disorders.[6]

Chronic pain poses a significant barrier to effective function for several reasons, most notably through the development of maladaptive behaviors that compromise later function. The experience of recurrent pain frequently manifests in patterns of avoidant behavior, such as discontinuation of exercise, work, or social activities. Development of maladaptive patterns of behavior is due to a complex interaction of internal and external factors. For example, there is a robust body of literature that the experience of pain functions as a punishment (i.e., reducing the likelihood of any behavior with which pain is associated).[7,8]

The process of adaptation to chronic pain is complex; coping responses to pain occur in the context of cognitions and affective states related to pain, social context, and trajectories of behavioral adjustment to pain.[9–11] Patterns of maladaptive cognitive appraisal related to pain, such as viewing pain as a catastrophic personal experience[12] or as both an irreparable and unjust circumstance,[13] can increase the likelihood of avoidant or ineffective coping efforts and contribute to long-term dysfunction. Notably, both pain catastrophizing and injustice beliefs related to pain also appear to be associated with an elevated degree of emotional distress, including more intense depressive and anxious symptoms and increased feelings of fear, loneliness, and anger.[14–17]

Positive characteristics also appear to be key determinants of chronic pain–related outcomes. Individuals who report greater levels of pain-related self-efficacy (i.e., beliefs that an individual can maintain meaningful function despite the presence of pain) appear to be more resistant to pain-related emotional distress and maladaptive pain coping strategies, which may buoy overall physical functioning.[18] Given that pain is a salient and distressing signal, the success of an individual's adaptation efforts to chronic pain is closely related to regulation of automatic cognitive, affective, and behavioral responses to pain. Indeed, psychological interventions for chronic pain (detailed in a later section) ameliorate automatic processes of avoidance and distress, from which more adaptive behavioral responses emerge.

SHARED NEURAL CORRELATES OF MENTAL DISORDERS, ACUTE PAIN, AND CHRONIC PAIN

Neuroimaging findings show that altered psychology and emotion in chronic pain are associated with myriad alterations in brain structure and function. It is currently unknown whether neuroimaging findings in chronic pain overlap with brain differences due to emotional changes, or conversely, whether the preexistence of emotional disruptions (and associated neurophysiological alterations) contributes or leads to chronic pain. Symptoms of depression are highly prevalent in chronic pain and are likely entangled in the structural magnetic resonance imaging (MRI) brain changes observed in imaging studies of chronic pain. A recent meta-analysis indicated that levels of depression among patients with fibromyalgia are correlated with, and moreover appear to account for, the majority of gray matter differences observed compared with healthy controls.[19] Additionally, pain processing is often altered in individuals diagnosed primarily with psychological conditions such as major depressive disorder[20] and post-traumatic stress disorder,[21] further underlining the connections between pain and emotions, behaviors, and social functioning. (See schematic of the main brain regions involved in psychological aspects of pain processing in Figure 9.1.)

Thus, confounds of brain changes due to depression and anxiety in chronic pain exist, and researchers are currently unable to explain with certainty neither the causality of these changes nor which predisposes to the other.

Neuroimaging findings indicate alterations in structure and activity within brain regions subserving the affective (e.g., pain unpleasantness) dimension of pain. Levels of unpleasantness and the context (e.g., positive or negative) of pain play a large role in how pain is perceived, as described previously. The anterior insula and anterior cingulate cortex (ACC) are two regions that are involved in the affective dimensions of pain processing. Brain structural differences (i.e., decreased gray matter) within the primary somatosensory cortex and brainstem in patients with chronic back pain are correlated with increased levels of pain intensity and unpleasantness.[22] In individuals with chronic pain, a region

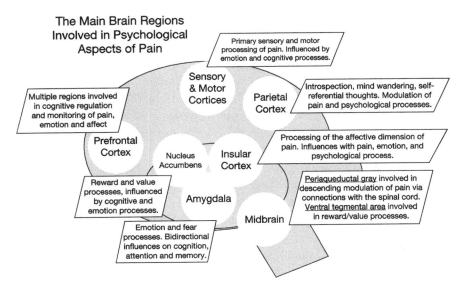

Figure 9.1. A Schematic of the Main Brain Regions Involved in Psychological Aspects of Pain. Multiple brain regions are involved in processing the psychological (or affective) aspects of pain. Psychological states have a profound effect on how pain is perceived, and this is relevant for both the acute pain and chronic pain experience.

within the ACC shows altered activity in response to viewed images of human hands and feet in painful or nonpainful positions.[23]

Neurophysiological evidence associated with emotional decision-making and cognitive impairment in chronic pain provides a framework for understanding how top-down cognitive modulation of emotion and pain processes are altered in chronic pain. The prefrontal cortex (PFC) is typically associated with higher order cognitive processes and the ability to cognitively inhibit pain. Dysregulation of activity within this region has been observed in multiple studies of chronic pain.[24,25] Changes within the ventromedial, dorsolateral, and orbitofrontal subregions of the PFC[25] are associated with altered pain regulation in chronic pain. Interestingly, evidence of impaired performance on emotional decision-making tasks occurs in fibromyalgia,[26] temporomandibular joint disorder,[27] and chronic low back pain.[28] In addition, neural circuits underlying these impairments have been investigated in arthritis rodent models, and these studies suggest that impaired decision-making may be related to altered relationships between the amygdala and PFC.[29]

The neurophysiological circuits processing various psychological constructs such as anxiety, depression, fear, and catastrophizing are altered in chronic pain, as evidenced by neuroimaging research. Altered amygdala function in children with complex regional pain syndrome is correlated with altered processing of emotion and fear.[30] Amygdala structure and connectivity to other pain-related brain networks and regions is altered in patients with chronic low back pain.[31,32] Studies of fear avoidance (of movement) in chronic pain indicate that neurophysiological changes are due not simply to fear of pain but also to rather more generalized psychological alterations.[33] Altered amygdala activity may influence pain through the spino-parabrachio-amygdaloid pathway, which influences emotional and affective aspects of the pain experience.[34] Altered opioid-related activity within the amygdala is associated with anxiety levels in chronic pain.[35] Additionally, in patients with irritable bowel syndrome (IBS), altered fear-related learning is related to altered activity (in response to visual cues) within the amygdala and PFC.[36] Further, increased measures of catastrophizing and anxiety in women with provoked vestibulodynia are associated with altered brain structure in pain-relevant brain areas as observed by neuroimaging.[37] During pain anticipation in fibromyalgia, catastrophizing-induced increases in pain sensitivity are mediated by activity in the lateral PFC.[38] Among females with IBS undergoing rectal distension, anxiety scores are associated with pain-induced activation of the ACC, while depression scores are associated with pain-induced activation of PFC and cerebellum.[39] Additionally, depression scores are correlated with increased periaqueductal gray–thalamus functional connectivity in fibromyalgia.[40] Furthermore, decreased parietal cortex cortical thickness and decreased ventral striatum activity are correlated with depression in fibromyalgia.[41]

Altered neural circuits involved in the processes of mood, affect and introspection in chronic pain appear to be related to many of these behavioral constructs as they are observed in chronic pain. For example, in patients with chronic pelvic pain, brain morphology within the right primary somatosensory cortex is correlated with pain intensity and mood (anxiety).[42] Induction of negative mood in patients with chronic low back pain is associated with altered brain connectivity that appears to modulate pain.[43] Altered affective processing in migraine patients has been observed in response to the presentation of pain-associated adjectives; patients demonstrated significantly increased activity within the anterior insular cortex and the left orbitofrontal cortex to pain-associated adjectives (e.g., excruciating, grueling) compared with negative pain-unassociated adjectives (e.g., dirty, disgusting).[44] Brain reward systems are impaired in fibromyalgia, as indicated by reduced dopamine activity in the brain,[45] reduced brain response to anticipation of pain relief,[46] and altered response to anticipated rewards.[47]

Neurophysiological models integrating neuroimaging findings with behavioral data describe how emotion is dysregulated in states of chronic pain. Within the parietal cortex, regions involved in introspection and thoughts of self, such as the precuneus, posterior cingulate cortex, and temporoparietal junction, show altered connectivity to brain regions associated with emotion (e.g., amygdala) and memory formation (e.g., hippocampus) in chronic pain.[48] In a study of the effects of meditation on anxiety relief, individuals with greater levels of anxiety had higher levels of activity within certain brain regions (the posterior parietal cortex) related to self-referential thought processes, suggesting that these individuals may face greater challenges with meditation and mindfulness-based therapies.[49] Individuals with chronic back pain demonstrate altered activity within the medial PFC, a region involved in introspection, planning, and cognitive processes, which is correlated with levels of spontaneous chronic pain intensity. These findings suggest that this region is involved in monitoring and modulating levels of ongoing chronic pain.[50] Finally, a meta-analysis of several neuroimaging studies suggests that the transition from acute pain to chronic pain involves shifts in altered brain processes, from pain-specific brain activity to abnormal levels of integration of emotion-related brain activity.[51] These findings all suggest that emotion, introspection, and memory may be key to understanding the neurobiological alterations associated with chronic pain. As we continue to gain more information regarding the neural underpinnings of chronic pain and emotion, these models will continue to be updated.

NEUROIMAGING EVIDENCE OF THE EFFICACY
OF PSYCHOLOGICAL INTERVENTIONS IN PAIN

Psychology-based interventions for chronic pain "manage" (or reduce) pain symptoms, while also managing maladaptive behavioral, cognitive, and emotional responses to pain. These therapies modify brain activity in response to pain and may serve to reverse some of the maladaptive brain changes in chronic pain described previously.[52] Of the validated psychological interventions for chronic pain, cognitive behavioral therapy (CBT) for pain has the largest body of evidence for efficacy.[53,54] CBT for pain adopts a "toolbox" approach to pain management, including behavioral relaxation techniques (e.g., diaphragmatic breathing, progressive muscle relaxation, guided imagery), cognitive and behavioral strategies for sleep improvement, cognitive restructuring skills for maladaptive and unrealistic thoughts about pain, scheduling of pleasurable activities, activity pacing approaches to maximize physical activity while reducing pain flares, and assertive communication skills.[55] CBT reduces disability and pain-related catastrophizing, and somewhat reduces pain and improvements in mood.[56] However, the CBT approach carries the implicit assumption that the key mechanism of change in chronic pain is a lack of adaptive coping skills; it thus appears to have limited long-term benefits[56] as well as a poorer conceptual fit for some patients. For example, in individuals with chronic pain not yet psychologically prepared to adopt a management approach to their pain, the mismatch between the individual's goals of pain resolution and the use of management strategies may impair the degree of benefit experienced from the intervention.

In cases of preoccupation with pain as a source of personal injustice, coupled with typically low levels of pain-related acceptance,[57] management-focused approaches may be unpalatable for an individual with pain. In these cases, there may be greater benefit from acceptance and mindfulness-focused therapies, including acceptance and commitment therapy (ACT) and mindfulness-based stress reduction (MBSR). Together, these approaches have been termed *acceptance-based therapies*[58] and share a degree of overlap in both their clinical approach and their mechanisms of effect. (See summary of CBT, ACT, and MBSR therapies in Figure 9.2.)

Both therapies emphasize nonreactivity toward pain and resulting cognitive and emotional states through the promotion of nonjudgmental attitudes and mindful awareness. In the case of MBSR, acceptance of bodily sensations and psychological experiences is cultivated through daily practice of mindfulness meditation, including awareness training of breathing and other sensations; mindful engagement in everyday activities, including walking and eating; and fostering of kindness toward the self and others.[59] MBSR has shown benefits in

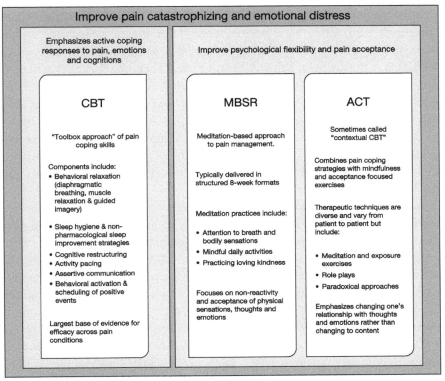

Figure 9.2. Comparison Chart between CBT, MBSR, and ACT. Cognitive Behavioral Therapy (CBT), Mindfulness Based Stress Reduction (MBSR), Acceptance and Commitment Therapy (ACT) all improve pain catastrophizing and emotional distress. The emphasis of CBT differs from the emphasis of MBSR and ACT as shown. Main concepts and practices for each type of therapy are shown in the individual boxes.

both reductions in pain intensity[60] and reductions in the negative psychological consequences of pain, such as depressive and anxiety symptoms and pain catastrophizing.[61]

Unlike MBSR, which follows both a structured training protocol and necessitates a daily meditation practice, ACT approaches in chronic pain are best defined as a set of principles that can be customized to the clinical characteristics of the patient. ACT approaches are flexible and are commonly made up of a combination of meditation, exposure exercises, role plays, and other therapeutic techniques, and they are adopted in an effort to help patients "defuse" from the experience of their pain, thoughts, and emotions, rather than needing to identify distortions in thought content, as in CBT.[62] This therapeutic goal is intended to help patients identify their own values and flexibly pursue more adaptive, personally meaningful goals.[62,63] Although there is a relatively smaller body of evidence for MBSR and ACT approaches in chronic pain compared with CBT, both interventions have demonstrated efficacy in improving psychological well-being, reduction of psychiatric symptoms, and a reduction in the degree of pain-related interference reported by patients in their everyday lives.[61] Notably, all of the extant psychological treatments for chronic pain (CBT, ACT, and MBSR) have demonstrated efficacy in reducing pain catastrophizing,[56,64,65] whereas both ACT and MBSR appear to affect outcomes through increased acceptance of pain and psychological flexibility.[64,66-68] Recent evidence of neurological change after psychological treatment includes changes in activity primarily within the PFC and brain regions implicated in emotion and memory processing.[69-71]

Neuroimaging investigations of these psychological therapies for chronic pain can help us to understand the neurological mechanisms subserving the effectiveness of these treatments. Neurophysiologically, the positive effects of psychological therapies, including CBT and ACT, are mediated by increased activity within the PFC, indicating enhanced processes of ("top-down") cognitive control of psychological processes[72] and further validating cortical mechanisms of pain control proposed more than a decade ago.[73] Additionally, reductions in resting-state functional MRI connectivity between the somatosensory cortex and anterior insular cortex are observed after 4 weeks of CBT and are associated with reduced catastrophizing.[74] The benefits of MBSR are also mediated by increases in mindfulness, reduced emotional reactivity to stress, and reductions in rumination and worry.[68] In all of these cases, however, reduction of pain intensity itself is a secondary goal, if achieved at all; rather, by reducing the emotional, cognitive, and behavioral impact of pain, these interventions appear to improve pain-related outcomes.[56,61,75] Similar brain mechanisms may be underlying the positive effects of MBSR on pain, as with mindfulness meditation on pain. Neuroimaging has shown that meditation reduces pain while decreasing PFC activity,[76,77] suggesting effects through decreased maladaptive cognitive processes such as rumination and catastrophizing. Mindfulness meditation reduces pain by increasing activity within regions of the ACC and the anterior insula, regions that are involved in the cognitive regulation of the pain experience.[78] Similarly, the neurophysiological changes associated with the effects of mindfulness meditation on anxiety include activation of the ACC, PFC, and anterior insula.[49] The neural correlates of these psychological therapies may be similar to changes in brain activity that occur during placebo interventions. Aspects of CBT, ACT, and MBSR that induce positive expectations for pain relief may, like the placebo effect, effectively harness the individual's psychology and reduce pain intensity and unpleasantness by influencing neurological processes of pain and emotion.[79,80] Personalization of these techniques according to characteristics of each individual patient may increase the potential benefits of these psychological treatments for pain. Meanwhile, future neuroimaging studies will continue to clarify how these therapies are harnessing the power of neural circuits to control pain.

CONCLUSION

The experience of chronic pain has complex neurophysiological and psychological consequences that can complicate most aspects of effective function in humans. Among the most salient problems faced by individuals with chronic pain is dysregulation of cognitive, affective, and behavioral responses, which contribute to greater dysfunction in the future. However, nonpharmacological treatment approaches have been developed that reduce these maladaptive responses. These treatments appear to share key mechanisms of effect, including enhanced regulation of behavioral, cognitive, and emotional processes related to pain, and the neurophysiological changes (as seen by neuroimaging studies) associated with these and related therapeutic techniques provide further support for their efficacy in treating chronic pain. The evidence for psychological interventions for chronic pain thus appears promising, and continued empirical study into the overlapping behavioral and neurophysiological changes that occur as a result of these interventions may yield greater information regarding both the broader understanding of pain and avenues for its effective treatment.

REFERENCES

1. Turk DC. A diathesis-stress model of chronic pain and disability following traumatic injury. *Pain Res Manage.* 2002;7(1):9–19.
2. Smith MT, Haythornthwaite JA. How do sleep disturbance and chronic pain inter-relate? Insights from the longitudinal and cognitive-behavioral clinical trials literature. *Sleep Med Rev.* 2004;8(2):119–132.
3. Arnow BA, Hunkeler EM, Blasey CM, et al. Comorbid depression, chronic pain, and disability in primary care. *Psychosom Med.* 2006;68(2):262–268.
4. McWilliams LA, Cox BJ, Enns MW. Mood and anxiety disorders associated with chronic pain: An examination in a nationally representative sample. *Pain.* 2003;106(1–2):127–133.
5. Feldman SI, Downey G, Schaffer-Neitz R. Pain, negative mood, and perceived support in chronic pain patients: A daily diary study of people with reflex sympathetic dystrophy syndrome. *J Consult Clin Psych.* 1999;67(5):776–785.
6. Martell BA, O'Connor PG, Kerns RD, et al. Systematic review. Opioid treatment for chronic back pain: Prevalence, efficacy, and association with addiction. *Ann Intern Med.* 2007;146(2):116–127.

7. Apkarian AV, Baliki MN, Geha PY. Towards a theory of chronic pain. *Prog Neurobiol*. 2009;87(2):81–97.

8. Baliki MN, Geha PY, Fields HL, Apkarian AV. Predicting value of pain and analgesia: Nucleus accumbens response to noxious stimuli changes in the presence of chronic pain. *Neuron*. 2010;66(1):149–160.

9. Smith BW, Zautra AJ. Vulnerability and resilience in women with arthritis: Test of a two-factor model. *J Consult Clin Psychol*. 2008;76(5):799–810.

10. Sturgeon JA, Zautra AJ. Resilience: A new paradigm for adaptation to chronic pain. *Curr Pain Headache Rep*. 2010;14(2):105–112.

11. Sturgeon JA, Zautra AJ. Psychological resilience, pain catastrophizing, and positive emotions: Perspectives on comprehensive modeling of individual pain adaptation. *Curr Pain Headache Rep*. 2013;17(3):317.

12. Quartana PJ, Campbell CM, Edwards RR. Pain catastrophizing: A critical review. *Exp Rev Neurotherapeut*. 2009;9(5):745–758.

13. Sullivan MJ, Scott W, Trost Z. Perceived injustice: A risk factor for problematic pain outcomes. *Clin J Pain*. 2012;28(6):484–488.

14. Scott W, Trost Z, Bernier E, Sullivan MJL. Anger differentially mediates the relationship between perceived injustice and chronic pain outcomes. *Pain*. 2013;154(9):1691–1698.

15. Sullivan MJ, Rodgers WM, Kirsch I. Catastrophizing, depression and expectancies for pain and emotional distress. *Pain*. 2001;91(1):147–154.

16. Wolf LD, Davis MC, Yeung EW, Tennen HA. The within-day relation between lonely episodes and subsequent clinical pain in individuals with fibromyalgia: Mediating role of pain cognitions. *J Psychosom Res*. 2015;79(3):202–206.

17. Sturgeon JA, Carriere JS, Kao M-CJ, Rico T, Darnall BD, Mackey SC. social disruption mediates the relationship between perceived injustice and anger in chronic pain: A Collaborative Health Outcomes Information Registry Study. *Ann Behav Med*. 2016:1–11.

18. Arnstein P, Caudill M, Mandle CL, Norris A, Beasley R. Self efficacy as a mediator of the relationship between pain intensity, disability and depression in chronic pain patients. *Pain*. 1999;80(3):483–491.

19. Smallwood RF, Laird AR, Ramage AE, et al. Structural brain anomalies and chronic pain: A quantitative meta-analysis of gray matter volume. *J Pain*. 2013;14(7):663–675.

20. Strigo IA, Simmons AN, Matthews SC, Arthur D, Paulus MP. Association of major depressive disorder with altered functional brain response during anticipation and processing of heat pain. *Arch Gen Psychiatry*. 2008;65(11):1275–1284.

21. Klossika I, Flor H, Kamping S, et al. Emotional modulation of pain: A clinical perspective. *Pain*. 2006;124(3):264–268.

22. Schmidt-Wilcke T, Leinisch E, Gänssbauer S, et al. Affective components and intensity of pain correlate with structural differences in gray matter in chronic back pain patients. *Pain*. 2006;125(1):89–97.

23. Noll-Hussong M, Otti A, Wohlschlaeger AM, et al. Neural correlates of deficits in pain-related affective meaning construction in patients with chronic pain disorder. *Psychosom Med*. 2013;75(2):124–136.

24. Apkarian AV, Thomas PS, Krauss BR, Szeverenyi NM. Prefrontal cortical hyperactivity in patients with sympathetically mediated chronic pain. *Neurosci Lett.* 2001;311(3):193–197.

25. Bechara A, Damasio H, Damasio AR. Emotion, decision making and the orbitofrontal cortex. *Cereb Cortex.* 2000;10(3):295–307.

26. Walteros C, Sánchez-Navarro JP, Muñoz MA, Martínez-Selva JM, Chialvo D, Montoya P. Altered associative learning and emotional decision making in fibromyalgia. *J Psychosom Res.* 2011;70(3):294–301.

27. Weissman-Fogel I, Moayedi M, Tenenbaum H, Goldberg M, Freeman B, Davis K. Abnormal cortical activity in patients with temporomandibular disorder evoked by cognitive and emotional tasks. *Pain.* 2011;152(2):384–396.

28. Apkarian AV, Sosa Y, Krauss BR, et al. Chronic pain patients are impaired on an emotional decision-making task. *Pain.* 2004;108(1):129–136.

29. Ji G, Sun H, Fu Y, et al. Cognitive impairment in pain through amygdala-driven prefrontal cortical deactivation. *J Neurosci.* 2010;30(15):5451–5464.

30. Simons LE, Moulton EA, Linnman C, Carpino E, Becerra L, Borsook D. The human amygdala and pain: Evidence from neuroimaging. *Human Brain Mapp.* 2014;35(2):527–538.

31. Jiang Y, Oathes D, Hush J, et al. Perturbed connectivity of the amygdala and its subregions with the central executive and default mode networks in chronic pain. *Pain.* 2016;157(9):1970–1978.

32. Mao CP, Yang HJ. Smaller amygdala volumes in patients with chronic low back pain compared with healthy control individuals. *J Pain.* 2015;16(12):1366–1376.

33. Barke A, Baudewig J, Schmidt-Samoa C, Dechent P, Kroner-Herwig B. Neural correlates of fear of movement in high and low fear-avoidant chronic low back pain patients: An event-related fMRI study. *Pain.* 2012;153(3):540–552.

34. Bernard J, Bester H, Besson J. Involvement of the spino-parabrachio-amygdaloid and hypothalamic pathways in the autonomic and affective emotional aspects of pain. *Prog Brain Res.* 1996;107:243–255.

35. Narita M, Kaneko C, Miyoshi K, et al. Chronic pain induces anxiety with concomitant changes in opioidergic function in the amygdala. *Neuropsychopharmacology.* 2006;31(4):739–750.

36. Icenhour A, Langhorst J, Benson S, et al. Neural circuitry of abdominal pain-related fear learning and reinstatement in irritable bowel syndrome. *Neurogastroenterol Motil.* 2015;27(1):114–127.

37. Sutton K, Pukall C, Wild C, Johnsrude I, Chamberlain S. Cognitive, psychophysical, and neural correlates of vulvar pain in primary and secondary provoked vestibulodynia: A pilot study. *J Sex Med.* 2015;12(5):1283–1297.

38. Loggia ML, Berna C, Kim J, et al. The lateral prefrontal cortex mediates the hyperalgesic effects of negative cognitions in chronic pain patients. *J Pain.* 2015;16(8):692–699.

39. Elsenbruch S, Rosenberger C, Enck P, Forsting M, Schedlowski M, Gizewski ER. Affective disturbances modulate the neural processing of visceral pain stimuli in irritable bowel syndrome: An fMRI study. *Gut.* 2010;59(4):489–495.

40. Cifre I, Sitges C, Fraiman D, et al. Disrupted functional connectivity of the pain network in fibromyalgia. *Psychosom Med.* 2012;74(1):55–62.

41. Jensen KB, Srinivasan P, Spaeth R, et al. Overlapping structural and functional brain changes in patients with long-term exposure to fibromyalgia pain. *Arthritis Rheum.* 2013;65(12):3293–3303.

42. Kairys AE, Schmidt-Wilcke T, Puiu T, et al. Increased brain gray matter in the primary somatosensory cortex is associated with increased pain and mood disturbance in patients with interstitial cystitis/painful bladder syndrome. *J Urol.* 2015;193(1):131–137.

43. Letzen JE, Robinson ME. Negative mood influences default mode network functional connectivity in chronic low back pain patients: Implications for functional neuroimaging biomarkers. *Pain.* 2016;158(1):48–57.

44. Eck J, Richter M, Straube T, Miltner WH, Weiss T. Affective brain regions are activated during the processing of pain-related words in migraine patients. *Pain.* 2011;152(5):1104–1113.

45. Wood PB, Patterson JC 2nd, Sunderland JJ, Tainter KH, Glabus MF, Lilien DL. Reduced presynaptic dopamine activity in fibromyalgia syndrome demonstrated with positron emission tomography: A pilot study. *J Pain.* 2007;8(1):51–58.

46. Loggia ML, Berna C, Kim J, et al. Disrupted brain circuitry for pain-related reward/ punishment in fibromyalgia. *Arthritis Rheum.* 2013;66(1):203–212.

47. Martucci KT, Borg N, MacNiven KH, Knutson B, Mackey SC. Altered prefrontal correlates of monetary anticipation and outcome in chronic pain. *Pain.* 2018;159(9):1495–1507.

48. Martucci KT, Shirer WR, Bagarinao E, et al. The posterior medial cortex in urologic chronic pelvic pain syndrome: Detachment from default mode network. A resting-state study from the MAPP Research Network. *Pain.* 2015;156(9):1755–1764.

49. Zeidan F, Martucci KT, Kraft RA, McHaffie JG, Coghill RC. Neural correlates of mindfulness meditation-related anxiety relief. *Social Cogn Affect Neurosci.* 2014;9(6):751–759.

50. Baliki MN, Chialvo DR, Geha PY, et al. Chronic pain and the emotional brain: Specific brain activity associated with spontaneous fluctuations of intensity of chronic back pain. *J Neurosci.* 2006;26(47):12165–12173.

51. Hashmi JA, Baliki MN, Huang L, et al. Shape shifting pain: Chronification of back pain shifts brain representation from nociceptive to emotional circuits. *Brain.* 2013;136(Pt 9):2751–2768.

52. Bushnell MC, Čeko M, Low LA. Cognitive and emotional control of pain and its disruption in chronic pain. *Nat Rev Neurosci.* 2013;14(7):502–511.

53. Day MA, Thorn BE, Burns JW. The continuing evolution of biopsychosocial interventions for chronic pain. *J Cogn Psychother.* 2012;26(2):114–129.

54. Sturgeon JA. Psychological therapies for the management of chronic pain. *Psychol Res Behav Manag.* 2014;7:115–124.

55. Keefe FJ. Cognitive behavioral therapy for managing pain. *Clin Psychol.* 1996;49(3):4–5.

56. Williams AC, Eccleston C, Morley S. Psychological therapies for the management of chronic pain (excluding headache) in adults. *Cochrane Database Syst Rev.* 2012;11:CD007407.

57. Martel M-E, Dionne F, Scott W. The mediating role of pain acceptance in the relation between perceived injustice and chronic pain outcomes in a community sample. *Clin J Pain.* 2016;33(6):509–516.

58. McCracken LM, Vowles KE. Acceptance and commitment therapy and mindfulness for chronic pain: Model, process, and progress. *Am Psychologist.* 2014;69(2):178–187.

59. Kabat-Zinn J. An outpatient program in behavioral medicine for chronic pain patients based on the practice of mindfulness meditation: Theoretical considerations and preliminary results. *Gen Hosp Psychiatry.* 1982;4(1):33–47.

60. Reiner K, Tibi L, Lipsitz JD. Do mindfulness-based interventions reduce pain intensity? A critical review of the literature. *Pain Med.* 2013;14(2):230–242.

61. Veehof M, Trompetter H, Bohlmeijer E, Schreurs K. Acceptance- and mindfulness-based interventions for the treatment of chronic pain: A meta-analytic review. *Cogn Behav Therapy.* 2016;45(1):5–31.

62. Yu L, McCracken LM. Model and processes of acceptance and commitment therapy (ACT) for chronic pain including a closer look at the self. *Curr Pain Headache Rep.* 2016;20(2):1–7.

63. Wicksell RK, Vowles KE. The role and function of acceptance and commitment therapy and behavioral flexibility in pain management. *Pain Manag.* 2015;5(5):319–322.

64. Trompetter HR, Bohlmeijer ET, Fox J-P, Schreurs KM. Psychological flexibility and catastrophizing as associated change mechanisms during online Acceptance & Commitment Therapy for chronic pain. *Behav Res Ther.* 2015;74:50–59.

65. Turner JA, Anderson ML, Balderson BH, Cook AJ, Sherman KJ, Cherkin DC. Mindfulness-based stress reduction and cognitive-behavioral therapy for chronic low back pain: Similar effects on mindfulness, catastrophizing, self-efficacy, and acceptance in a randomized controlled trial. *Pain.* 2016;157(11):2434–2444.

66. Kabat-Zinn J. *Full Catastrophe Living: The Program of the Stress Reduction Clinic at the University of Massachusetts Medical Center.* New York, NY: Delta; 1990.

67. Scott W, Hann KE, McCracken LM. A comprehensive examination of changes in psychological flexibility following acceptance and commitment therapy for chronic pain. *J Contemp Psychother.* 2016;46:139–148.

68. Gu J, Strauss C, Bond R, Cavanagh K. How do mindfulness-based cognitive therapy and mindfulness-based stress reduction improve mental health and wellbeing? A systematic review and meta-analysis of mediation studies. *Clin Psychol Rev.* 2015;37:1–12.

69. Deckersbach T, Peters AT, Shea C, et al. Memory performance predicts response to psychotherapy for depression in bipolar disorder: A pilot randomized controlled trial with exploratory functional magnetic resonance imaging. *J Affect Disord.* 2018;229:342–350.

70. Fonzo GA, Goodkind MS, Oathes DJ, et al. Selective effects of psychotherapy on frontopolar cortical function in PTSD. *Am J Psychiatry.* 2017;174(12):1175–1184.

71. Walsh E, Carl H, Eisenlohr-Moul T, et al. Attenuation of frontostriatal connectivity during reward processing predicts response to psychotherapy in major depressive disorder. *Neuropsychopharmacology.* 2017;42(4):831–843.

72. Jensen KB, Kosek E, Wicksell R, et al. Cognitive behavioral therapy increases pain-evoked activation of the prefrontal cortex in patients with fibromyalgia. *Pain.* 2012;153(7):1495–1503.
73. Lorenz J, Minoshima S, Casey K. Keeping pain out of mind: The role of the dorsolateral prefrontal cortex in pain modulation. *Brain.* 2003;126(5):1079–1091.
74. Lazaridou A, Kim J, Cahalan CM, et al. Effects of cognitive-behavioral therapy (CBT) on brain connectivity supporting catastrophizing in fibromyalgia. *Clin J Pain.* 2017;33(3):215–221.
75. Hughes LS, Clark J, Colclough JA, Dale E, McMillan D. Acceptance and commitment therapy (ACT) for chronic pain: A systematic review and meta-analyses. *Clin J Pain.* 2017;33(6):552–568.
76. Grant JA, Courtemanche J, Rainville P. A non-elaborative mental stance and decoupling of executive and pain-related cortices predicts low pain sensitivity in Zen meditators. *Pain.* 2011;152(1):150–156.
77. Gard T, Hölzel BK, Sack AT, et al. Pain attenuation through mindfulness is associated with decreased cognitive control and increased sensory processing in the brain. *Cerebral Cortex.* 2012;22(11):2692–2702.
78. Zeidan F, Martucci KT, Kraft RA, Gordon NS, McHaffie JG, Coghill RC. Brain mechanisms supporting the modulation of pain by mindfulness meditation. *J Neurosci.* 2011;31(14):5540–5548.
79. Petersen GL, Finnerup NB, Grosen K, et al. Expectations and positive emotional feelings accompany reductions in ongoing and evoked neuropathic pain following placebo interventions. *Pain.* 2014;155(12):2687–2698.
80. Lui F, Colloca L, Duzzi D, Anchisi D, Benedetti F, Porro CA. Neural bases of conditioned placebo analgesia. *Pain.* 2010;151(3):816–824.

PART III

Pain Syndromes and Psychiatric Comorbidities

10

Navigating the Pain and Suicide Conundrum

MARTIN D. CHEATLE, SIMMIE L. FOSTER, AND NICOLE K. Y. TANG ■

INTRODUCTION

There has been a great deal of scholarly activity devoted to the burgeoning rate of opioid misuse/abuse and opioid-related fatalities, particularly in the United States. However, this has overshadowed the silent epidemic of suicidal ideation (SI) and suicidal behavior (SB). Suicide has become a global problem. The World Health Organization published an executive summary, *Preventing Suicide, A Global Imperative*.[1] In this summary, there were some alarming facts: Every 40 seconds, someone in the world dies of suicide; an estimated 804,000 suicide deaths occurred worldwide in 2012; the annual global suicide rate was 11.4/100,000 population (15.0 male and 8.0 female); and in the age group of 15 to 29 years, suicide is the second leading cause of death. Suicide constitutes 54% of the 1.5 million violent deaths per year globally. More than 75% of suicides occur in low- and middle-income families, and all of these numbers continue to grow annually.

PAIN AND SUICIDE

A robust literature underscores that there is a high prevalence of SI and SB in patients with pain, ranging anywhere from 18 to 50%.[2-7] A systematic review by Tang and Crane[5] revealed that the risk for successful suicide was doubled in patients with chronic pain compared with nonpain controls. Ilgen et al.[2] discovered in a large cohort from the US Veterans Affairs database ($N = 260,254$) that veterans experiencing severe pain were more likely to end their life by suicide than veterans with no, mild, or moderate pain. Cheatle et al.[3] evaluated 466 patients with chronic nonmalignant pain treated in a behaviorally based pain program. Results revealed a high rate of SI (26%), and a logistic regression indicated that history of sexual abuse, family history of depression, and being socially withdrawn were predictive of SI.

SUICIDAL IDEATION AND BEHAVIOR AND SUBSTANCE USE DISORDER

Compared with the general population, individuals with an alcohol use disorder are almost 10 times more likely to die by suicide, and those who inject drugs are approximately 14 times more likely to die by suicide.[8] These individuals tend to have multiple risk factors for SB, including having depressive symptoms and enduring a significant number of severe stressors, such as loss of relationships, jobs, or health and financial problems. Patients with co-occurring pain and substance use disorder (SUD) are particularly at high risk for attempting and ending their lives by suicide.

PAIN AND SUICIDAL IDEATION AND BEHAVIOR: RISK FACTORS

There are general, non–pain-specific risk factors and pain-specific risk factors for suicidality. General, non–pain-specific risk factors include gender (female); age (>45 years old); co-occurring mental disorders (especially depression and SUD); acute losses and stressors (relationships, job, finances); chronic medical illnesses; experiences of conflict, disaster, or discrimination; past psychiatric hospitalizations; frequency of SI; severity of psychiatric disorder; poor social support; and, the strongest predictor of suicide, a previous suicide attempt.[1,9] While patients with pain commonly have a number of these risk factors,[10] pain-specific risk factors include pain duration, pain intensity, sleep disturbance, catastrophizing, mental defeat, and opioid dosing. General and pain-specific risk factors for SI and SB are outlined in Box 10.1.

Box 10.1

RISK FACTORS FOR SUICIDE

- Gender (female)
- Age (>45 years old)
- Acute losses and stressors
- Chronic medical illnesses
- Previous suicide attempts
- Concomitant mental health history (especially depression and SUD)
- Social isolation/poor social support
- Experiences conflict, discrimination
- Frequency of suicidal ideation
- Severity of psychiatric disease
- Past psychiatric hospitalizations
- Past suicide attempt
- Pain type*
- Pain intensity*
- Pain duration*
- Sleep disturbance*
- Opioid dosing*

* Pain-specific risk factors.

Pain Duration and Intensity

There is generally convincing evidence that pain intensity[5,6] and pain duration[5] are predictive of SI and SB. In a large cohort study, Ilgen et al.[6] analyzed data from the Veterans Affairs medical records database and the National Death Index (N = 260,254) evaluating the association between self-assessed pain severity and SB in veterans. They discovered after controlling for demographic and psychiatric factors that veterans with severe pain were more likely to die by suicide than ones with mild or moderate pain.

Sleep Disturbance

Sleep disturbance is very common in patients with chronic pain, with the prevalence ranging from 50 to 80%,[11,12,14] and has been postulated as a potential mediator of suicidal ideation in this patient population. Racine et al.[13] examined data of 88 patients with chronic pain who completed a number of self-administered questionnaires at intake to three pain clinics in Canada.

They discovered that 24% of these patients endorsed experiencing SI. Poor sleep quality was the only significant physical variable predictor of SI. There is also persuasive evidence that pain and sleep are bidirectional (pain leading to poorer sleep quality and sleep deprivation causing increased pain), which potentially could synergistically increase the risk for SI and SB. Although sleep disturbance is common in patients with pain, it is often not evaluated or effectively treated.[14]

Opioid Dosing

Ilgen et al.[15] performed a retrospective data analysis on the risk for suicide by different opioid doses in veterans with chronic nonmalignant pain. After controlling for demographic and other clinical features (e.g., depression, post-traumatic stress disorder), results indicated that higher opioid doses were associated with increased risk for suicide mortality. These results suggest that when a patient is on higher doses of opioids, clinicians should be more cognizant of an increased risk for SI and SB, especially if a patient has one or more of the known risk factors.

PAIN AND SUICIDAL IDEATION AND BEHAVIOR: POSSIBLE MEDIATORS

There are a number of postulated mediators for suicide in patients with chronic pain. These include catastrophizing, burdensomeness/social isolation, and mental defeat.

Catastrophizing

Patients with chronic pain tend to engage in pain-related catastrophizing, which can be conceptualized as a magnified, exaggerated negative focus on pain that can contribute to depression and disability and in turn exacerbate an individual's experience of pain and suffering.[16] The association between SI and individual differences in the use of pain-related coping strategies and pain catastrophizing was assessed in a large cohort of 1515 patients with chronic pain. In this sample, 32% reported recent SI. It was revealed that the extent of depression and pain catastrophizing best predicted the occurrence and the degree of SI.[4]

Burdensomeness and Social Isolation

A prevailing theory of SI and SB is based on the interpersonal theory of suicide by Joyner and colleagues.[17] This theory proposes that thwarted belongingness (unfulfilled need for social interaction and connectedness) and perceived burdensomeness (perceiving oneself as a burden or a liability to others, particularly family members) are two primary factors that significantly contribute to the context that leads to SI and possible SB. In a study by Kranzler et al.,[18] 113 patients with chronic nonmalignant pain were evaluated, and a logistic regression model revealed that one question measuring perceived burdensomeness was the only predictor of suicidal ideation. Cheatle et al.[3] also discovered that social withdrawal and isolation were predictive of SI in a cohort of 466 patients undergoing treatment at a pain center.

According to the interpersonal theory of suicide, the desire for suicide is caused by the confluence of thwarted belongingness and perceived burdensomeness, and the capability for SB and attempts develop in response to repeated exposure to physically or emotionally painful or fear-inducing experiences. This is very pertinent to patients with chronic pain because two strong risk factors for suicide are pain duration and pain intensity.

Mental Defeat

A novel construct for increased risk for suicidal ideation in chronic pain is mental defeat, which has been defined as a state of mind marked by a loss of autonomy, agency, and human integrity.[19-22]

The link between mental defeat and suicide intent has been investigated in a study with 62 patients seeking specialist treatment from a hospital chronic pain self-management service.[23] Among these patients, 22.6% had a history of past suicide attempts, with 69% indicating that their wish to die during the last attempt was moderate to high. All participants completed a set of questionnaires assessing factors that have been linked to suicidality. Two hierarchical linear regression analyses were subsequently carried out to examine the effect of mental defeat—in competition with the remaining significant correlates of suicidality (pain intensity, anxiety, depression, and pain catastrophizing)—on worst-ever suicide intent, as measured with the 21-item Beck Scale of Suicide Ideation.[24] Both regression models controlled for the effect of pain intensity (step 1), but in the first model mental defeat was entered to the equation first (step 2) before the three psychological predictors, namely anxiety, depression, and pain catastrophizing (step 3); whereas in the second model, the entry order was reversed so that mental defeat (step 3) was added to a full model of pain intensity (step 1), anxiety, depression, and pain catastrophizing (step 2) last. As expected, pain intensity alone was a significant predictor of worst-ever suicide intent in both models. When mental defeat was added to the model next, it improved the predictor by increasing the total amount of variance explained from 11% to 23%. In contrast, the combined power of anxiety, depression, and pain catastrophizing was weaker and did not significantly improve the model's prediction of suicide intent. Also, none of the psychological predictors included in the model, except mental defeat, was found to be a significant predictor of suicide intent. These findings suggest that the effect of mental defeat on suicide intent is independent of pain intensity and that mental defeat may be a better predictor of suicide intent than anxiety, depression, and pain catastrophizing, both as an individual and a combined set of predictors.

SCREENING FOR RISK FOR SUICIDE

Screening for risk for suicide in patients with chronic pain should include general mental health screening, SUD screening, sleep disturbance assessment, and use of specific tools to assess SI and SB.

Mental Health Screening

There are a number of self-administered measures of depression, for example, the Beck Depression Inventory (BDI),[24] Profile of Mood States (POMS),[25] and Patient Health Questionnaire (PHQ-9).[26] Two measures of anxiety that are highly valid and reliable are the Beck Anxiety Inventory (BAI)[27] and the State–Trait Anxiety Inventory.[28] There are also tools that assess both depression and anxiety, such as the Hospital Anxiety and Depression Scale.[29]

Substance Use Disorder Assessment

While patients with pain have an elevated risk for SI, those patients with both pain and SUD are particularly vulnerable to the risk for SI and SB. Assessing the presence of a SUD, therefore, is critical in this patient population.

Examples of assessment tools for SUDs include the CAGE-AID (Cut down, Annoyed, Guilty, Eye-opener Tool),[30] which assesses for both alcohol and drug abuse, and the DAST (Drug Abuse Screening Test).[31]

Risk assessment tools for potential prescription opioid misuse and abuse include the Opioid Risk Tool (ORT) [32] and the Screener and Opioids Assessment for Patients With Pain (SOAPP).[33] These two instruments are examples of assessing risk for potential aberrant drug-related behavior (ADRB) before the initiation of long-term opioid therapy. Examples of assessment tools to monitor misuse after opioid treatment has been initiated include the Current Opioid Misuse Measure (COMM)[34] and the Prescription Drug Use Questionnaire(PDUQ).[35] A recently developed tool, the ORT-OUD, has been demonstrated to predict the risk for developing an opioid use disorder with good specificity and sensitively.[36]

Screening Tools for Sleep Disturbance

Measures for insomnia predominantly include patient self-report in questionnaire and daily sleep diary to capture the subjective experience of sleep disturbance, but they may also include objective measures such as actigraphy and polysomnography to provide objective estimates of sleep patterns and for the assessment of possible concomitant sleep disorders (e.g., sleep apnea, restless leg syndrome/period limb movement disorder, narcolepsy). Self-report measures assess different aspects of sleep disturbance. Moul et al. provide a review of the various sleep assessment scales.[37]

Screening Tools for Mental Defeat

The Pain Self-Perception Scale (PSPS) has been developed to assess the sense of mental defeat in relation to pain experiences.[19] The PSPS contains 24 items that describe negative thoughts and feelings people may have about themselves due to a specified recent episode of intense pain. All items begin with the referent "Because of the pain. . . ," followed by statements such as, "I felt defeated by life," or "I felt destroyed as a person." Respondents rate the extent to which each item applied to their specified recent episode of pain on a 5-point scale (0–4), where 0 is anchored with "not at all/never" and 4 "very strongly." Scores of each item are then summed to give a total score that ranges from 0 to 96, with higher scores indicating higher levels of mental defeat in relation to pain.

Screening Tools for Suicide

The Columbia Suicide Severity Rating Scale (C-SSRS) has been frequently used for clinical trials on new medications and in clinical practice. The C-SSRS assesses a number of domains, including ideation, intensity, behaviors, severity of self-injury, and potential lethality of suicide attempts.[38] The C-SSRS provides greater precision in the assessment of SB and SI, but owing to its length, it can be cumbersome in clinical practice.

Another example of a commonly used assessment for risk for suicide is the Suicide Assessment Five-Step Evaluation and Triage (SAFE-T) tool that was developed in collaboration with the Substance Abuse and Mental Health Services Administration (SAMHSA).[39] The SAFE-T includes assessment of risk factors such as suicidal behavior, current and past psychiatric disorders, family history, change in treatment, and access to fire arms; protective factors, both internal, such as the ability to cope with stress, spiritual or religious beliefs, and frustration tolerance, and external, such as responsibility to children or others and having a positive therapeutic relationship and good social supports; and suicidal inquiry, which asks specific questions about thoughts, plans, behaviors, intents, risk level, and intervention. The SAFE-T assesses the risk level based on the clinical judgment after completing the first three steps. Patients are stratified into low, moderate, and high risk, with specific interventions indicated for each risk level.

PREVENTION AND TREATMENT STRATEGIES

Preventative Measures

Patients who present with moderate to severe depression with or without endorsing SI or plans should be comanaged with a behavioral health specialist. Patients who acknowledge active SI may require inpatient treatment depending on certain factors such as depression and SI severity and whether they have vague or specific plans for completing suicide, including having access to means (potentially lethal medications or own a gun), a history of past SB, or impulsivity. During an acute phase, the patient will require meaningful treatment consisting of both pharmacotherapy and intensive psychotherapy. The pharmacotherapy strategy should include managing depressive symptoms, sleep disturbance, and pain. If opioid or benzodiazepine use is necessary, these medications should be prescribed cautiously, in small amounts, and held and administered by a family member.[10]

Interventions and Treatment

There are a number of pharmacological and nonpharmacological interventions to mitigate the risk for SI/SB.

PHARMACOLOGICAL TREATMENTS

For suicidal patients with or without pain, the general pharmacological strategy is to treat comorbid illness that leads to increased suicide risk, including depression, anxiety, sleep disorder, psychosis, and uncontrolled pain.

Medications That Show Benefit for Reducing Suicidality

Four medications have been shown to decrease risk for suicide: lithium, clozapine, and ketamine, and buprenorphine. Lithium is a first-line treatment for bipolar depression and also may be used to augment antidepressants in treatment-resistant depression. It has been shown to decrease suicidality in patients with mood disorders.[40] Clozapine is an atypical antipsychotic frequently used for treatment-resistant schizophrenia and schizoaffective disorders and has also been shown to decrease suicides in these populations.[41] Ketamine is an N-methyl-D-aspartate (NMDA) receptor antagonist that has recently been shown to have potent and rapid antidepressant and pain-relieving effect. In several small studies, ketamine has shown promise in rapidly reducing SI.[42] Most recently, buprenorphine has shown promise in abating even acute SI.[43]

Medications That Treat Comorbid Risk Factors for Suicidality: Depression, Sleep, and Anxiety

Patients with pain often have comorbid anxiety and sleep and mood disturbance, which can increase risk for SI/SB. Many of these comorbidities may be treated with antidepressants. Augmenting strategies, including anxiolytics, sleep aids, and antiepileptics, may also be employed.

Antidepressants. For suicidal patients with comorbid depression, anxiety, and pain, treating with an antidepressant should be considered. There is no clear data showing that any single antidepressant works better than another, so the choice of antidepressant depends on the patient's comorbidities, the side-effect profile, and the whether the goal is to add additional pain control. Selective serotonin reuptake inhibitors (SSRIs) and serotonin/norepinephrine reuptake inhibitors (SNRIs) are first-line agents for treating depression and anxiety disorders. SSRIs may be better tolerated, while SNRIs also treat pain. For SNRIs and SSRIs, it is often good to start at a low dose, even half of the typical recommended starting dose, because initial side effects can include elevated anxiety, prompting anxious patients to discontinue the drug before it has a chance to take effect. Other side effects can include sexual dysfunction, nausea and diarrhea, insomnia, and weight gain. Of note, SSRIs and SNRIs, while effective for depression, anxiety, and pain, have been shown to disrupt and fragment sleep.[44]

Tricyclic antidepressants (TCAs), such as amitriptyline and doxepin, are a good choice for patients with depression, anxiety, and sleep disorder and also have benefit for pain.[14] However, this benefit must be carefully weighed against their risk in suicidal patients because they are extremely lethal in overdose.[45] Other significant side effects include anticholinergic and adrenergic effects and cardiac conduction delay.

Anxiolytics. Although many clinicians avoid benzodiazepines, a long-acting benzodiazepine such as clonazepam can be useful in the short-term to reduce anxious agitation in a suicidal patient because such agitation potentially contributes to completed suicide.[46] These drugs should not be combined with opioids, and as with TCAs, should be given in small or observed doses. Other medications potentially useful for anxiety include buspirone, hydroxyzine, and antiepileptic drugs.

Anticonvulsants. Like antidepressants, antiepileptics may be used to treat not just pain but also anxiety and sleep disturbance. Gabapentin and pregabalin both have some benefit for pain, sleep and anxiety.[47]

Sleep aids. As mentioned previously, the TCAs can be effective for treating sleep. Many patients may need additional assistance to fall asleep and stay asleep, so adding a dedicated sleep aid is an option. Eszopiclone treats not only sleep but also anxiety. Trazodone is an antidepressant that at low doses is indicated for sleep. Mirtazapine similarly is an antidepressant that improves sleep.[14]

Special Consideration: Risk of Suicidality With Antidepressants and Anticonvulsants

Antidepressants (of all classes) and antiepileptic drugs have the additional complication of possibly leading to SI/SB in some patients. In 2004, the US Food and Drug Administration issued a black box warning regarding an increased risk for SI/SB in children and adolescents, which was extended to young adults (ages 18–25 years) in 2006.[48] This warning was based on a meta-analysis showing an approximately two-fold increase in risk for SI/SB in these populations. Of note, there were no completed suicides and no distinctions among class of antidepressant. Antidepressants in older patients (65 years and older) are actually protective against SI/SB. A similar analysis of antiepileptic drugs showed an increased risk for SI/SB in patients with various disorders taking any antiepileptic drug, again showing an approximately two-fold increased risk in those taking anticonvulsants over placebo, with no distinction among age.[49]

On balance, the risk of untreated depression leading to suicide in a general population outweighs the risk of treating with an antidepressant.[48]

BEHAVIORAL INTERVENTIONS

Cognitive Behavioral Therapy

Cognitive behavioral therapy (CBT) has been highly efficacious in treating mood and anxiety disorders, and the basic principles of CBT have been applied to other conditions, including pain, sleep, and SUD.

Treatment of pain. CBT can include various techniques to assist and support the patient in identifying maladaptive behaviors and/or dysfunctional thought patterns that may diminish the patient's ability to adjust to and cope with their chronic pain, thus contributing to their related depression and anxiety.

The process of CBT typically involves the patient acquiring specific skills, which can include mindfulness-based stress reduction, progressive muscle relaxation training, pacing, effective communication, and cognitive restructuring, which is followed by skill consolidation, rehearsal, and relapse training.[50]

There is a robust literature supporting the clinical efficacy and cost-effectiveness of CBT in improving mood, anxiety, and functionality in a number of chronic pain disorders.

Treatment of insomnia. CBT tailored to insomnia has also been effective in improving sleep disturbance. As noted previously, sleep disturbance is highly prevalent in patients with chronic pain, pain and sleep are bidirectional, and sleep disturbance is a known risk factor for SI/SB in patients with chronic nonmalignant pain.

There is evidence that CBT for insomnia (CBT-I) in patients with chronic primary insomnia is equally effective or even superior to pharmacotherapy in multiple outcomes.[51]

A course of CBT-I typically includes psychoeducation about sleep and insomnia; stimulus control; sleep restriction; sleep hygiene; relaxation training; and cognitive restructuring.

Treatment of pain and substance use disorder. There is emerging evidence that CBT can reduce the risk for prescription opioid misuse and abuse in high-risk patients indirectly by improving mood, anxiety, sleep, and pain coping skills and also in improving outcomes in patients with pain who have a history of a SUD. In a recently published pilot study,[52] patients with hepatitis C who also experienced chronic pain and had a history of SUD were enrolled in an eight-session integrated group CBT program for chronic pain and SUD. Results revealed improvement in key outcomes, including pain-related interference, reduction in cravings for alcohol and other substances, and a decrease in past-month alcohol and substance use.

CONCLUSION

Patients suffering from persistent pain often present with complicating medical and psychiatric comorbidities, including mood and anxiety disorders, and a substantial subgroup of this patient population experience SI and engage in SB. A number of risk factors for SI/SB have been identified in the general population, including gender, age, social isolation, and past history of suicide attempts, and there are several risk factors more specific to the pain population, such as sleep disturbance, pain intensity and duration, and opioid dosing, as well as potential mediators of pain and SI/SB, such as burdensomeness, sleep disturbance, pain catastrophizing, and mental defeat. Many of these risk factors and mediators are modifiable, thus reducing the potential of SI and SB in this vulnerable patient population. Clinicians need to be cognizant of the potential of SI/SB when managing patients with chronic nonmalignant pain, routinely screen for and treat or refer for treatment of concomitant mood, anxiety, sleep, and substance use disorders, and develop a plan of action if patients endorse active SI/SB.

ACKNOWLEDGMENTS

MDC would like to acknowledge the support from Grant 1R01DA032776-01 from the National Institute on Drug Abuse, National Institutes of Health in the writing of this manuscript.

REFERENCES

1. World Health Organization. *Preventing Suicide: A Global Imperative.* 2014. http://apps.who.int/iris/bitstream/10665/131056/1/9789241564779_eng.pdf?ua=1&ua=1. Accessed December 18, 2016.
2. Ilgen MA, Zivin K, McCammon RJ, Valenstein M. Pain and suicidal thoughts, plans and attempts in the United States. *Gen Hosp Psychiatry.* 2008;30:521–527.
3. Cheatle M, Wasser T, Foster C, Olugbodi A, Bryan J. Prevalence of suicidal ideation in patients with chronic noncancer pain referred to a behaviorally based pain program. *Pain Phys.* 2014;17(3):E359–E367.
4. Edwards RR, Smith MT, Kudel I, Haythornthwaite J. Pain-related catastrophizing as a risk factor for suicidal ideation in chronic pain. *Pain.* 2006;126:272–279.
5. Tang NK, Crane C. Suicidality in chronic pain: A review of the prevalence, risk factors and psychological links. *Psychol Med.* 2006;36:575–586.
6. Ilgen MA, Zivin K, Austin KL, Bohnert AS, Czyz EK, Valenstein M, Kilbourne AM. Severe pain predicts greater likelihood of subsequent suicide. *Suicide Life Threat Behav.* 2010;40(6):597–608.
7. Campbell G, Darke S, Bruno R, Degenhardt L. The prevalence and correlates of chronic pain and suicidality in a nationally representative sample. *Aust N Z J Psychiatry.* 2015;49(9):803–811.
8. Wilcox HC, Conner KR, Caine ED. Association of alcohol and drug use disorders and completed suicide: An empirical review of cohort studies. *Drug Alcohol Depend.* 2004;76:S11–S19.

9. Centers for Disease Control and Prevention (CDC). National Center for Injury Prevention and Control; 2010. www.cdc.gov/violenceprevention/suicide/statistics. Accessed December 18, 2016.

10. Cheatle MD. Depression, chronic pain, and suicide by overdose: On the edge. *Pain Med.* 2011;12(suppl 2):S43–S48.

11. Tang NK, Wright KJ, Salkovskis PM. Prevalence and correlates of clinical insomnia co-occurring with chronic back pain. *J Sleep Res.* 2007;16(1):85–95.

12. McCracken LM, Williams JL, Tang NK. Psychological flexibility may reduce insomnia in persons with chronic pain: A preliminary retrospective study. *Pain Med.* 2011;12(6):904–912.

13. Racine M, Choinière M, Nielson WR. Predictors of suicidal ideation in chronic pain patients: An exploratory study. *Clin J Pain.* 2014;30(5):371–378.

14. Cheatle MD, Foster S, Pinkett A, Lesneski M, Qu D, Dhingra L. Assessing and managing sleep disturbance in patients with chronic pain. *Anesthesiol Clin.* 2016;34(2):379–393.

15. Ilgen MA, Bohnert AS, Ganoczy D, Bair MJ, McCarthy JF, Blow FC. Opioid dose and risk of suicide. *Pain.* 2016;157(5):1079–1084.

16. Turner JA, Aaron LA. Pain-related catastrophizing: What is it? *Clin J Pain.* 2001;17(1):65–71.

17. Van Orden KA, Witte TK, Cukrowicz KC, Braithwaite SR, Selby EA, Joiner TE. The Interpersonal Theory of Suicide. *Psychol Rev.* 2010;117:575–600.

18. Kanzler KE, Bryan CJ, McGeary DD, Morrow CE. Suicidal ideation and perceived burdensomeness in patients with chronic pain. *Pain Pract.* 2012;12:602–609.

19. Tang NK, Salkovskis PM, Hanna M. Mental defeat in chronic pain: Initial exploration of the concept. *Clin J Pain.* 2007;23(3):222–232.

20. Tang NK, Salkovskis PM, Hodges A, Soong E, Hanna MH, Hester J. Chronic pain syndrome associated with health anxiety: A qualitative thematic comparison between pain patients with high and low health anxiety. *Br J Clin Psychol.* 2009;48(part 1):1–20.

21. Tang NK, Goodchild CE, Hester J, Salkovskis PM. Mental defeat is linked to interference, distress and disability in chronic pain. *Pain.* 2010;149(3):547–554.

22. Taylor PJ, Gooding PA, Wood AM, Johnson J, Pratt D, Tarrier N. Defeat and entrapment in schizophrenia: The relationship with suicidal ideation and positive psychotic symptoms. *Psychiatry Res.* 2010;178(2):244–248.

23. Tang NK, Beckwith P, Ashworth P. Mental defeat is associated with suicide intent in patients with chronic pain. *Clin J Pain.* 2016;32(5):411–419.

24. Beck A, Ward C, Mendelson M, Mock J, Erbaugh J. An inventory for measuring depression. *Arch Gen Psychiatry.* 1961;4:561–571.

25. McNair D, Lorr M, Droppleman L. *Profile of Mood States.* San Diego, CA: Educational and Industrial Testing Service; 1971.

26. Kroenke K, Spitzer RL, Williams JB. The PHQ-9: Validity of a brief depression severity measure. *J Gen Intern Med.* 2001;16(9):606–613.

27. Beck AT, Epstein N, Brown G, Steer RA. An inventory for measuring clinical anxiety: Psychometric properties. *J Consult Clin Psychol.* 1988;56(6):893–897.

28. Spielberg C, Gorsuch R, Lushene R. *Manual for the State-Trait Anxiety Inventory.* Palo Alto, CA: Consulting Psychologists; 1970.

29. Bjelland L, Dahl AA, Haug TT, Neckelmann D. The validity of the Hospital Anxiety and Depression Scale. An updated literature review. *J Psychosom Res.* 2002;52(2):69–77.

30. Brown RL, Rounds LA. Conjoint screening questionnaires for alcohol and other drug abuse: Criterion validity in a primary care practice. *Wis Med J.* 1995;94(3):135–140.

31. Cocco KM, Carey KB. Psychometric properties of the Drug Abuse Screening Test in psychiatric outpatients. *Psych Assess.* 1998;10(4):681–691.

32. Webster LR, Webster RM. Predicting aberrant behaviors in opioid-treated patients: Preliminary validation of the Opioid Risk Tool. *Pain Med.* 2005;6:432–442.

33. Butler SF, Fernandez K, Benoit C, Budman SH, Jamison RN. Validation of the revised Screener and Opioid Assessment for Patients with Pain (SOAPP-R). *J Pain.* 2008;9:360–372.

34. Butler SF, Budman SH, Fernandez KC, et al. Development and validation of the Current Opioid Misuse Measure. *Pain.* 2007;130:144–156.

35. Compton PA, Wu SM, Schieffer B, Pham Q, Naliboff BD. Introduction of a self-report version of the Prescription Drug Use Questionnaire and relationship to medication agreement noncompliance. *J Pain Symptom Manage.* 2008;36:383–395.

36. Cheatle MD, Compton PA, Dhingra L, Wasser T, O'Brien CP. Development of the revised Opioid Risk Tool to predict opioid use disorder in patients with chronic nonmalignant pain. *J Pain.* 2019;20(7):843–851.

37. Moul DE, Hall M, Pilkonis PA, Buysse DJ. Self-report measures of insomnia in adults: Rationales, choices, and needs. *Sleep Med Rev.* 2004;8(3):177–198.

38. Posner K, Brown GK, Stanley B, et al. The Columbia-Suicide Severity Rating Scale: Initial validity and internal consistency findings from three multisite studies with adolescents and adults. *Am J Psychiatry.* 2011;168(12):1266–1277.

39. SAMSHA. Suicide Assessment Five-Step Evaluation and Triage (SAFE-T). http://store.samhsa.gov/shin/content//SMA09-4432/SMA09-4432.pdf. Accessed December 19, 2016.

40. Cipriani A, Hawton K, Stockton S, Geddes JR. Lithium in the prevention of suicide in mood disorders: Updated systematic review and meta-analysis. *BMJ.* 2013;346:f3646–f3646.

41. Meltzer HY, Alphs L, Green AI, et al.; International Suicide Prevention Trial Study Group. Clozapine treatment for suicidality in schizophrenia: International Suicide Prevention Trial. *Arch Gen Psychiatry.* 2003;60:82–91.

42. Wilkinson ST, Sanacora G. Ketamine: A potential rapid-acting antisuicidal agent. *Depress Anxiety.* 2016;33:711–717.

43. Yovell Y, Bar G, Mashiah M, et al. Ultra-low-dose buprenorphine as a time-limited treatment for severe suicidal ideation: A randomized controlled trial. *Am J Psychiatry.* 2016;173(5):491–498.

44. Gursky JT, Krahn LE. The effects of antidepressants on sleep: A review. *Harv Rev Psychiatry.* 2000;8:298–306.

45. Rosenbaum JF. *Handbook of Psychiatric Drug Therapy.* Philadelphia: Lippincott Williams & Wilkins; 2009.

46. Sani G, Tondo L, Koukopoulos A, et al. Suicide in a large population of former psychiatric inpatients. *Psychiatry Clin Neurosci.* 2011;65:286–295.

47. Argoff C. The coexistence of neuropathic pain, sleep, and psychiatric disorders: A novel treatment approach. *Clin J Pain*. 2007;23:15–22.

48. Pereira A, Conwell Y, Gitlin MJ, Dworkin RH. Suicidal ideation and behavior associated with antidepressant medications: Implications for the treatment of chronic pain. *Pain*. 2014;155:2471–2475.

49. Pereira A, Gitlin MJ, Gross RA, Posner K, Dworkin RH. Suicidality associated with antiepileptic drugs: Implications for the treatment of neuropathic pain and fibromyalgia. *Pain*. 2013;154:345–349.

50. Turk DC, Flor H. Etiological theories and treatments for chronic back pain. II. Psychological models and interventions. *Pain*. 1984;19(3):209–233.

51. Sivertsen B, Omvik S, Pallesen S, et al. Cognitive behavioral therapy vs zopiclone for treatment of chronic primary insomnia in older adults: A randomized controlled trial. *JAMA*. 2006;295(24):2851–2858.

52. Morasco BJ, Greaves DW, Lovejoy TI, Turk DC, Dobscha SK, Hauser P. Development and preliminary evaluation of an integrated cognitive-behavior treatment for chronic pain and substance use disorder in patients with the hepatitis c virus. *Pain Med*. 2016;17(12):2280–2290.

11

Considering Depression and Anxiety as Risk Factors for Temporomandibular Joint Disorder

A German Perspective

STEFAN KINDLER AND MARIKE BREDOW-ZEDEN ■

INTRODUCTION

Chronic pain is a large and rapidly growing public health problem.[1,2] Lower back, joint, head, and facial pain are frequent types of chronic pain.[3] Painful functional disorders of the temporomandibular joint, masticatory muscles, and associated musculoskeletal structures of the head and neck are called temporomandibular joint disorder (TMD).[4] TMD is a type of chronic pain[5] and are widely used as a model for chronic pain.[6] The etiology of TMD pain is multifactorial.[4] Biological, behavioral, environmental, social, emotional, and cognitive factors can contribute to TMD.[7] TMD can manifest with musculoskeletal facial pain complaints and with different forms of jaw dysfunction.[5] Typical signs of TMD are temporomandibular joint pain and masticatory muscle pain on palpation. The prevalence of at least one sign or symptom of TMD was reported to range between 40 and 75% among adults in the United States.[4] In Finland, a prevalence of temporomandibular joint pain on palpation and muscle pain on palpation was 5.1%, and 18.9% in women, and 2.4%, and 7.2% in men.[8]

The etiology of TMD, however, still is not completely understood.[4] Parafunctional habits such as tooth grinding and clenching,[9] trauma,[10] and genetic factors[6,11] may initiate TMD. The importance of psychological disorders as risk factors for TMD pain is discussed. Several studies described an association between TMD pain and coexisting psychopathology, including depression, anxiety, and post-traumatic stress disorder (PTSD).[12-14] Mongini et al. recommend careful screening for depression and anxiety in facial pain patients,[15] despite the fact that the causal relationship between depression, anxiety, and TMD pain is not clear.[16]

Methodological differences may be a possible explanation for divergent findings. Most studies have selected relatively small numbers of participants from treatment facilities,[17] whereas in observational studies, a clinical examination has not been performed.[18,19] Moreover, patients who sought treatment for TMD pain are often not willing to accept depression and anxiety as possible reasons for their TMD pain complaints. Only a few studies analyzed the role of depression[17] and anxiety[19] using a prospective cohort design. In most patient studies, the research diagnostic criteria for TMD are based on clusters of signs and symptoms that may not define a common pathophysiology.[20]

In this chapter, we describe the results of a population-based study of depression and anxiety as risk factors for TMD pain. We also present our treatment strategy used at the University Medicine of Greifswald Germany for TMD. Clinically relevant case reviews are presented to offer guidelines for evaluation and treatment of TMD pain.

OUR STUDY ON DEPRESSION AND ANXIETY AS RISK FACTORS FOR TEMPOROMANDIBULAR JOINT DISORDER

The Study of Health in Pomerania (SHIP) is a longitudinal population-based follow-up investigation in West Pomerania, the northeastern region of Germany, with a total population of 212,157 inhabitants. Our aim was to identify the incidence of signs and symptoms of TMD in adults 20 years or older. In this study 4289 participants aged 20 to 81 years were clinically examined; 49.9% had one or more clinical signs of TMD, but only 2.7% were subjectively aware of temporomandibular joint pain symptoms.[21]

Symptoms of depression and anxiety emerged as risk factors for TMD pain. We found moderate to strong relationships that were independent of relevant confounders. Depressive symptoms were more strongly related to joint pain compared with muscle pain, whereas anxiety symptoms were more strongly related to muscle pain compared with joint pain.[22] In our study, we used the Composite International Diagnostic Screener for detecting depression and anxiety symptoms.[23]

Proposed Link Between Psychopathology and Temporomandibular Joint Disorder

A relationship between depression, anxiety symptoms, and the increased risk for muscle or joint pain could be explained by the following reasons. Depression and anxiety may induce muscular hyperactivity and altered muscle mechanics, which lead to muscle pain.[4] Joint inflammation could be induced by biomechanical alterations and may lead to joint pain.[4] TMD also might be linked to abnormal pain processing in the trigeminal system.[4] Imbalances of the neurotransmitters serotonin and catecholamines may lead to painful TMD.[1,4,24,25] TMD may also be a physical manifestation of anxiety or depression.[26]

Anxiety and depression are the most frequent mental disorders in Europe[27]— hence the importance of the association of TMD with depression and anxiety.[28,29] The causality of that relation has not been demonstrated.[28]

Interestingly, patients with complete temporomandibular joint intracapsular disorder have a low proportion of accompanying psychological symptoms and usually have a normal personality profile. Depression and anxiety symptoms may differently alter the stress and alarm systems of the body as a result of differential regulations of the hypothalamus-pituitary-adrenal axis.[30]

Case Vignettes

TEMPOROMANDIBULAR JOINT DISORDER WITH PHYSICAL TRAUMA

A 45-year-old woman was referred to the clinic of oral maxillofacial surgery with orofacial pain. She was suffering from this pain for 8 months. She reported a stair fall that resulted in the injury of her right mandible, and described a loosening of her teeth in the right side and complaints in the left temporomandibular joint. She also described parafunctional habits and a tendency to have locked joints. After the stair fall, she experienced a left-sided temporomandibular joint clicking. Eventually, she developed full-fledged TMD pain. The patient received multiple treatment modalities, including manual therapy of the masticatory muscles, an unadjusted occlusal appliance, and later, an occlusal appliance in centric relation. She was prescribed ibuprofen and metamizole.

The clinical functional analysis and screening revealed signs of TMD. There was both-sided myogelosis in the neck muscles, the masseter muscles, the temporalis muscles, and the pterygoid muscles. Joint clicking could be objectified in the left temporomandibular joint. The opening of the mouth was of 36 mm width at the beginning of the therapy; after 1 year, the incisal edge distance returned to normal values. The initial therapy with splints, physiotherapy and transcutaneous electrical nerve stimulation (TENS) was not successful.

Computed tomography was performed and revealed no signs of trauma, and subsequent magnetic resonance imaging showed a partial anterior disk dislocation without reposition. In parallel, she was treated by an orthopedist. However, even though Composite International Diagnostic Screener screening questions ("Did you ever suffer from feelings of sadness or depressed mood for a period of at least 2 weeks?" and "Did you ever suffer from lack of interest, tiredness, or loss of energy for a period of at least 2 weeks?") were positive and she complained of suffering from stress, she rejected a consultation with a psychiatrist or psychologist. After the death of her mother, she had an acute exacerbation of TMD pain, and she was in poor general condition. Now, she agrees to receive parallel psychological treatment. The patient is undergoing periodic follow-up examinations, and her TMD pain complaints have improved significantly.

Because the number and severity of traumatic events are also a risk factor for TMD pain, appropriately estimating the confounding effect of the number of traumatic events on the relationship between TMD pain and PTSD is crucial.[14]

TEMPOROMANDIBULAR JOINT DISORDER WITHOUT PHYSICAL TRAUMA

A 55-year-old woman was referred to the oral maxillofacial surgery clinic because of pain in the right neck and facial region that was present for 1 year. The initial examination revealed a pressure pain in the right tragus and mastoid. The subsequent conventional radiograph and computed tomography scan showed no signs of a mastoiditis and sinusitis. As a clinical differential diagnosis, TMD and occlusion disorders were considered. She was given a self-observation form to monitor and document her pain. After 1 month, her self-reports were analyzed, and the evaluation hinted at bruxism without occlusion disorders. The initial therapy comprised physiotherapy and the preparation and insertion of a centric splint. A pain medication (metamizole) was prescribed, to be taken on demand. However, she still described ear noises and was therefore referred to the ear, nose, and throat specialist with the diagnosis of presbyacusis. The patient was undergoing periodic follow-up examinations, and her TMD pain complaints gradually resolved. The initial psychosocial anamnesis had revealed occupational stress in her work as a teacher that was considered to be the trigger for depression and TMD. After a combined psychological and a clinical functional therapy, stabilization of the general medical condition and TMD pain reduction were achieved.

Successfully Managing Temporomandibular Joint Disorder Pain

In our department, the first step in examining an orofacial pain patient is to take a pain anamnesis. Next, the medical history—with all relevant general diseases, including psychiatric disorders such as depression, anxiety, and PTSD—is evaluated. We consider it necessary to ask about physical trauma in the maxillofacial region. An oral examination of teeth and mucosa should be performed. Dental and gingival origins of orofacial pain should be excluded. A current panoramic radiography is necessary to screen for radiological findings that may contribute to orofacial pain. In cases of physical trauma, further radiographic examinations are needed to exclude fractures in the maxillofacial region.

If pain anamnesis and oral examination show signs or symptoms of TMD pain, a clinical functional analysis is indicated. A dentist or maxillofacial surgeon who is experienced in treatment and therapy of TMD should conduct a clinical functional analysis.

For the definition of TMD pain in daily clinical practice, we use the clinical examination tool for TMD of the German Society of Craniomandibular Function and Disorders 2012.

We focus only on clinical signs of TMD rather than on subjective symptoms. Clinical signs are joint pain on lateral pressure and pressure pain referred cranially. Pain in the masseter and temporalis muscles could be assessed bilaterally. Typical subjective TMD symptoms are joint sounds, temporomandibular joint pain, and pain of facial muscles. Individual perception of these symptoms differs considerably during diagnosis between diagnosticians.[21]

Therapeutic Recommendations

If TMD pain in the clinical functional analysis of an orofacial pain patient is diagnosed, we start the initial therapy, which includes self-monitoring of habits like clenching and grinding and physiotherapy of the painful masticatory and neck muscles. Depending on the intensity of TMD pain, pain treatment with nonsteroidal anti-inflammatory drugs may also be indicated. If necessary, a treatment with occlusal splints is started. If this treatment is not successful, further imaging and consultations to other specialists are recommended. In the imaging diagnostic workup, it is important to exclude relevant general diseases like tumors and to look for pathologies that may contribute to orofacial pain. Systemic inflammatory diseases that may affect the maxillofacial region, such as rheumatoid arthritis, must also be evaluated.

After the exclusion of all these case-specific relevant diseases, we focus on psychiatric diseases. Therefore, the Composite International Diagnostic Screener could be used as screening tool for psychological disorders in clinical practice. Eight questions of the Composite International Diagnostic Screener are designed to assess lifetime occurrence of somatoform, anxiety, and depressive disorders. The screening questions for depressive disorders ("Did you ever suffer from feelings of sadness or depressed mood for a period of at least 2 weeks?" and "Did you ever suffer from lack of interest, tiredness, or loss of energy for a period of at least 2 weeks?") and for anxiety (panic attacks, generalized anxiety, agoraphobia, social phobia, specific phobia) can be used to screen TMD pain patients in clinical practice. Cognitive behavioral treatment,[12] biopsychosocial intervention, biofeedback, and minimal therapist contact interventions[31] are among the nonpharmacological options to treat TMD pain.

Pharmacological treatment options include the use of tricyclic antidepressants and serotonin reuptake inhibitors.[4] TMD pain is generally understood to be related to abnormal pain processing in the trigeminal system,[24] caused by serotonin and catecholamine neurotransmitter imbalances.[1,4] In the therapy of PTSD patients, randomized clinical trials have demonstrated the benefit of treatment with tricyclic antidepressants, serotonin reuptake inhibitors, and monoamine oxidase inhibitors.[1,4]

CONCLUSION

Depressive and anxiety symptoms should be considered as risk factors for TMD pain. It is important to identify depression and anxiety disorders during patient assessment. Accurate diagnosis and adequate treatment of depression and anxiety in TMD pain help improve outcomes, patient satisfaction, and quality of care. We hope that the guideposts offered in this chapter will support interdisciplinary management of TMD pain that include psychiatrists, pain medicine specialists, and other health professionals. These results also should encourage dental practitioners to screen TMD patients in clinical practice.

ACKNOWLEDGMENTS

SHIP is part of the Community Medicine Research net of the University of Greifswald, Germany, which is funded by the Federal Ministry of Education and Research (grants 01ZZ9603, 01ZZ0103, and 01ZZ0403), the Ministry of Cultural Affairs, and the Social Ministry of the Federal State of Mecklenburg–West Pomerania.

I would like to thank all the colleagues and patients who have contributed significantly to this work. Especially, I would like to thank Mrs. Bredow-Zeden, Mrs. Mksoud, Prof. Bernhardt, and Prof. Metelmann for their contributions to this book chapter.

REFERENCES

1. Apkarian AV, Baliki MN, Geha PY. Towards a theory of chronic pain. *Prog Neurobiol.* 2009;87(2):81–97.
2. Sharp TJ, Harvey AG. Chronic pain and posttraumatic stress disorder: Mutual maintenance? *Clin Psychol Rev.* 2001;21(6):857–877.
3. Grabe HJ, Meyer C, Hapke U, et al. Specific somatoform disorder in the general population. *Psychosomatics.* 2003;44(4):304–311.
4. Scrivani SJ, Keith DA, Kaban LB. Temporomandibular disorders. *N Engl J Med.* 2008;359(25):2693–2705.
5. Goldstein BH. Temporomandibular disorders: A review of current understanding. *Oral Surg Oral Med Oral Pathol Oral Radiol Endod.* 1999;88(4):379–385.
6. Schwahn C, Grabe HJ, Meyer zu Schwabedissen H, et al. The effect of catechol-O-methyltransferase polymorphisms on pain is modified by depressive symptoms. *Eur J Pain.* 2012;16(6):878–889.
7. Dworkin SF, Massoth DL. Temporomandibular disorders and chronic pain: Disease or illness? *J Prosthet Dent.* 1994;72(1):29–38.
8. Tuuliainen L, Sipila K, Maki P, Kononen M, Suominen AL. Association between clinical signs of temporomandibular disorders and psychological distress among an adult Finnish population. *J Oral Facial Pain Headache.* 2015;29(4):370–377.
9. Michelotti A, Cioffi I, Festa P, Scala G, Farella M. Oral parafunctions as risk factors for diagnostic TMD subgroups. *J Oral Rehabil.* 2010;37(3):157–162.
10. Zhang ZK, Ma XC, Gao S, Gu ZY, Fu KY. Studies on contributing factors in temporomandibular disorders. *Chin J Dent Res.* 1999;2(3–4):7–20.
11. Oakley M, Vieira AR. The many faces of the genetics contribution to temporomandibular joint disorder. *Orthod Craniofac Res.* 2008;11(3):125–135.
12. Litt MD, Shafer DM, Ibanez CR, Kreutzer DL, Tawfik-Yonkers Z. Momentary pain and coping in temporomandibular disorder pain: Exploring mechanisms of cognitive behavioral treatment for chronic pain. *Pain.* 2009;145(1–2):160–168.
13. Gameiro GH, da Silva Andrade A, Nouer DF, Ferraz de Arruda Veiga MC. How may stressful experiences contribute to the development of temporomandibular disorders? *Clin Oral Invest.* 2006;10(4):261–268.
14. Kindler S, Schwahn C, Bernhardt O, et al. Association between symptoms of posttraumatic stress disorder and signs of temporomandibular disorders in the general population. *J Oral Facial Pain Headache.* 2019;33(1):67–76.
15. Mongini F, Ciccone G, Ceccarelli M, Baldi I, Ferrero L. Muscle tenderness in different types of facial pain and its relation to anxiety and depression: A cross-sectional study on 649 patients. *Pain.* 2007;131(1–2):106–111.

16. Yap AU, Chua EK, Tan KB, Chan YH. Relationships between depression/somatization and self-reports of pain and disability. *J Orofacial Pain*. 2004;18(3):220–225.
17. Slade GD, Diatchenko L, Bhalang K, et al. Influence of psychological factors on risk of temporomandibular disorders. *J Dent Res*. 2007;86(11):1120–1125.
18. Sipila K, Veijola J, Jokelainen J, et al. Association of symptoms of TMD and orofacial pain with alexithymia: An epidemiological study of the Northern Finland 1966 birth cohort. *Cranio*. 2001;19(4):246–251.
19. Aggarwal VR, Macfarlane GJ, Farragher TM, McBeth J. Risk factors for onset of chronic oro-facial pain: Results of the North Cheshire oro-facial pain prospective population study. *Pain*. 2010;149(2):354–359.
20. Kim H, Clark D, Dionne RA. Genetic contributions to clinical pain and analgesia: Avoiding pitfalls in genetic research. *J Pain*. 2009;10(7):663–693.
21. Gesch D, Bernhardt O, Alte D, et al. Prevalence of signs and symptoms of temporomandibular disorders in an urban and rural German population: Results of a population-based study of health in Pomerania. *Quintessence Int*. 2004;35(2):143–150.
22. Kindler S, Samietz S, Houshmand M, et al. Depressive and anxiety symptoms as risk factors for temporomandibular joint pain: A prospective cohort study in the general population. *J Pain*. 2012;13(12):1188–1197.
23. Wittchen HU, Höfler M, Gander F, et al. Screening for mental disorders: Performance of the Composite International Diagnostic—Screener (CID-S). *Int J Meth Psychiat Res*. 1999;8(2):59–70.
24. McEwen BS. Physiology and neurobiology of stress and adaptation: Central role of the brain. *Physiol Rev*. 2007;87(3):873–904.
25. Bair MJ, Robinson RL, Katon W, Kroenke K. Depression and pain comorbidity: A literature review. *Arch Intern Med*. 2003;163(20):2433–2445.
26. van der Windt DA, Dunn KM, Spies-Dorgelo MN, Mallen CD, Blankenstein AH, Stalman WA. Impact of physical symptoms on perceived health in the community. *J Psychosom Res*. 2008;64(3):265–274.
27. Wittchen HU, Jacobi F. Size and burden of mental disorders in Europe: A critical review and appraisal of 27 studies. *Eur Neuropsychopharmacol*. 2005;15(4):357–376.
28. Sipila K, Veijola J, Jokelainen J, et al. Association between symptoms of temporomandibular disorders and depression: An epidemiological study of the Northern Finland 1966 birth cohort. *Cranio*. 2001;19(3):183–187.
29. Vimpari SS, Knuuttila ML, Sakki TK, Kivela SL. Depressive symptoms associated with symptoms of the temporomandibular joint pain and dysfunction syndrome. *Psychosom Med*. 1995;57(5):439–444.
30. Heim C, Newport DJ, Mletzko T, Miller AH, Nemeroff CB. The link between childhood trauma and depression: Insights from HPA axis studies in humans. *Psychoneuroendocrinology*. 2008;33(6):693–710.
31. Sherman JJ, Turk DC. Nonpharmacologic approaches to the management of myofascial temporomandibular disorders. *Curr Pain Headache Rep*. 2001;5(5):421–431.

12

Recognizing the Psychiatric Burden of Anxiety and Depression in Children With Headache, Chest Pain, and Abdominal Pain

SUSAN T. TRAN, ANA B. GOYA ARCE,
AND ANJANA JAGPAL ■

Pain is a common problem among children and adolescents,[1] frequently associated with substantial functional disability.[2,3] Pediatric chronic pain is best viewed through a biopsychosocial model in which biological, psychological, and sociocultural factors interact and influence one's experience of chronic pain.[4,5] Youths with chronic pain often have difficulty attending school,[6] participating in social and physical activities, and getting sufficient sleep[7] and have problems with emotional functioning[2,3] and peer relationships.[8] These difficulties are compounded when chronic pain coexists with depression[9–11] and anxiety.[12–15] In children and adolescents, developmental stage plays an important role, and family members may aid in reporting symptoms and in treatment.[16,17] Thus, pediatric chronic pain should be considered in terms of developmental and biopsychosocial factors within the family and broader environment.[18]

Depression is strongly related to functional disability, well-being,[9,11] and school-related impairments[19] in youths with chronic pain. Even mild depressive symptoms predict persistence of pain and functional disability 1 year later in youths with pain.[10] Comorbid anxiety is also related to difficulty in functioning across domains. Higher anxiety is related to lower quality of life in general[14] and with school impairments in youths with chronic pain.[12] Anxiety moderates the relationship between social, physical, and school functioning and pain. Pain typically predicts functioning; however, when anxiety is high, functioning is impaired regardless of pain intensity.[13,20] Developmentally, anxiety and fear of pain play a more significant role in the daily functioning and avoidance of activities in adolescents with chronic pain compared with younger children, perhaps owing to more complex cognitive abilities and more varied roles and responsibilities.[14,21] The comorbidity of these conditions warrants attention from researchers and clinicians alike.

COMORBIDITY OF ANXIETY AND DEPRESSION WITH CHRONIC PAIN

Anxiety and depression commonly co-occur with chronic pain. Data across studies indicate that children experiencing chronic pain are more likely to endorse higher levels of psychiatric symptoms than their healthy peers,[22] and adolescents with anxiety and depressive symptoms have higher rates of comorbid widespread pain compared with youths without anxiety or depression.[23] In the primary care setting, approximately two-thirds of children reporting recurrent nonspecific aches and pains also endorse symptoms of anxiety and depression.[24] Of children presenting to pain clinics with unexplained chronic pain, 40 to 53% meet criteria for one or more psychiatric disorder, with as many as 21 to 29% experiencing clinically significant psychiatric symptoms that impair the child in more than one area of life.[25]

Given the data suggesting high comorbidity between pain, anxiety, and depression, it has been proposed that these conditions share underlying etiologies.[26,27] Common genetic factors[28] and biological processes may predispose individuals to the development of pain, depression, and anxiety disorders. Individuals with any one of these conditions demonstrate higher sensitivity to stress and dysfunction of the stress response system, which manifests both physiologically (i.e., increased anticipation and activation of the stress response with minor stressors) and psychologically (i.e., maladaptive cognitions and problem-solving patterns).[26,29] The hypothalamic-pituitary-adrenal (HPA) axis, which regulates the stress response, may be chronically activated in youths with depression and pain, ultimately maintaining symptoms over time.[29,30] Given that medication management may successfully aid in reducing both pain and depressive symptoms,[31,32] shared neurobiological mechanisms have been examined. Dysregulation of serotonin and norepinephrine has been implicated in anxiety, depression, and pain processing.[29] Thus, anxiety, depression, and somatic symptoms may all be symptoms of one underlying internalizing disorder rather than three distinct disorders.[28]

Furthermore, there is a dynamic bidirectional relationship between pain, depression, and anxiety. Symptoms fluctuate over time, and changes in psychological symptoms may correspond to changes in pain over time.[27] When anxiety or depression and chronic pain coexist, they increase the negative effects of one another. For example, pain and fear of pain may increase stress and worrying, and the resulting muscle tension associated with stress may increase pain.[33,34] This downward cycle also has implications for functioning. Fear of pain and pain's negative consequences, such as discomfort and disability, lead to avoidance of activities that may flare pain, resulting in deconditioning and loss of reinforcing activities, thus resulting in higher pain sensitivity, pain, depression, and disability.[21] Although not exhaustive of pain types amongst the pediatric population, abdominal pain, chest pain, and headaches are common sources of pain among youths.

Abdominal Pain Comorbidity

Youths with recurrent abdominal pain have some of the highest rates of reported comorbid psychiatric disorders, ranging from 67 to 85%. The majority of children with abdominal pain meet criteria for at least one anxiety disorder (60–79%), and about 40% meet criteria for depression.[35,36] Another study found slightly lower prevalence rates in youths with functional abdominal pain, with 9% meeting criteria for generalized anxiety disorder, 11% for obsessive-compulsive disorder, 24% for separation anxiety disorder, and 16% for major depressive disorder.[37] Overall, children with abdominal pain are more likely to report internalizing emotional symptoms than their healthy counterparts.[38,39] Anxiety disorders are a heterogeneous group of disorders with distinct symptom profiles, including generalized anxiety disorder, panic disorder, and specific phobias. Some research suggests that there is a particular relationship between pediatric abdominal pain and the physical symptoms of anxiety, such as those characteristic of panic disorder (e.g., increased heart rate, sweating).[20,40]

Gastrointestinal (GI) disorders resulting in abdominal pain are influenced by the brain–gut axis. This bidirectional communication through the autonomic nervous system between the brain and the GI system influences functioning in the GI tract such that emotional and psychological functioning may affect physiological processes.[41] In particular, chronic elevations in the body's stress response, through anxiety or depression, may result in prolonged activation of the autonomic nervous system, disrupting GI functioning and resulting in visceral hypersensitivity to benign processes.[29,41] Given the bidirectionality of these pathways, anxiety and depression may worsen with increased pain, and may also flare pain symptoms. Over time, this cycle may produce chronically heightened pain sensitivity.[29,41]

Chest Pain Comorbidity

Understanding the relation and comorbidity between noncardiac chest pain (NCCP) and psychiatric concerns is particularly difficult. Of pediatric patients seen for chest pain, it is estimated that 2.2 to 20% have a "psychiatric" origin for pain, such as a stressful event.[42,43] NCCP may also arise from organic causes, such as musculoskeletal, hematological, or gastrointestinal problems; as a result, there is much variation regarding chest pain nomenclature across disciplines.[44] For the purpose of this chapter, NCCP will be defined as pain or discomfort in the chest with an underlying cause other than angina. Overall, patients presenting with NCCP endorsed higher symptoms of anxiety than patients with benign heart murmurs and healthy controls.[45] In a study investigating 100 consecutive referrals to a pediatric cardiology department for chest pain, 92% of the causes were idiopathic.[46] Of those evaluated for psychiatric symptoms, 74% endorsed significant symptoms, most often anxiety, conversion disorder, and depression.[46] In another study, 16 out of 17 patients referred to a pediatric cardiology practice for NCPP received a *Diagnostic and Statistical Manual of Mental Disorders* (DSM) psychiatric diagnosis. Of those diagnosed with a psychiatric disorder, 56% met criteria for an anxiety disorder, 60% of whom had a current diagnosis of panic disorder.[45] NCCP may also be influenced by the brain–gut axis, particularly for cases in which NCCP is related to esophageal-related disorders (e.g., gastroesophageal reflux disease).[29] Just as with abdominal pain, emotional and psychological factors, such as anxiety and depression, may influence autonomic nervous system functioning and pain processing for youths with NCCP.

Headache Comorbidity

Children with headaches and migraines endorse higher levels of family problems, somatic concerns, anxiety, and depressive symptoms than their headache-free counterparts.[47–49] Some studies equate the rates and profiles of psychiatric comorbidity in children with headache with those found in children with abdominal pain,[39,50] while other studies estimate that 29.6% of youths with chronic daily headache have a current comorbid psychiatric diagnosis, and 34.9% have a lifetime comorbidity.[51] Some literature suggests that individuals with migraine are at increased higher risk for affective disorders, anxiety,[49] and oppositional defiant disorders[51]; while other evidence suggests that individuals experiencing chronic daily headaches are at higher risk for anxiety, affective disorders, and substance abuse disorders than those experiencing migraines.[49,52] Evidence from longitudinal studies suggests that anxiety may predispose one to headaches, and that headaches may cause stress and anxiety, resulting in a bidirectional relationship between anxiety and headaches.[27,53] Finally, children who experience comorbid anxiety and depression with headaches utilize the health care system frequently and incur significantly greater direct medical costs compared with their healthy peers.[54]

SCREENING CONSIDERATIONS

Because of the high comorbidity of psychiatric disorders, particularly anxiety and depression, in youths with chronic pain, it is important to capture these patients early in an effort to prevent further impairment. Implementing brief screening protocols for depression and anxiety in primary care, pain, and specialty clinics (e.g., gastroenterology) may aid in identifying children with depression and anxiety.[55-57] Many different measures of child anxiety exist and have been used in pediatric chronic pain samples (e.g., the Revised Children's Manifest Anxiety Scale). However, the Screen for Child Anxiety and Related Emotional Disorders (SCARED) is one of the only anxiety measures that has been validated for use in pediatric chronic pain populations.[14,58] The SCARED, a brief measure commonly used in both medical and psychiatric settings, is normed in many languages for youths ages 8 to 18 years[55,58,59] and predicts poor functioning in pediatric chronic pain.[14] Items on anxiety screeners should be carefully considered given that many screeners include items that represent overlapping symptoms of both anxiety and pain conditions (i.e., "I get headaches when I am at school"). These items reflect the presence of pain symptoms; thus, their presence on anxiety screeners may artificially inflate anxiety scores.[14,58]

Regarding depression, Logan and colleagues examined the appropriateness of the widely used, well-validated Children's Depression Inventory (CDI) for use in youths with chronic pain. In a multisite study of 1043 youths, the CDI was validated as a tool for assessing mood in pediatric chronic pain. Similar to anxiety screening, some items regularly used for assessing depression should be interpreted with caution because of their occurrence in both pain and depression. Among youths with chronic pain, symptoms common in chronic pain—sleep difficulties, fatigue, and somatic concerns—are the most commonly endorsed symptoms on depression screeners.[56] Thus, in pediatric chronic pain samples, these items may not indicate depression or anhedonia to the same extent that they would in a non–chronic pain sample.

Because of different clinics utilizing a myriad of assessment tools, efforts have been made to implement standardized tools. The Patient-Reported Outcomes Measurement Information System (PROMIS) project is an initiative to gather patient-reported outcomes associated with chronic diseases. The primary goal of PROMIS is to provide the clinical research community with the same set of measures to be employed across health disciplines.[60] Specifically within the pediatric pain community, the Collaborative Health Outcomes Information Registry (CHOIR) was created to establish consistent screening measures (patient and caregiver reports) for pediatric pain patients to facilitate collaboration across research clinics.[61]

During assessment, youths and their parents are often asked to complete measures of the child's symptoms and functioning. Obtaining parents' perspectives on their child's health and functioning is important and can provide insight that a child may not have; however, obtaining parent-proxy reports of children's symptoms of anxiety and depression in addition to the child's self-report may not necessarily improve detection of psychiatric symptoms. Studies have found that parents tend to underreport symptoms of anxiety and depression compared with their children's reports. Parents may be unaware of their child's psychological distress, or families may underreport symptoms of anxiety and depression to minimize the presence of psychological factors in order to highlight the "realness" of their pain.[20,40]

MULTIDIMENSIONAL TREATMENT OF COMORBID PAIN AND ANXIETY/DEPRESSION

Psychopharmacological Therapy

Given the shared neurobiology between anxiety, depression, and pain, specifically regarding serotonin and noradrenaline,[31,32] pharmacological therapies are one treatment option for comorbid pediatric pain and anxiety/depression. Pharmacological treatments for functional abdominal pain in children include antispasmodics, antireflux agents, antihistaminic agents, laxatives, and antidepressants.[62] Selective serotonin reuptake inhibitors and tricyclic antidepressants, such as amitriptyline, have both been used to treat functional abdominal pain in children. Tricyclic antidepressants are believed to work by inducing pain tolerance through peripheral or central antinociceptive properties and anticholinergic effects.[63] Children given amitriptyline report overall improvements in quality of life but do not report changes in pain.[64] Meta-analyses of pharmacological treatments for pediatric functional abdominal pain reveal a lack of adequately powered, placebo-controlled trials; thus, caution should be taken when prescribing medications in this population.[62,65]

Pharmacological treatment of pediatric migraines and chronic headaches have faced similar challenges—findings from the adult literature are often extrapolated to children without properly powered placebo-controlled trials.[66] Two main groups of medications have been used to treat migraines or chronic headache in children: abortive, or rescue, medications and prophylactics, or preventative, medications.[67] Abortive medications, typically anti-inflammatories, are used after the pain has started, and their goal is to provide pain relief. Maintenance or prophylactic therapies for migraine have been recommended in children who have more than one headache per week in order to help reduce the overall frequency of headaches.[67] The most commonly prescribed maintenance medications for migraine include the anticonvulsants valproate, topiramate, and gabapentin; the antidepressant amitriptyline; and beta blockers such as propranolol.[67] A recent multicenter study, the Childhood and Adolescent Migraine Prevention (CHAMP) trial, tested the effects that topiramate, amitriptyline, and a placebo had on pediatric migraine.[68] This trial found that neither amitriptyline nor topiramate was more effective in reducing migraine frequency than the placebo. In addition, patients who received the prophylactic medications had higher rates of adverse events (including altered mood, suicide attempt, and syncope).[68] Because of concerns about the effects of psychopharmacological interventions with youths and the effectiveness of psychological therapies (see following section), it is frequently recommended that youths prescribed these medications also engage in cognitive behavioral therapy (CBT) to obtain optimal benefits.[69] In a study examining the use of amitriptyline and CBT versus amitriptyline plus headache education, results showed that CBT in combination with amitriptyline resulted in greater reductions in days with headache and migraine-related disability than the other group.[69] Integrating pharmacological and psychological therapies seems to supersede outcomes for medication alone[69] and for medication combined with education about migraines.[70,71]

Cognitive Behavioral Therapy

Psychological therapies, particularly pain-focused CBT, are effective for treating chronic pain in children and adolescents.[72] CBT is a group of treatments based on the interrelationships between thoughts, feelings, and behaviors. Specific interventions may target a number of different conditions, including anxiety, depression, and pain. The effectiveness of an intervention may depend on choosing an appropriate target of treatment and focusing on teaching relevant skills and coping strategies. Pain-focused CBT typically involves psychoeducation about the gate-control theory of pain, parent guidelines for helping manage children's pain, relaxation training (e.g., diaphragmatic breathing), behavioral management strategies (i.e., reinforcing functioning), challenging maladaptive thoughts about pain and functioning, and fostering problem-solving.[16,73] The average length of most treatment protocols is between 6 and 8 weeks.[72] In a review of psychological therapies for chronic pain in children and adolescents, including a considerable number of intervention trials for abdominal pain and headache, pain-focused psychological therapies (primarily CBT) were effective in reducing pain and pain-related disability; there were mixed results for anxiety outcomes, and pain-focused CBT was not effective in reducing depression in youths.[72]

Although there are many overlapping features between CBT for pain and CBT for anxiety and depression (e.g., behavioral relaxation strategies, challenging maladaptive thinking patterns, exposure procedures, and building problem-solving skills),[74–78] CBT designed to treat *only* pain, depression, or anxiety has limited effectiveness for youths with comorbid pain and psychiatric conditions.[72,79,80] It may be prudent to utilize a tailored behavioral intervention for those with comorbid anxiety or depression. Thus, there are several recent efforts to offer intervention modalities targeting pain *with* comorbid anxiety or depression. Given the considerable overlap between components of CBT for chronic pain, depression, and anxiety, there is promise for a well-designed, integrated intervention.[26] Transdiagnostic interventions have been developed to target this "internalizing cluster" of comorbid depression, anxiety, and pain and the theorized underlying causes such as biological sensitivity to stress, maladaptive thoughts and behaviors, and emotion regulation difficulties.[26,81] Brief "toolbox" behavioral intervention approaches have been proposed to target underlying stress reactivity and maladaptive thoughts and behaviors. To specifically address comorbid pain and anxiety, interventions emphasize relaxation techniques, exposure to and coping with stress and pain to reduce avoidance behaviors, and problem-solving and self-management techniques to prevent relapse.[26] Another approach is rooted in the perspective that comorbid pain problems and anxiety or depression stem from underlying emotion regulation difficulties.[81] This intervention includes identifying and modifying maladaptive emotional responses to pain, anxiety, depression, anger, and so forth across contexts and situations. Treatment focuses on education regarding the awareness of emotions and pain, flexible thinking strategies, and modifying maladaptive behavioral responses.[81] Both approaches have demonstrated feasible and preliminary results through case study reports[26,81]; further investigation and replication would benefit the field.

A novel intervention approach integrating the behavioral skills taught in CBT for pain, depression, and anxiety is the Treatment for Anxiety and Physical Symptoms Program (TAPS). TAPS combines pain-focused CBT and an adapted version of a commonly used anxiety protocol, the Coping Cat, to treat children with anxiety and unexplained somatic complaints, primarily pain. The program emphasizes the relationships between physical and anxiety symptoms, instruction on relaxation techniques to reduce anxiety and physical discomfort, and expansion of cognitive restructuring and exposure techniques to target thoughts and behaviors related to pain.[57] A preliminary trial of the TAPS program included seven youths (ages 8–15 years) with comorbid abdominal pain and anxiety disorders (most had more than one anxiety diagnosis). Results showed all participants were classified as treatment responders, with reductions in diagnosis severity, anxiety, and pain. Despite encouraging results, a small sample and lack of control group and follow-up limit the conclusions about effectiveness.[82]

Related Therapies

Other psychological therapies have offered promising results in treating pain and comorbid anxiety/depression; however, these have typically been evaluated in smaller studies. Biofeedback is an increasingly common modality to teach relaxation skills and demonstrate to patients the relationship between their physical and mental functioning. Youths are particularly savvy using technology and often benefit from "seeing" how practicing relaxation skills influences physiological changes with the help of biofeedback technology. In a small retrospective study of children and adolescents who were referred for biofeedback to treat migraines, chronic headache, and chronic abdominal pain (5–7 sessions), patients reported significant decreases in pain, depression, physical symptoms of anxiety (e.g., restlessness, somatic symptoms), and social anxiety after treatment. Patients with severe symptoms of depression and anxiety in particular seemed to benefit from biofeedback intervention.[83]

Acceptance and commitment therapy (ACT) is another therapeutic approach that can be adapted to treat chronic pain, depression, and anxiety. The focus of ACT is on acceptance of the presence of symptoms (pain, depression, anxiety), setting goals, and improving functioning while coping with symptoms.[84,85] Even brief interventions may offer therapeutic effects. A 1-day ACT Training and Migraine Education workshop was conducted for individuals with migraine and depression. The intervention was associated with improvements in depression, overall functioning, and pain-related disability at 3-month follow-up compared with a waitlist control.[86] Research of ACT-based programs to treat pediatric pain and comorbid depression and anxiety is scarcer; however, there is preliminary evidence that acceptance-based programming may be beneficial. Treatment outcomes of a 3-week intensive outpatient interdisciplinary pain program, including physical therapy, occupational therapy, recreational therapy, and group-based therapy focusing on functioning despite symptoms (consistent with ACT theory), demonstrated that increased acceptance of pain predicted decreases in depressive symptoms and functional disability.[87]

CONCLUSION

Youths with comorbid chronic pain and anxiety/depression are at increased risk for severe symptoms and negative consequences such as difficulties with physical and academic activities and social and emotional functioning. Because pain is a biopsychosocial phenomenon, a variety of contributing factors need to be addressed in assessment and treatment of pain, and a multidisciplinary team approach is best. Early identification and treatment of anxiety and depression in youths with chronic pain are imperative. It would be wise to implement brief screening protocols for anxiety and depression in routine clinical practice, especially when patients are reporting unremitting pain. Clinics that frequently service children with pain complaints such as gastroenterology, neurology, and pain clinics would especially benefit from these protocols. Combined treatment approaches, using appropriate psychopharmacological and targeted CBT interventions, may provide optimal relief from symptoms and facilitate return to premorbid functioning. While research has established the efficacy of CBT for pediatric chronic pain, further studies on tailored psychological therapies for youths with chronic pain and comorbid anxiety/depression are likely to better inform our evaluation of these transdiagnostic interventions—in particular, their effectiveness in producing lasting improvement for youths with chronic pain and comorbid psychiatric burden.[72]

REFERENCES

1. King S, Chambers CT, Huguet A, et al. The epidemiology of chronic pain in children and adolescents revisited: A systematic review. *Pain*. 2011;152(12):2729–2738.
2. Palermo TM. Impact of recurrent and chronic pain on child and family daily functioning: A critical review of the literature. *J Dev Behav Pediatr*. 2000;21(1):58–69.

3. Roth-Isigkeit A, Thyen U, Stoven H, Schwarzenberger J, Schmucker P. Pain among children and adolescents: Restrictions in daily living and triggering factors. *Pediatrics*. 2005;115(2):e152–e162.
4. Flor H, Hermann C. Biopsychosocial models of pain. *Prog Pain Res Manage*. 2004;27:47–78.
5. Gatchel RJ, Peng YB, Peters ML, Fuchs PN, Turk DC. The biopsychosocial approach to chronic pain: Scientific advances and future directions. *Psychol Bull*. 2007;133(4):581.
6. Logan DE, Simons LE, Carpino EA. Too sick for school? Parent influences on school functioning among children with chronic pain. *Pain*. 2012;153(2):437–443.
7. Long AC, Krishnamurthy V, Palermo TM. Sleep disturbances in school-age children with chronic pain. *J Pediatr Psychol*. 2008;33(3):258–268.
8. Forgeron PA, King S, Stinson JN, McGrath PJ, MacDonald AJ, Chambers CT. Social functioning and peer relationships in children and adolescents with chronic pain: A systematic review. *Pain Res Manage*. 2010;15(1):27–41.
9. Kashikar-Zuck S, Goldschneider KR, Powers SW, Vaught MH, Hershey AD. Depression and functional disability in chronic pediatric pain. *Clin J Pain*. 2001;17(4):341–349.
10. Palermo TM, Hoff A, Schluchter M, Drotar D, Zebracki K. Depressive symptoms predict persistence of pain and disability in children with disease-related pain. *J Pain*. 2005;6(3):S1.
11. Tarakci E, Yeldan I, Mutlu EK, Baydogan SN, Kasapcopur O. The relationship between physical activity level, anxiety, depression, and functional ability in children and adolescents with juvenile idiopathic arthritis. *Clin Rheumatol*. 2011;30(11):1415–1420.
12. Anderson Khan K, Tran ST, Jastrowski Mano KE, Simpson PM, Cao Y, Hainsworth KR. Predicting multiple facets of school functioning in pediatric chronic pain: Examining the direct impact of anxiety. *Clin J Pain*. 2015;31(10):867–875.
13. Cohen LL, Vowles KE, Eccleston C. The impact of adolescent chronic pain on functioning: Disentangling the complex role of anxiety. *J Pain*. 2010;11(11):1039–1046.
14. Tran ST, Jastrowski Mano KE, Hainsworth KR, et al. Distinct influences of anxiety and pain catastrophizing on functional outcomes in children and adolescents With chronic pain. *J Pediatr Psychol*. 2015;40(8):744–755.
15. Wendland M, Jackson Y, Stokes LD. Functional disability in paediatric patients with recurrent abdominal pain. *Child*. 2010;36(4):516–523.
16. Kashikar-Zuck S. Treatment of children with unexplained chronic pain. *Lancet*. 2006;367(9508):380–382.
17. Palermo TM, Holley AL. The importance of the family environment in pediatric chronic pain. *JAMA Pediatr*. 2013;167(1):93–94.
18. Palermo TM, Valrie CR, Karlson CW. Family and parent influences on pediatric chronic pain: A developmental perspective. *Am Psychol*. 2014;69(2):142.
19. Logan DE, Simons LE, Kaczynski KJ. School functioning in adolescents with chronic pain: The role of depressive symptoms in school impairment. *J Pediatr Psychol*. 2009;34(8):882–892.
20. Simons LE, Sieberg CB, Claar RL. Anxiety and functional disability in a large sample of children and adolescents with chronic pain. *Pain Res Manage*. 2012;17(2):93–97.

21. Simons LE, Kaczynski KJ. The Fear Avoidance Model of chronic pain: Examination for pediatric application. *J Pain.* 2012;13(9):827–835.
22. Pinquart M, Shen Y. Depressive symptoms in children and adolescents with chronic physical illness: An updated meta-analysis. *J Pediatr Psychol.* 2011;36(4):375–384.
23. Hoftun GB, Romundstad PR, Rygg M. Factors associated with adolescent chronic non-specific pain, chronic multisite pain, and chronic pain with high disability: The Young–HUNT Study 2008. *J Pain.* 2012;13(9):874–883.
24. Campo JV, Comer DM, Jansen-McWilliams L, Gardner W, Kelleher KJ. Recurrent pain, emotional distress, and health service use in childhood. *J Pediatr.* 2002;141(1):76–83.
25. Knook LM, Konijnenberg AY, van der Hoeven J, et al. Psychiatric disorders in children and adolescents presenting with unexplained chronic pain: What is the prevalence and clinical relevancy? *Eur Child Adolesc Psychiatry.* 2011;20(1):39–48.
26. Weersing VR, Rozenman MS, Maher-Bridge M, Campo JV. Anxiety, depression, and somatic distress: Developing a transdiagnostic internalizing toolbox for pediatric practice. *Cogn Behav Pract.* 2012;19(1):68–82.
27. Ligthart L, Gerrits MM, Boomsma DI, Penninx BW. Anxiety and depression are associated with migraine and pain in general: An investigation of the interrelationships. *J Pain.* 2013;14(4):363–370.
28. Ask H, Waaktaar T, Seglem KB, Torgersen S. Common etiological sources of anxiety, depression, and somatic complaints in adolescents: A multiple rater twin study. *J Abnorm Child Psychol.* 2016;44(1):101–114.
29. Mayer EA, Tillisch K. The brain-gut axis in abdominal pain syndromes. *Annu Rev Med.* 2011;62:381–396.
30. Vinall J, Pavlova M, Asmundson GJ, Rasic N, Noel M. Mental health comorbidities in pediatric chronic pain: A narrative review of epidemiology, models, neurobiological mechanisms and treatment. *Children.* 2016;3(4):40.
31. Bair MJ, Robinson RL, Katon W, Kroenke K. Depression and pain comorbidity: A literature review. *Arch Intern Med.* 2003;163(20):2433–2445.
32. Robinson MJ, Edwards SE, Iyengar S, Bymaster F, Clark M, Katon W. Depression and pain. *Front Biosci.* 2009;14(1):5031–5051.
33. Beesdo K, Hoyer J, Jacobi F, Low NC, Hofler M, Wittchen HU. Association between generalized anxiety levels and pain in a community sample: Evidence for diagnostic specificity. *J Anxiety Disord.* 2009;23(5):684–693.
34. Radat F, Mekies C, Geraud G, et al. Anxiety, stress and coping behaviours in primary care migraine patients: Results of the SMILE study. *Cephalalgia.* 2008;28(11):1115–1125.
35. Campo JV, Bridge J, Ehmann M, et al. Recurrent abdominal pain, anxiety, and depression in primary care. *Pediatrics.* 2004;113(4):817–824.
36. Dufton LM, Dunn MJ, Compas BE. Anxiety and somatic complaints in children with recurrent abdominal pain and anxiety disorders. *J Pediatr Psychol.* 2009;34(2):176–186.
37. Ghanizadeh A, Moaiedy F, Imanieh MH, et al. Psychiatric disorders and family functioning in children and adolescents with functional abdominal pain syndrome. *J Gastroenterol Hepatol.* 2008;23(7 part 1):1132–1136.

38. Garber J, Zeman J, Walker LS. Recurrent abdominal pain in children: Psychiatric diagnoses and parental psychopathology. *J Am Acad Child Adolesc Psychiatry.* 1990;29(4):648–656.

39. Galli F, D'Antuono G, Tarantino S, et al. Headache and recurrent abdominal pain: A controlled study by the means of the Child Behaviour Checklist (CBCL). *Cephalalgia.* 2007;27(3):211–219.

40. Tran ST, Jastrowski Mano KE, Anderson Khan K, Davies W, Hainsworth KR. Patterns of anxiety symptoms in pediatric chronic pain as reported by youth, mothers, and fathers. *Clin Pract Pediatr Psychol.* 2016;4(1):51.

41. Reed-Knight B, Maddux MH, Deacy AD, Lamparyk K, Stone AL, Mackner L. Brain-gut interactions and maintenance factors in pediatric gastroenterological disorders: Recommendations for clinical care. *Clin Pract Pediatr Psychol.* 2017;5(1):93–105.

42. Cava JR, Sayger PL. Chest pain in children and adolescents. *Pediatr Clin North Am.* 2004;51(6):1553–1568.

43. Eslick GD. Epidemiology and risk factors of pediatric chest pain: A systematic review. *Pediatr Clin North Am.* 2010;57(6):1211–1219.

44. McDonnell CJ, White KS, Grady RM. Noncardiac chest pain in children and adolescents: A biopsychosocial conceptualization. *Child Psychiatry Hum Dev.* 2012;43(1):1–26.

45. Lipsitz JD, Masia-Warner C, Apfel H, et al. Anxiety and depressive symptoms and anxiety sensitivity in youngsters with noncardiac chest pain and benign heart murmurs. *J Pediatr Psychol.* 2004;29(8):607–612.

46. Tunaoglu F, Olguntürk R, Akcabay S, Oguz D, Gücüyener K, Demirsoy S. Chest pain in children referred to a cardiology clinic. *Pediatr Cardiol.* 1995;16(2):69–72.

47. Anttila P, Sourander A, Metsähonkala L, Aromaa M, Helenius H, Sillanpää M. Psychiatric symptoms in children with primary headache. *J Am Acad Child Adolesc Psychiatry.* 2004;43(4):412–419.

48. Andrasik F, Kabela E, Quinn S, Attanasio V, Blanchard EB, Rosenblum EL. Psychological functioning of children who have recurrent migraine. *Pain.* 1988;34(1):43–52.

49. Antonaci F, Nappi G, Galli F, Manzoni GC, Calabresi P, Costa A. Migraine and psychiatric comorbidity: A review of clinical findings. *J Headache Pain.* 2011;12(2):115–125.

50. Liakopoulou-Kairis M, Alifieraki T, Protagora D, et al. Recurrent abdominal pain and headache. *Eur Child Adolesc Psychiatry.* 2002;11(3):115–122.

51. Pakalnis A, Gibson J, Colvin A. Comorbidity of psychiatric and behavioral disorders in pediatric migraine. *Headache.* 2005;45(5):590–596.

52. Mazzone L, Vitiello B, Incorpora G, Mazzone D. Behavioural and temperamental characteristics of children and adolescents suffering from primary headache. *Cephalalgia.* 2006;26(2):194–201.

53. Powers SW, Gilman DK, Hershey AD. Headache and psychological functioning in children and adolescents. *Headache.* 2006;46(9):1404–1415.

54. Pesa J, Lage MJ. The medical costs of migraine and comorbid anxiety and depression. *Headache.* 2004;44(6):562–570.

55. Cunningham NR, Lynch-Jordan A, Mezoff AG, Farrell MK, Cohen MB, Kashikar-Zuck S. Importance of addressing anxiety in youth with functional abdominal pain: Suggested guidelines for physicians. *J Pediatr Gastroenterol Nutr.* 2013;56(5):469–474.

56. Logan DE, Claar RL, Guite JW, et al. Factor structure of the children's depression inventory in a multisite sample of children and adolescents with chronic pain. *J Pain.* 2013;14(7):689–698.

57. Reigada LC, Fisher PH, Cutler C, Warner CM. An innovative treatment approach for children with anxiety disorders and medically unexplained somatic complaints. *Cogn Behav Pract.* 2008;15(2):140–147.

58. Jastrowski Mano KE, Evans JR, Tran ST, Anderson Khan K, Weisman SJ, Hainsworth KR. The psychometric properties of the screen for child anxiety related emotional disorders in pediatric chronic pain. *J Pediatr Psychol.* 2012;37(9):999–1011.

59. Birmaher B, Khetarpal S, Brent D, et al. The screen for child anxiety related emotional disorders (SCARED): Scale construction and psychometric characteristics. *J Am Acad Child Adolesc Psychiatry.* 1997;36(4):545–553.

60. Irwin DE, Stucky B, Langer MM, et al. An item response analysis of the pediatric PROMIS anxiety and depressive symptoms scales. *Quality of Life Research.* 2010;19(4):595–607.

61. Bhandari RP, Feinstein AB, Huestis SE, et al. Pediatric-Collaborative Health Outcomes Information Registry (Peds-CHOIR): A learning health system to guide pediatric pain research and treatment. *Pain.* 2016;157(9):2033–2044.

62. Korterink JJ, Rutten JMTM, Venmans L, Benninga MA, Tabbers MM. Pharmacologic treatment in pediatric functional abdominal pain disorders: A systematic review. *J Pediatr.* 2015;166(2):424–431, e426.

63. Rajagopalan M, Kurian G, John J. Symptom relief with amitriptyline in the irritable bowel syndrome. *J Gastroenterol Hepatol.* 1998;13(7):738–741.

64. Bahar RJ, Collins BS, Steinmetz B, Ament ME. Double-blind placebo-controlled trial of amitriptyline for the treatment of irritable bowel syndrome in adolescents. *J Pediatr.* 2008;152(5):685–689.

65. Huertas-Ceballos A, Logan S, Bennett C, Macarthur C. Pharmacological interventions for recurrent abdominal pain (RAP) and irritable bowel syndrome (IBS) in childhood. *Cochrane Database Syst Rev.* 2008;(1):CD003071.

66. Lewis D, Ashwal S, Hershey A, Hirtz D, Yonker M, Silberstein S. Practice parameter: Pharmacological treatment of migraine headache in children and adolescents. Report of the American Academy of Neurology Quality Standards Subcommittee and the Practice Committee of the Child Neurology Society. *Neurology.* 2004;63(12):2215–2224.

67. Merison K, Jacobs H. Diagnosis and treatment of childhood migraine. *Curr Treat Options Neurol.* 2016;18(11):48.

68. Powers SW, Coffey CS, Chamberlin LA, et al. Trial of amitriptyline, topiramate, and placebo for pediatric migraine. *N Engl J Med.* 2017;376(2):115–124.

69. Powers SW, Kashikar-Zuck SM, Allen JR, et al. Cognitive behavioral therapy plus amitriptyline for chronic migraine in children and adolescents: A randomized clinical trial. *JAMA.* 2013;310(24):2622–2630.

70. Kroner JW, Hershey AD, Kashikar-Zuck SM, et al. Cognitive behavioral therapy plus amitriptyline for children and adolescents with chronic migraine reduces headache days to ≤4 per month. *Headache.* 2016;56(4):711–716.

71. Kroner JW, Peugh J, Kashikar-Zuck SM, et al. Trajectory of improvement in children and adolescents with chronic migraine: Results from the Cognitive-Behavioral Therapy and Amitriptyline Trial. *J Pain.* 2017;18(6):637–644.

72. Eccleston C, Palermo TM, Williams AC, et al. Psychological therapies for the management of chronic and recurrent pain in children and adolescents. *Cochrane Database Syst Rev.* 2014;2014(5).

73. Palermo TM. *Cognitive-behavioral therapy for chronic pain in children and adolescents.* New York, NY: Oxford University Press; 2012.

74. Klein JB, Jacobs RH, Reinecke MA. Cognitive-behavioral therapy for adolescent depression: A meta-analytic investigation of changes in effect-size estimates. *J Am Acad Child Adolesc Psychiatry.* 2007;46(11):1403–1413.

75. Curry JF, Reinecke MA. Modular therapy for adolescents with major depression. *Cogn Ther Child Adolesc.* 2003:95–128.

76. In-Albon T, Schneider S. Psychotherapy of childhood anxiety disorders: A meta-analysis. *Psychother Psychosom.* 2006;76(1):15–24.

77. Borkovec TD, Roemer L. Generalized anxiety disorder. In: Ammerman RT, Hersen M, eds. *Handbook of Prescriptive Treatments for Adults.* New York, NY: Springer; 1994:261–281.

78. Walker LS, Beck J, Anderson J. Functional abdominal pain and separation anxiety: Helping the child return to school. *Pediatr Ann.* 2009;38(5).

79. van der Veek SM, Derkx BH, Benninga MA, Boer F, de Haan E. Cognitive behavior therapy for pediatric functional abdominal pain: A randomized controlled trial. *Pediatrics.* 2013;(peds):2013–0242.

80. Cunningham NR, Jagpal A, Tran ST, et al. Anxiety adversely impacts response to cognitive behavioral therapy in children with chronic pain. *J Pediatr.* 2016;171:227–233.

81. Allen LB, Tsao JC, Seidman LC, Ehrenreich-May J, Zeltzer LK. A unified, transdiagnostic treatment for adolescents with chronic pain and comorbid anxiety and depression. *Cogn Behav Pract.* 2012;19(1):56–67.

82. Warner CM, Reigada LC, Fisher PH, Saborsky AL, Benkov KJ. CBT for anxiety and associated somatic complaints in pediatric medical settings: An open pilot study. *J Clin Psychol Medical Settings.* 2009;16(2):169–177.

83. Rotkis LN, Abelon R, Breuner CC. The effect of biofeedback therapy on depression and anxiety in the pediatric and adolescent when used to treat migraines, chronic headaches and chronic abdominal pain. *J Adolesc Health.* 2014;54(2):S42.

84. Dahl J, Wilson KG, Nilsson A. Acceptance and commitment therapy and the treatment of persons at risk for long-term disability resulting from stress and pain symptoms: A preliminary randomized trial. *Behav Ther.* 2004;35(4):785–801.

85. Hayes SC, Strosahl KD, Wilson KG. *Acceptance and Commitment Therapy: An Experiential Approach to Behavior Change.* New York, NY: Guilford Press; 1999.

86. Dindo L, Recober A, Marchman JN, Turvey C, O'Hara MW. One-day behavioral treatment for patients with comorbid depression and migraine: A pilot study. *Behav Res Ther*. 2012;50(9):537–543.
87. Weiss KE, Hahn A, Wallace DP, Biggs B, Bruce BK, Harrison TE. Acceptance of pain: Associations with depression, catastrophizing, and functional disability among children and adolescents in an interdisciplinary chronic pain rehabilitation program. *J Pediatr Psychol*. 2013;38(7):756–765.

13

Exploring Pain Conditions in Schizophrenia and Bipolar Disorder

MAËL GAGNON-MAILHOT, JANIE DAMIEN,
VINCENT PELLAND, AND SERGE MARCHAND ■

SCHIZOPHRENIA

According to the *Diagnostic and Statistical Manual of Mental Disorders,* fifth edition (DSM-V), schizophrenia is characterized by a large spectrum of positive symptoms, including hallucinations, delirious ideation, disorganized speech, and disorganized behavior, and negative symptoms, such as avolition (decrease in the motivation to initiate and perform self-directed purposeful activities), anhedonia (inability to feel pleasure), and diminished emotional expression.[1] Onset usually occurs when the patient is in their early 20s and follows a chronic course characterized by acute episodes of psychosis and remissions. The patient usually does not return to premorbid functioning.

Pharmacology of Schizophrenia

In 2005, a study attempted to find which type of medication was most effective at treating the symptoms of psychosis, but 74% of the subjects stopped taking the medications because of side effects, inefficacy, or other personal choices.[2] These worrying results indicate the magnitude of the side effects associated with drugs used for the treatment of schizophrenia and the difficulties patients suffering from psychosis face when they try to get adequate treatment. Considering these results, drugs that may control psychosis more effectively and precisely are being researched to this day.[3,4] It should be noted that a glutamatergic dysregulation is now also being targeted by a few drugs to potentially alleviate symptoms of schizophrenia.[5] The role of glutamate receptors in schizophrenia is interesting considering that N-methyl-D-aspartate (NMDA) receptors are implicated in the central sensitization of pain.[6]

Schizophrenia and Pain

The literature generally supports a reduced sensitivity to pain in individuals with schizophrenia, as revealed by increased tolerance and endurance to pain induced by thermal, mechanical, and electrical stimuli.[7]

Case reports about patients affected by schizophrenia inflicting various kinds of extreme pain upon themselves or putting themselves in hazardous situations, in which they would normally suffer atrocious pain, are frequent in the scientific literature. For example, Virit et al.[8] reported a patient who suffered severe third-degree burns on the arm after being exposed to the flame of a liquefied petroleum gas cylinder. Despite the severity of his wounds, the patient did not complain of any pain during this episode. Moreover, Nielsen et al.[9] found an increased prevalence of unrecognized heart attacks in individuals with schizophrenia compared with the general population.

Despite the clinical evidence of decreased sensitivity to pain in this particular population, only a few studies have been conducted using experimental paradigms that aim at unveiling the mechanisms behind this phenomenon, and their results are conflicting. However, a few studies have even observed increased pain sensitivity in patients suffering from schizophrenia. For instance, Girard et al.[10] found an increased sensitivity to pain caused by ischemia and pressure. The patients with schizophrenia needed less pressure and a shorter duration of ischemia than healthy controls to report pain. Moreover, Lévesque et al.[11] also observed an increased sensitivity to acute pain. Considering the relatively low prevalence of schizophrenia in epidemiological studies on chronic pain, the authors suggest a unique experimental pain profile in schizophrenics characterized by high sensitivity to acute pain and decreased sensitivity to prolonged pain. However, this conclusion does not account for the numerous case report studies on schizophrenia describing absence of pain in acute medical conditions.

Also, the efficacy of diffuse noxious inhibitory control (DNIC), an endogenous system regulating ascending pain signals, seems to be intact in people with schizophrenia.[12] However, a lack of sensitization is observed in these subjects. Lévesque et al.[11] confirmed that schizophrenic subjects did not show an increase in response to persistent pain as the healthy subjects did when a continuous painful electrical stimulation was applied. Furthermore, in the same study, the authors observed that the spinal nociceptive reflex activated by a painful stimulus is similar in schizophrenic and healthy subjects. This, along with the finding of an intact DNIC in people with schizophrenia, suggests that the difference in pain perception might arise from supraspinal mechanisms. The brain imaging study of de la Fuente-Sandoval et al.[13] supports this supraspinal theory, showing an increased primary somatosensory cortex activity but a decreased cingulate cortex activation. These results suggest that it is the affective pain component that is reduced in schizophrenia.

The discrepancy of results in the literature might arise from methodological issues and differences in inclusion criteria among studies. Overall, it appears that decreased pain sensitivity could be an endophenotype of schizophrenia, as demonstrated by a meta-analysis conducted by Stubbs et al.,[7] although the underlying mechanisms are still unclear.

Neurophysiology and Brain Imaging

In the schizophrenic population, there is a diminished connectivity between the sensorimotor, visual, and auditory cortices, although all of these areas are largely connected to the thalamus.[15] The thalamus also shows a hypoconnectivity with the frontal and prefrontal cortices.[16,17] Together, these results suggest poor communication between sensory areas of the brain. There is also an impact on the integration of those signals (from the hypothalamus) in the frontal and prefrontal cortices. This hypoconnectivity between sensory areas and the frontal lobe may result in the patients' inability to interpret adequately the affective component of pain and other sensory stimuli. It has been reported that patients suffering from schizophrenia tend to focus on some perceptual modalities while completely ignoring others. This could interfere with their abilities to recognize pain and report it to health professionals and caregivers.

A study by Linnman et al.[18] observed a decreased response to aversive electrical stimulus in the insula that is correlated with the intensity of positive symptomsin patients with schizophrenia. In healthy individuals, the insula is implicated in the processing of emotional and sensory stimuli, and in interoception (awareness of one's body).[19] Altered function of the insula in schizophrenia might be responsible for several of the observed symptoms, notably difficulties in recognizing emotions in facial and vocal expressions, a distorted perception of self, and difficulties in distinguishing self, versus nonself, inputs.[20] Moreover, insula is part of the acute pain–processing network.[21] It is thus possible that a dysfunction of this brain structure leads some patients to not interpret nociceptive signals as originating from themselves. It could also be possible that, because of the lack of reactivity of the insula, negative emotions in response to the nociceptive stimulus are not processed, leading to an apparent diminished reactivity to pain and its expression even though the nociceptive signal remains intact.

The basal ganglia network is another brain area characterized by hypoconnectivity in patients suffering from schizophrenia.[22,23] This area is closely involved in pain perception; it is reported to play a key role in the integration of cognitive, motor, emotional, and autonomic responses to painful stimuli.[24,25] A diminution of the activation pattern may disrupt pain perception. In addition, patients suffering from schizophrenia have generally below average cognitive skills, which can lead to communication difficulties.[26]

Neurotransmitters

The neurotransmitter glutamate, which binds to NMDA receptors, is now one of the main neurotransmitters thought to be involved in schizophrenia.[27] It was found that noncompetitive antagonists to NMDA receptors, such as phencyclidine and ketamine, produce symptoms similar to psychosis.[28,29] In animals, NDMA receptor blockade causes nervous system degradation similar to what is seen in patients with schizophrenia. This lack of NMDA receptors may cause glutamate to be released excessively, which could result in excitotoxicity (degradation of the nervous system through glutamate overactivation).[30] It has been suggested that a decrease in NMDA receptor transmission might be responsible for the pain insensitivity observed in the schizophrenic population.[31]

Glutamate plays an important role in inducing central sensitization, which in general is decreased in schizophrenia.[32,33] Furthermore, glutamate levels in some key brain areas are correlated with pain sensitivity.[34] It has been reported that areas involved in pain perception, such as the basal ganglia, the anterior cingulate cortex, and the thalamus, have abnormal glutamate levels in the schizophrenic population.[35,36] Studies report both increased and decreased levels of glutamate in individuals with schizophrenia, sometimes contradicting each other. It is still too early to draw a definitive conclusion from those studies, but considering the involvement of glutamate in both pain perception and schizophrenia, future research may help deepen our understanding of this relationship.

Dopamine, serotonin, norepinephrine, gamma-aminobutyric acid (GABA), and the opioid system are also possible candidates in explaining the altered pain perception in the schizophrenic population.[4,37-41] However, these various hypotheses are not mutually exclusive and thus may coexist in the physiopathology of this disease.

Conclusion

Considering the complexity of both pain and schizophrenia, a definitive conclusion concerning the mechanisms underlying pain sensitivity and insensitivity in the schizophrenic population is hard to determine. Many brain areas affected by schizophrenia are also involved in pain-processing and cognition. No single brain area seems to be responsible for all aspects of the disorder and the diminished sensitivity of patients with schizophrenia to painful stimuli in clinical settings. The cumulative evidence, however, suggests that schizophrenia leads to decreased pain sensitivity partly because of poor connectivity in specific brain areas involved in perception, emotions, cognition, and integration processes.

We hypothesize that two conditions engendered by schizophrenia may interfere with pain perception. In the first case, patients may have a distorted perception or difficulties interpreting what they are feeling. In the other more rare and extreme case, patients may be completely dissociated from what happens to them, as demonstrated in the shocking case report mentioned earlier.[8] In general, patients with schizophrenia should be treated with special care considering their cognitive difficulties and reduced pain perception.[7,42] Clinicians should always be on the lookout for extreme cases that may endanger the lives of patients who are completely unaware of their situation because of pain insensitivity.

BIPOLAR DISORDER

Bipolar disorder, once named *manic depression*, has similar features to schizophrenia.[43] As defined by the DSM-V, episodes of mania consist of elevated, irritable, or expansive moods as well as abnormal and persistent increased goal-directed activity.[1] Manic episodes are sometimes accompanied by psychotic symptoms like delusions or hallucinations. Hypomanic episodes are very similar to manias, but less intense. Major depressive episodes are characterized by depressed mood and/or decreased pleasure.

Psychological, behavioral, and physiological symptoms in bipolar disorder seem to be related to dysregulated reinforcement–reward functions, psychomotor activity, and central pain mechanisms.[43] During depression, cognitive stimuli that previously were neutral or nonaversive are experienced as distressing. On the other hand, during manic phases, patients might not experience aversion to negative stimuli, and they might not think about the painful consequences of their behavior.[43]

Pharmacology of Bipolar Disorder

Considering that chronic pain disorders have a high incidence among patients with bipolar disorder, it is important to determine whether monotherapy can be an efficient and safe treatment for both conditions. In the general population, antidepressants, cyclobenzaprine, milnacipran, and tramadol can be used to treat chronic pain. However, they may precipitate manic states in bipolar disorder patients and increase the risk for suicide, especially if not administered with mood-stabilizing medication.[14,44] Other analgesic drugs, such as nonsteroidal anti-inflammatory drugs, may impair renal excretion of lithium taken by patients with bipolar disorder, thus increasing their serum lithium levels and possibly eliciting lithium toxicity.[44]

The efficacy and safety of these drugs in patients affected by bipolar disroderare not currently well established.[45] According to data of the American Psychiatric Association treatment guidelines for bipolar mood disorder and the 2012 Cochrane database for pain disorders, no single drug seemed to efficiently treat the comorbidity of chronic pain and bipolar disorder. Carbamazepine was mentioned in both guidelines as an evidence-based treatment for each condition separately.[45] These results should be interpreted with caution considering that the meta-analysis by Miura et al.[46] found carbamazepine to be less effective than a placebo when treating mood disorders. It should be noted that, in addition to pharmacological treatment, some form of cognitive treatment is recommended.[47]

Bipolar Disorder and Pain

A systematic review and meta-analysis of studies on pain conditions in adults with bipolar disorder (N = 171,352) reported a prevalence of 24% for chronic pain, which is comparable to the general population.[14] Other studies report an even higher prevalence (40–46%) of chronic pain or regular pain interfering with daily functioning in patients with bipolar disorder.[48,49] Migraine and chronic headaches, the most prevalent pain conditions in adults with bipolar disorder, affect approximately 14% of them and are considered three times more frequent than in the general population.[14,49] In a sample of patients with bipolar disorder experiencing a depressive phase, the pain was most frequently located in the back, and the most common cause of chronic pain was musculoskeletal disease.[44] Fibromyalgia is also a common chronic pain condition in individuals with a diagnosis of bipolar disorder or with lifetime manic and depressive spectrum symptoms (but no diagnosis of bipolar disorder).[50]

Pain interference, restriction of work, life roles, and interpersonal relationship in the last month due to pain was significantly greater in individuals with bipolar disorder (24.8%) than with major depressive disorder (20.3%), anxiety (19.3%), or none of these conditions (11.0%), according to an epidemiological study of Goldstein et al.[51]

Individuals with bipolar disorder sometimes demonstrate atypical responses to pain depending on the phase of the disorder, but there are some inconsistencies in the literature.[52] Some studies have found that the positive affect observed in manias may reduce pain, while the negative affect of depressive episodes may intensify the perceived pain.[53] For instance, Mel'nikova[54] noted lower pain thresholds to painful electric pulses in patients diagnosed with unipolar and bipolar depression than in healthy subjects, but increased pain thresholds after antidepressive therapy.

Some psychotic patients with bipolar disorder may even seem insensitive to pain.[53] For instance, in a report published by Fishbain,[55] a woman diagnosed with psychotic depressive reaction was brought to the hospital after attempting suicide by jumping from a second-story balcony, and did not complain of pain until the second day of hospitalization. Her radiograph test revealed fractures of the left superior pubic ramus, left inferior ischial ramus, coccyx, anterior wedge L2 and T12, and long-segment pedicle. The patient recovered after appropriate medical care and the improvement of her manic-depressive symptoms. This case illustrates the complexity of evaluating the medical condition of patients with mania especially in the absence of pain complaints. Boggero and Cole[52] report that a majority of patients with bipolar I or bipolar II and comorbid chronic lower back pain recalled a reduced intensity of pain during their most recent manic or hypomanic episodes. Patients may engage in activities that could aggravate their pain levels after the manic symptoms resolve. Over time, their lack of care may contribute to the high prevalence of acute and chronic pain in bipolar disorder reported by most epidemiological studies.

These findings of altered responses to experimental pain are also found in healthy relatives of individuals (first- to third-degree of relatedness) with bipolar disorder or schizophrenia, who indicated greater pain tolerance, greater maximum pain tolerance, and less frequent pain intolerance during an 8-minute pain test, than healthy subjects without a family history of psychopathology.[53]

It is important for clinicians performing their pain assessments to take into consideration the phase of cycle of patients affected by bipolar disorder. Certain pain procedures (e.g., spinal cord stimulator surgery) require a trial period to assess the intensity of pain reduction. If during the trial period, patients in manic or hypomanic states report decreased levels of pain, then the results of the trial may lead to false-positive results and unnecessary surgeries or treatments afterward.[52]

Neuroanatomical Changes in Bipolar Disorder

During painful stimulations, the amygdala and the right thalamic and prefrontal regions show an increased activation, while the periaqueductal gray matter and the rostral anterior cingulate and prefrontal cortices show a decreased activation in patients with bipolar disorder.[45] In cases of chronic pain comorbid with bipolar disorder, the anterior cingulate cortex, amygdala, and prefrontal cortex show some dysregulated brain activation.[56]

To a lesser extent than patients with schizophrenia, individuals with bipolar I demonstrate dysregulations in the activity of both the sensory–discriminative and the affective–motivational pathways. More precisely, a hypoactivity of the secondary somatosensory cortex S2 and the anterior cingulate and anterior insular cortices is seen in response to pain. These results suggest pain-processing abnormalities in psychosis spectrum disorders.[57]

Neurotransmitters

A wide array of neurotransmitters and other neurochemicals are thought to be involved in bipolar disorder.[58,59] Abnormalities of serotonin, norepinephrine, and dopamine neurotransmission in the brain and within the peripheral nervous system have been noted in both pain and psychiatric conditions.[49] Indeed, the activity of the serotonergic and adrenergic antinociceptive systems has been found to be diminished in this comorbidity. The activity of the noradrenergic system, which is known to be involved in pain modulation, might be specifically decreased in depression and increased in mania.[60,61] The activity of the opioid system is also found to be diminished in this population; there is a decreased concentration of endogenous opioids in the central nervous system.[62] Since the endogenous opioids and norepinephrine are neurotransmitters involved in pain modulation,[63,64] their interaction with bipolar disorder may influence the altered pain perception observed in these patients.

Conclusion

Even though studies have accumulated results with considerable heterogeneity, mania generally seems to be associated with a decreased perception of pain, whereas depression seems to be associated with an amplified experience of pain. Their experience or pain-processing mechanisms might be altered, but current studies do not allow us to advance strong conclusions. The issue of pain condition in psychiatric conditions, such as bipolar disorder, requires critical judgment and further experimentation. The comorbidity of pain and bipolar disorder is linked to delayed recovery, greater functional disability, lower quality of life, and increased risk for suicide compared with healthy subjects.[14] Therefore, it would be beneficial to identify and treat early pain conditions among patients with bipolar disorder because it could lead to reduced pain interference, reduced health care costs, and improved mood and anxiety treatment outcomes.[51] The assessment and treatment of pain should form an integral part of the management of bipolar disorder. Clinicians need to be very careful when assessing pain in people with comorbid psychiatric and pain conditions.[14]

REFERENCES

1. American Psychiatric Association. *Diagnostic and Statistical Manual of Mental Disorders.* 5th ed. Washington, DC: Author; 2013.
2. Lieberman JA, Stroup TS, McEvoy JP, et al. Effectiveness of antipsychotic drugs in patients with chronic schizophrenia. *N Engl J Med.* 2005;353(12):1209–1223. doi:10.1056/NEJMoa1214609.
3. Borroto-Escuela DO, Pintsuk J, Schäfer T, et al. Multiple D2 heteroreceptor complexes: New targets for treatment of schizophrenia. *Ther Adv Psychopharmacol.* 2016;6(2):77–94. doi:10.1177/2045125316637570.
4. Howes O, McCutcheon R, Stone J. Glutamate and dopamine in schizophrenia: An update for the 21st century. *J Psychopharmacol.* 2015;29(2):97–115. doi:10.1177/0269881114563634.
5. Stone JM. Glutamatergic antipsychotic drugs: A new dawn in the treatment of schizophrenia? *Ther Adv Psychopharmacol.* 2011;1(1):5–18. doi:10.1177/2045125311400779.
6. Woolf CJ. Central sensitization: Implications for the diagnosis and treatment of pain. *Pain.* 2011;152(3 suppl):S2–S15. doi:10.1016/j.pain.2010.09.030.

7. Stubbs B, Thompson T, Acaster S, Vancampfort D, Gaughran F, Correll CU. Decreased pain sensitivity among people with schizophrenia. *Pain.* 2015;156(11):2121–2131. doi:10.1097/j.pain.0000000000000304.

8. Virit O, Savas HA, Altindag A. Lack of pain in schizophrenia: A patient whose arm was burned and amputated. *Gen Hosp Psychiatry.* 2017;30(4):384–385. doi:10.1016/j.genhosppsych.2008.01.005.

9. Nielsen J, Juel J, Al Zuhairi KSM, et al. Unrecognised myocardial infarction in patients with schizophrenia. *Acta Neuropsychiatr.* 2015;27(2):106–112. doi:10.1017/neu.2014.41.

10. Girard M, Plansont B, Bonnabau H, Malauzat D. Experimental pain hypersensitivity in schizophrenic patients. *Clin J Pain.* 2011;27(9):790–795. doi:10.1097/AJP.0b013e31821d904c.

11. Lévesque M, Potvin S, Marchand S, et al. Pain perception in schizophrenia: Evidence of a specific pain response profile. *Pain Med.* 2012;13(12):1571–1579. doi:10.1111/j.1526-4637.2012.01505.x.

12. Potvin S, Stip E, Tempier A, et al. Pain perception in schizophrenia: No changes in diffuse noxious inhibitory controls (DNIC) but a lack of pain sensitization. *J Psychiatr Res.* 2008;42(12):1010–1016. doi:10.1016/j.jpsychires.2007.11.001.

13. de la Fuente-Sandoval C, Favila R, Gómez-Martin D, Pellicer F, Graff-Guerrero A. Functional magnetic resonance imaging response to experimental pain in drug-free patients with schizophrenia. *Psychiatry Res.* 2010;183(2):99–104. doi:10.1016/j.pscychresns.2010.05.003.

14. Stubbs B, Eggermont L, Mitchell AJ, et al. The prevalence of pain in bipolar disorder: A systematic review and large-scale meta-analysis. *Acta Psychiatr Scand.* 2015;131(2):75–88. doi:10.1111/acps.12325.

15. Damaraju E, Allen EA, Belger A, et al. Dynamic functional connectivity analysis reveals transient states of dysconnectivity in schizophrenia. *NeuroImage Clin.* 2014;5(July):298–308. doi:10.1016/j.nicl.2014.07.003.

16. Woodward ND, Karbasforoushan H, Heckers S. Thalamocortical dysconnectivity in schizophrenia. *Am J Psychiatry.* 2012;169(10):1092–1099. doi:10.1176/appi.ajp.2012.12010056.

17. Cheng W, Palaniyappan L, Li M, et al. Voxel-based, brain-wide association study of aberrant functional connectivity in schizophrenia implicates thalamocortical circuitry. *NPJ Schizophr.* 2015;1(Dec 2014):15016. doi:10.1038/npjschz.2015.16.

18. Linnman C, Coombs G, Goff DC, Holt DJ. Lack of insula reactivity to aversive stimuli in schizophrenia. *Schizophr Res.* 2013;143(1):150–157. doi:10.1016/j.schres.2012.10.038.

19. Craig AD. Interoception: The sense of the physiological condition of the body. *Curr Opin Neurobiol.* 2003;13(4):500–505. http://www.ncbi.nlm.nih.gov/pubmed/12965300.

20. Wylie KP, Tregellas JR. The role of the insula in schizophrenia. *Schizophr Res.* 2010;123(2–3):93–104. doi:10.1016/j.schres.2010.08.027.

21. Apkarian AV, Bushnell MC, Treede R-D, Zubieta J-K. Human brain mechanisms of pain perception and regulation in health and disease. *Eur J Pain.* 2005;9(4):463–484. doi:10.1016/j.ejpain.2004.11.001.

22. Solé-Padullés C, Castro-Fornieles J, De La Serna E, et al. Altered cortico-striatal connectivity in offspring of schizophrenia patients relative to offspring of bipolar patients and controls. *PLoS One.* 2016;11(2):1–14. doi:10.1371/journal. pone.0148045.

23. Bernard JA, Russell CE, Newberry RE, Goen JRM, Mittal VA. Patients with schizophrenia show aberrant patterns of basal ganglia activation: Evidence from ALE meta-analysis. *NeuroImage Clin.* 2017;14:450–463. doi:10.1016/j.nicl.2017.01.034.

24. Borsook D, Upadhyay J, Chudler EH, Becerra L. A key role of the basal ganglia in pain and analgesia: Insights gained through human functional imaging. *Mol Pain.* 2010;6:27. doi:10.1186/1744-8069-6-27.

25. Chudler EH, Dong WK. The role of the basal ganglia in nociception and pain. *Pain.* 1995;60(1):3–38. doi:10.1016/0304-3959(94)00172-B.

26. Mosiolek A, Gierus J, Koweszko T, Szulc A. Cognitive impairment in schizophrenia across age groups: A case-control study. 2016;16:37. doi:10.1186/ s12888-016-0749-1.

27. Wei H, Matthew LM, Daniel EE, Robert AS. The glutamate hypothesis of schizophrenia: Evidence from human brain tissue studies. 2016;8(5):583–592. doi:10.1002/aur.1474.Replication.

28. Coyle JT. NMDA receptor and schizophrenia: A brief history. *Schizophr Bull.* 2012;38(5):920–926. doi:10.1093/schbul/sbs076.

29. Javitt DC. Glutamatergic theories of schizophrenia. *Isr J Psychiatry Relat Sci.* 2010;47(1):4–16.

30. Miladinovic T, Nashed MG, Singh G. Overview of glutamatergic dysregulation in central pathologies. *Biomolecules.* 2015;5(4):3112–3141. doi:10.3390/biom5043112.

31. Dworkin RH. Pain insensitivity in schizophrenia: A neglected phenomenon and some implications. *Schizophr Bull.* 1994;20(2):235–248. http://www.ncbi.nlm.nih. gov/pubmed/8085127.

32. Gruber O, Santuccione AC, Aach H. Magnetic resonance imaging in studying schizophrenia, negative symptoms, and the glutamate system. *Front Psychiatry.* 2014;5(Apr):1–11. doi:10.3389/fpsyt.2014.00032.

33. Latremoliere A, Woolf C. Central sensitization: A generator of pain hypersensitivity by central neural plasticity. *J Pain.* 2010;10(9):895–926. doi:10.1016/ j.jpain.2009.06.012.Central.

34. Zunhammer M, Schweizer LM, Witte V, Harris RE, Bingel U, Schmidt-Wilcke T. Combined glutamate and glutamine levels in pain-processing brain regions are associated with individual pain sensitivity. *Pain.* 2016;157(10):2248–2256. doi:10.1097/j.pain.0000000000000634.

35. Gallinat J, McMahon K, Kühn S, Schubert F, Schaefer M. Cross-sectional study of glutamate in the anterior cingulate and hippocampus in schizophrenia. *Schizophr Bull.* 2016;42(2):425–433. doi:10.1093/schbul/sbv124.

36. Merritt K, Egerton A, Kempton MJ, Taylor MJ, McGuire PK. Nature of glutamate alterations in schizophrenia: A meta-analysis of proton magnetic resonance spectroscopy studies. *JAMA Psychiatry.* 2016;73(7):665–674. doi:10.1001/ jamapsychiatry.2016.0442.

37. Sadock Bj, Sadock VA, Ruiz P. *Kaplan and Sadock's Synopsis of Psychiatry: Behavioral Sciences/Clinical Psychiatry.* Philadelphia, PA; Wolters Kluwer; 2014:1472.

38. Emrich HM, Cording C, Pirée S, Kölling A, von Zerssen D, Herz A. Indication of an antipsychotic action of the opiate antagonist naloxone. *Pharmakopsychiatr Neuropsychopharmakol.* 1977;10(5):265–270. doi:10.1055/s-0028-1094547.

39. Watson SJ, Berger PA, Akil H, Mills MJ, Barchas JD. Effects of naloxone on schizophrenia: reduction in hallucinations in a subpopulation of subjects. *Science.* 1978;201(4350):73–76. http://www.ncbi.nlm.nih.gov/pubmed/351804.

40. Davis GC, Buchsbaum MS, van Kammen DP, Bunney WE. Analgesia to pain stimuli in schizophrenics and its reversal by naltrexone. *Psychiatry Res.* 1979;1(1):61–69. http://www.ncbi.nlm.nih.gov/pubmed/298339.

41. Pickar D, Bunney WE, Douillet P, et al. Repeated naloxone administration in schizophrenia: A phase II world health organization study. *Biol Psychiatry.* 1989;25(4):440–448. doi:10.1016/0006-3223(89)90197-2.

42. Green MF, Kern RS, Braff DL, Mintz J. Neurocognitive deficits and functional outcome in schizophrenia: Are we measuring the "right stuff"? *Schizophr Bull.* 2000;26(1):119–136. doi:10.1093/oxfordjournals.schbul.a033430.

43. Carroll BJ. Brain mechanisms in manic depression. *Clin Chem.* 1994;40(2):303–308.

44. Failde I, Dueñas M, Agüera-Ortíz L, Cervilla JA, Gonzalez-Pinto A, Mico JA. Factors associated with chronic pain in patients with bipolar depression: A cross-sectional study. *BMC Psychiatry.* 2013;13(1):112. doi:10.1186/1471-244X-13-112.

45. Rahman T, Campbell A, O'Connell CR, Nallapula K. Carbamazepine in bipolar disorder with pain: Reviewing treatment guidelines. *Prim Care Companion CNS Disord.* 2014;16(5). doi:10.4088/PCC.14r01672.

46. Miura T, Noma H, Furukawa TA, et al. Comparative efficacy and tolerability of pharmacological treatments in the maintenance treatment of bipolar disorder: A systematic review and network meta-analysis. *Lancet Psychiatry.* 2014;1(5):351–359. doi:10.1016/S2215-0366(14)70314-1.

47. Mirabel-Sarron C, Giachetti R. Les thérapies non-médicamenteuses dans les troubles bipolaires. *Encephale.* 2012;38:S160–S166. doi:10.1016/S0013-7006(12)70094-5.

48. Cerimele JM, Chan Y-F, Chwastiak LA, Unützer J. Pain in primary care patients with bipolar disorder. *Gen Hosp Psychiatry.* 2014;36(2):228. doi:10.1016/j.genhosppsych.2013.11.004.

49. Nicholl BI, Mackay D, Cullen B, et al. Chronic multisite pain in major depression and bipolar disorder: Cross-sectional study of 149,611 participants in UK Biobank. *BMC Psychiatry.* 2014;14:350. doi:10.1186/s12888-014-0350-4.

50. Dell'Osso B, Mundo E, D'Urso N, et al. Augmentative repetitive navigated transcranial magnetic stimulation (rTMS) in drug-resistant bipolar depression. *Bipolar Disord.* 2009;11(1):76–81. doi:10.1111/j.1399-5618.2008.00651.x.

51. Goldstein BI, Houck PR, Karp JF. Factors associated with pain interference in an epidemiologic sample of adults with bipolar I disorder. *J Affect Disord.* 2009;117(3):151–156. doi:10.1016/j.jad.2009.01.011.

52. Boggero IA, Cole JD. Mania reduces perceived pain intensity in patients with chronic pain: Preliminary evidence from retrospective archival data. *J Pain Res.* 2016;9:147–152. doi:10.2147/JPR.S88120.

53. Hooley JM, Chung RJ. Pain insensitivity in relatives of patients with schizophrenia and bipolar disorder. In: Lenzenweger MF, Hooley JM, Lenzenweger MF, Hooley

JM, eds. *Principles of Experimental Psychopathology: Essays in Honor of Brendan A. Maher.* Washington, DC: American Psychological Association; 2003:157–171.

54. Mel'nikova TS. [Thresholds of pain responses to electric stimuli in patients with endogenous depressions]. *Patol Fiziol Eksp Ter.* 1993;(4):19–21. http://www.ncbi. nlm.nih.gov/pubmed/8183608.

55. Fishbain DA. Pain insensitivity in psychosis. *Ann Emerg Med.* 1982;11(11):630–632. doi:10.1016/S0196-0644(82)80210-2.

56. Ciaramella A. Mood spectrum disorders and perception of pain. *Psychiatr Q.* 2017;88:687–700. doi:10.1007/s11126-017-9489-8.

57. Minichino A, Delle Chiaie R, Cruccu G, et al. Pain-processing abnormalities in bipolar I disorder, bipolar II disorder, and schizophrenia: A novel trait marker for psychosis proneness and functional outcome? *Bipolar Disord.* 2016;18(7):591–601. doi:10.1111/bdi.12439.

58. Rapoport SI, Basselin M, Kim H-W., Rao JS. Bipolar disorder and mechanisms of action of mood stabilizers. *Brain Res Rev.* 2009;61(2):185–209. doi:10.1016/ j.brainresrev.2009.06.003.BIPOLAR.

59. Manji HK, Quiroz JA, Payne JL, et al. The underlying neurobiology of bipolar disorder. *World Psychiatry.* 2003;2(3):136–146. http://www.ncbi.nlm.nih.gov/ pubmed/16946919%0Ahttp://www.pubmedcentral.nih.gov/articlerender. fcgi?artid=PMC1525098%0Ahttp://www.pubmedcentral.nih.gov/articlerender.fcg i?artid=1525098&tool=pmcentrez&rendertype=abstract.

60. Ossipov MH, Dussor GO, Porreca F. Central modulation of pain. *J Clin Invest.* 2010;120(11):3779–3787. doi:10.1172/JCI43766.reduced.

61. Pertovaara A. The noradrenergic pain regulation system: A potential target for pain therapy. *Eur J Pharmacol.* 2013;716(1-3):2–7. doi:10.1016/j.ejphar.2013.01.067.

62. Szechiński M, Sidorowicz S, Małyszczak K. Characteristics of pain experienced in major depression. *Arch Psychiatry Psychother.* 2006;8(2):41–53.

63. Holden JE, Jeong Y, Forrest JM. The endogenous opioid system and clinical pain management. *AACN Clin Issues.* 2005;16(3):291–301. http://www.ncbi.nlm.nih. gov/pubmed/16082232.

64. Pertovaara A. Noradrenergic pain modulation. *Prog Neurobiol.* 2006;80(2):53–83. doi:10.1016/j.pneurobio.2006.08.001.

14

Post-traumatic Stress Disorder and Chronic Pain in the Military

JORDANA L. SOMMER, RACHEL ROY, PAMELA L. HOLENS, AND RENÉE EL-GABALAWY ■

Military personnel experience higher rates of psychiatric and physical conditions than the general population.[1-8] In active duty and veteran samples, prevalence estimates for psychiatric conditions range from 15 to 44%,[4,9,10] and an estimated 66% report at least one chronic physical condition.[7] Post-traumatic stress disorder (PTSD) and chronic pain conditions are particularly prevalent among military personnel[5,11] and often co-occur.[8,12] This chapter aims to provide an overview of PTSD and chronic pain among military populations, including a description of prevalence, risk factors, correlates, and intervention strategies.

TRAUMA EXPOSURE AND TRAUMA-RELATED DISORDERS IN THE MILITARY

Military personnel are frequently exposed to trauma, with an estimated 70% or more exposed to multiple traumatic events.[12-15] Elevated trauma exposure leaves military personnel at risk for stress-related sequelae, including acute stress disorder, PTSD, complex PTSD, and disorder of extreme stress not otherwise specified.[13,16-20] Acute stress disorder is characterized by symptoms of intrusion (e.g., flashbacks), negative mood, dissociation (e.g., altered sense of reality), avoidance (e.g., of external reminders), and hyperarousal (e.g., hypervigilance) that persist for at least 3 days and no longer than 1 month following trauma exposure.[21] Relatedly, PTSD is characterized by symptoms of intrusion, avoidance, negative mood and cognition, and hyperarousal that persist for longer than 1 month following a traumatic event.[21] Disorders of extreme stress, including complex PTSD, are typically characterized by affective dysregulation, impulsivity, dissociation, somatization, and impairments in identity and interpersonal functioning[16,22] alongside other trauma-related symptoms. These disorders are typically associated with the experience of prolonged traumatic events, such as repeated childhood sexual assault.[20,23] PTSD will remain the focus of the current chapter because of the limited body of literature examining acute stress disorder and disorders of extreme stress among military personnel.

Post-traumatic Stress Disorder Prevalence in the Military

Population-based estimates of PTSD among military populations vary greatly, ranging from 1 to 35% across Canada, the United States (US), and the United Kingdom (UK)[4,13,24-28] with highest rates generally among veterans.[29] The variability in estimates likely stems from differences in assessment methods (e.g., differing cut scores on screening measures),[30] timeframes (e.g., past-month vs. lifetime),[31] and subpopulations examined (e.g., active duty versus veteran).[26]

Risk Factors, Comorbidities, and Outcomes of Post-traumatic Stress Disorder in the Military

Considering sociodemographics, studies suggest that among military personnel, females, younger adults, members of ethnic or racial minority groups, and those with lower education or income experience higher rates of PTSD.[13,19,25,26,29,32-34] Psychological factors such as perceived threat to life during trauma, psychiatric history, previous trauma exposure, and a greater number of lifetime exposures to trauma are also associated with increased risk of PTSD.[19,29,32,34] Certain military-specific factors also increase the risk of PTSD, including history, number, and cumulative length of deployments; combat exposure; and either personal injury or witnessing the injury or death of others during combat.[25,29,32-36]

PTSD is associated with various adverse comorbidities and outcomes. Extant research demonstrates high rates of psychiatric comorbidity among military personnel with PTSD.[25,31,37–40] For example, a recent study of two national samples of US military veterans found rates of comorbidities ranging from 24 to 77% for depression, drug and alcohol use disorders, and social phobia.[31] PTSD is also commonly comorbid with physical conditions among military personnel, including respiratory, gastrointestinal, and cardiovascular conditions, sleep disorders, and, of relevance to this chapter, chronic pain conditions and traumatic brain injury (TBI).[8,12,34,41] PTSD among military personnel is also associated with disability and functional impairment.[6,34,42–45] At the extreme, PTSD can result in suicidality (ideation, attempts), death by suicide, and all-cause mortality in this population.[34,37,39,46,47]

CHRONIC PAIN IN THE MILITARY

Chronic pain is defined as pain that persists for longer than 3 months.[48] Population-based research suggests that 44 to 73% of military personnel experience chronic pain, and estimates are typically elevated among veteran samples compared with active personnel.[8,49–52] Rates vary according to type of chronic pain condition; across military samples, some of the most prevalent chronic pain conditions are arthritis, back pain, other musculoskeletal pain, and migraines.[7,8,11,12,50–52] Recognizing its relevance and burden in this population, the US Veterans Health Administration designated pain as the "fifth vital sign."[53]

Risk Factors, Comorbidities, and Outcomes of Chronic Pain in the Military

Prior research has identified various risk factors or correlates of chronic pain among military personnel, including older age, lower education, higher body mass index, black race, and being married/previously married.[5,49,52] Research regarding sex differences has yielded disparate findings; different studies suggest that chronic pain is more prevalent among both females[49] and males.[52] This discrepancy may relate to variability in chronic pain definitions across studies. Similar to PTSD, a variety of military-related factors are associated with chronic pain,[54,55] including combat- or deployment-related injury,[49,51] presence and intensity of combat exposure,[5,51,54,55] greater length of military service,[52] and military sexual trauma and polytrauma (i.e., physical trauma to more than one organ or body system).[56–58]

Psychiatric comorbidity is also highly prevalent among military personnel with chronic pain.[5,8,49,51,52,59] In a population-based sample of active Canadian military personnel, chronic pain conditions were associated with major depressive episode, generalized anxiety disorder, panic disorder, and PTSD[8]; across chronic pain conditions, major depressive episode (11.3–17.4%) and PTSD (8.8–14.5%) were the most prevalent. Further, in a nationally representative sample of Canadian military veterans, 85% of individuals with a psychiatric condition had comorbid chronic pain.[52] This is corroborated by population-based research of US veterans, with estimates ranging from 6 to 34% for PTSD, substance use, anxiety, and mood disorders among those with chronic pain.[49] Chronic pain is also associated with increased opioid use among US active duty and veteran samples.[5,60] In addition to psychiatric comorbidity, unsurprisingly, research suggests that chronic pain among military personnel is associated with poorer physical health status[61] and disability.[62]

POST-TRAUMATIC STRESS DISORDER AND CHRONIC PAIN COMORBIDITY IN THE MILITARY

There is a well-established association between PTSD and chronic pain among military personnel.[8,12,24,49,58,63] In a population-based sample of regular Canadian Forces members, 9.0 to 14.5% of those with PTSD had comorbid chronic pain, with particularly elevated comorbidity rates for migraine.[8] Comorbidity was even greater in a population-based sample of US veterans, wherein 42.3% of those with PTSD had a comorbid chronic pain condition.[12]

TBI is often discussed in military research, particularly in literature surrounding PTSD and chronic pain.[64] TBI can be conceptualized as either a chronic pain condition, particularly if accompanied by migraine headaches, or independent of chronic pain.[65] A commonly referenced comorbid presentation among military populations is the polytrauma clinical triad (i.e., comorbid chronic pain, TBI, and PTSD).[66-70] Chronic pain, TBI, and PTSD may all occur as a result of one traumatic incident (e.g., during combat), which may explain the high prevalence estimates of the polytrauma clinical triad, ranging from 14 to 42%.[66,69,70]

Unsurprisingly, comorbid PTSD and chronic pain is associated with a compromised health-related profile. However, extant research examining correlates of comorbidity in military personnel is limited. With respect to pain-related correlates, comorbid PTSD and chronic pain is associated with increased pain severity, pain-related disability and activity limitation, and pain interference compared with chronic pain only[8,71]; these findings are consistent across active duty personnel and veterans, from both American and Canadian samples. This comorbidity is also associated with adverse psychological correlates, including greater affective distress, maladaptive cognitions, violent impulses,[66,71] and suicidal ideation and attempts.[66,68] Chronic pain and PTSD comorbidity is also associated with increased risk for medical discharge from the military.[24]

With respect to the temporal and causal relationship between PTSD and chronic pain, research has found that trauma and PTSD may precede chronic pain, but the reverse pathway is also supported.[72] In the military, PTSD and chronic pain can share a common cause, such as in the case of blast exposure and TBI.[65,73] Proposed theoretical models[74] include the shared vulnerability theory, which suggests several common predisposing factors for PTSD and chronic pain (e.g., anxiety sensitivity).[75] In contrast, the mutual maintenance model posits that aspects of chronic pain maintain or exacerbate PTSD, and vice versa[76]; for example, pain can trigger trauma memories, and the hyperarousal stemming from trauma-related memories may worsen pain.[74] Exacerbation of PTSD and chronic pain symptoms may worsen and increase the risk for associated correlates, including pain severity and psychiatric comorbidity.

USEFUL CLINICAL INTERVENTION STRATEGIES

The adverse correlates and comorbidities of PTSD and chronic pain outlined previously highlight the importance of clinical interventions aimed at improving the health, functionality, and overall quality of life of military personnel with PTSD and/or chronic pain. To this end, developed preventative interventions aim to mitigate the risk for PTSD and other psychiatric sequelae among military personnel.[77,78] For example, predeployment virtual reality interventions developed as a method of stress inoculation training have demonstrated preliminary effectiveness.[79] Secondary prevention initiatives, such as morphine administration following traumatic combat injury, may also be protective against the development of PTSD.[80,81] Pre-emptive and preventive analgesia may also protect against chronic pain in perioperative contexts.[82] In line with the mutual maintenance model, successful prevention or mitigation of PTSD symptoms may affect the incidence, severity, and adverse downstream sequelae of chronic pain, and vice versa.[74,76]

Adequate assessment of risk factors and early symptoms of PTSD and chronic pain is essential to identify vulnerable individuals and enable opportunities for early intervention. Current established initiatives, such as the US Department of Defense Pre-Deployment Health Assessment and Post-Deployment Health Assessment programs,[2,83] aim to improve screening of psychiatric and physical symptoms, including PTSD and chronic pain. The Post-Deployment Health

Assessment program, administered at 1 to 2 weeks and 3 to 6 months following return from deployment, includes various psychiatric screening measures, such as the Primary Care PTSD Screen,[84] and screens for physical conditions, including chronic pain. The Post-Deployment Health Assessment program has demonstrated good sensitivity for identifying PTSD and chronic pain,[85,86] which may support the implementation of similar programs in other countries. With respect to chronic pain assessment, the US Army Surgeon General's Pain Management Task Force initiated the development of the Pain Assessment Screening Tool and Outcomes Registry, a comprehensive system of patient-reported data to facilitate pain research and improve clinical practice.[87]

The identification of high rates of PTSD and chronic pain symptoms through assessment initiatives has highlighted the need for appropriate interventions for this population, particularly for veterans.[8,12] Recognizing these concerns, Veterans Affairs departments and agencies worldwide provide a range of specialized health care services to military veterans.[88] Interventions targeting comorbid PTSD and chronic pain have been developed and evaluated among military personnel, with promising results.[89-91] Such interventions are typically comprised of elements of trauma-focused exposure alongside behavioral activation, relaxation, psychoeducation, cognitive restructuring, and physical therapy. For example, the South Texas Research Organizational Network Guiding Studies on Trauma and Resilience Consortium developed and is evaluating a chronic pain–PTSD assessment and treatment intervention, which includes prolonged exposure and other cognitive behavioral elements.[91] Acceptance and commitment therapy is also being evaluated as a transdiagnostic intervention, which may be appropriate for targeting both PTSD and chronic pain in military personnel.[92]

Because of the limited number of interventions geared toward comorbid presentations, military personnel may receive targeted treatment for PTSD and chronic pain independently. For example, the Functional and Occupational Rehabilitation Treatment Program was developed as a functional restoration program for chronic pain among US military personnel.[91] This multidisciplinary intervention includes physical therapy, occupational therapy, cognitive behavioral therapy (CBT), and physical exercise. With respect to PTSD treatment, trauma-focused CBT interventions, including prolonged exposure[93] and cognitive processing therapy,[94] are among the most common and well-validated[95]; however, research has shown that cognitive processing therapy may be associated with greater improvement in physical symptoms compared with prolonged exposure,[96] suggesting that cognitive processing therapy may be more appropriate for individuals with comorbid PTSD and chronic pain. Although integrated interventions for comorbid PTSD and chronic pain may be preferable, treatment of either condition alone may result in reduction of comorbid symptoms through modification of mutually maintaining mechanisms (e.g., avoidant coping, maladaptive cognitions).

The mutual maintenance of PTSD and chronic pain also presents challenges to effective treatment. For example, fear (of pain-related and/or trauma-related stimuli) and the avoidance of feared stimuli are mutually maintaining mechanisms of both conditions.[89] Fear-induced hyperarousal may worsen pain, and the experience of pain may trigger distressing trauma memories. This synergy may render engagement in treatment challenging, particularly when pain and PTSD are a consequence of a single trauma (e.g., combat injury) and exposure to feared stimuli is a core component of treatment, such as in the case of PTSD.[93] Despite the various complications in comorbidity, effective treatment of both conditions is important because it may increase retention of active duty personnel and lead to greater improvements in physical, mental, and psychosocial health.[91]

CONCLUSION

PTSD and chronic pain are prevalent among military personnel and commonly co-occur. This comorbidity increases adverse outcomes in the domains of physical health, mental health, functionality, and overall quality of life. Progress has been made toward better understanding, assessing, and treating these comorbid conditions; however, the mutual maintenance of PTSD and chronic pain may further complicate effective management. Further investigation is warranted to continue to improve assessment, intervention, and, ideally, prevention strategies for these debilitating and co-occurring conditions.

REFERENCES

1. Boulos D, Zamorski MA. Deployment-related mental disorders among Canadian forces personnel deployed in support of the mission in Afghanistan, 2001–2008. *CMAJ*. 2013;185:E545–E552. doi:10.1503/cmaj.122120.
2. Hoge CW, Auchterloine JL, Milliken CS. Mental health problems, use of mental health services, and attrition from military services after returning from deployment to Iraq or Afghanistan. *JAMA*. 2006;295:1023–1032. doi:10.1001/jama.295.9.1023.
3. Riddle JR, Smith TC, Smith B, et al. Millennium cohort: The 2001–2003 baseline prevalence of mental disorders in the U.S. military. *J Clin Epidemiol*. 2007;60:192–201. doi:10.1016/j.jclinepi.2006.04.008.
4. Seal KH, Bertenthal D, Miner CR, Sen S, Marmar C. Bringing the war back home: Mental health disorders among 103 788 US veterans returning from Iraq

and Afghanistan seen at Department of Veterans Affairs facilities. *Arch Intern Med.* 2007;167:476–482. doi:10.1001/archinte.167.5.476.

5. Toblin RL, Quartana PJ, Riviere LA, Walper KC, Hoge CW. Chronic pain and opioid use in US soldiers after combat deployment. *JAMA Intern Med.* 2014;174:1400–1401. doi:10.1001/jamainternmed.2014.2726.

6. Thomas JL, Wilk JE, Riviere LA, McGurk D, Catro CA, Hoge CW. Prevalence of mental health problems and functional impairment among active component and national guard soldiers 3 and 12 months following combat in Iraq. *Arch Gen Psychiatry.* 2010;67:614–623. doi:10.1001/archgenpsychiatry.2010.54.

7. Thompson J, MacLean MB, Van Til L, et al. *Survey on Transition to Civilian Life: Report on Regular Force Veterans.* Charlottetown, PEI: Veterans Affairs Canada, National Defence; 2011.

8. Vun E, Turner S, Sareen J, Mota N, Afifi TO, El-Gabalawy R. Prevalence of comorbid chronic pain and mental health conditions in Canadian Armed Forces active personnel: Analysis of a cross-sectional survey. *CMAJ Open.* 2018;6:E528–E536. doi:10.9778/cmajo.20180093.

9. Ursano RJ, Colpe LJ, Heeringa SG, et al. The Army Study to Assess Risk and Resilience in Servicemembers (Army STARRS). *Psychiatry.* 2014;77:107–119. doi:10.1521/psyc.2014.77.2.107.

10. Zamorski MA, Bennett RE, Boulos D, Garber BG, Jetly R, Sareen J. The 2013 Canadian Forces Mental Health Survey: Backgrounds and methods. *Can J Psychiatry.* 2016;61:10S–25S.

11. Edlund MJ, Austen MA, Sullivan MD, et al. Patterns of opioid use for chronic noncancer pain the Veterans Health Administration from 2009–2011. *Pain.* 2014;155:2337–2343. doi:10.1016/j.pain.2014.08.033.

12. El-Gabalawy R, Blaney C, Tsai J, Sumner JA, Pietzak RH. Physical health conditions associated with full and subthreshold PTSD in U.S. military veterans: Results from the National Health and Resilience in Veterans Study. *J Affect Disord.* 2018;227:849–853. doi:10.1016/j.jad.2017.11.058.

13. Brunet A, Monson E, Liu A, Fikretoglu D. Trauma exposure and posttraumatic stress disorder in the Canadian military. *Can J Psychiatry.* 2015;60:488–496. doi:10.1177/070674371506001104.

14. Jakob JM, Lamp K, Rauch SA, Smith ER, Buchholz KR. The impact of trauma type or number of traumatic events on PTSD diagnosis and symptom severity in treatment seeking veterans. *J Nerv Ment Dis.* 2017;205:83–86. doi:10.1097/NMD.0000000000000581.

15. Russell DW, Cohen GH, Gifford R, Fullerton CS, Ursano RJ, Galea S. Mental health among a nationally representative sample of United States military reserve component personnel. *Soc Psychiatry Psychiatr Epidemiol.* 2015;50:639–651. doi:10.1007/s00127-014-0981-2.

16. Ford JD. Disorders of extreme stress following warzone military trauma: Associated features of post-traumatic stress disorder (PTSD) or comorbid but distinct syndromes? *J Consult Clin Psychol.* 1999;67:3–12.

17. Luterek JA, Bittinger JN, Simpson TL. Posttraumatic sequelae associated with military sexual trauma in female veterans enrolled in VA outpatient mental health clinics. *J Trauma Dissociation.* 2011;12:261–274. doi:10.1080/15299732.2011.551504.

18. Newman E, Orsillo SM, Herman DS, Niles BL, Litz BT. Clinical presentation of disorders of extreme stress in combat veterans. *J Nerv Ment Dis*. 1995;183:628–632.

19. Smith SM, Goldstein RB, Grant BF. The association between post-traumatic stress disorder and lifetime DSM-5 psychiatric disorders among veterans: Data from the National Epidemiologic Survey on Alcohol and Related Conditions-III (NESARC-III). *J Psychiatr Res*. 2016;82:16–22. doi:10.1016/j.jpsychires.2016.06.022.

20. Wolf EJ, Miller MW, Kilpatrick D, et al. ICD-11 complex PTSD in US national and veteran samples: Prevalence and structural associations with PTSD. *Clin Psychol Sci*. 2015;3:215–229. doi:10.1177/2167702614545480.

21. American Psychiatric Association. *Diagnostic and Statistical Manual of Mental Disorders*. 5th ed. Washington, DC: Author; 2013.

22. Maercker A, Brewin CR, Bryant RA, et al. Proposals for mental disorders specifically associated with stress in the International Classification of Diseases-11. *Lancet*. 2013;381:11–17. doi:10.1016/S0140-6736(12)62191-5.

23. Herman JL. Complex PTSD: A syndrome in survivors of prolonged repeated trauma. *J Trauma Stress*. 1992;5:377–391. doi:10.1002/jts.2490050305.

24. Benedict TM, Singleton MD, Nitz AJ, Shing TL, Kardouni JR. Effect of chronic low back pain and post-traumatic stress disorder on the risk for separation from the US army. *Mil Med*. 2019;185(9–10):431–439. doi:10.1093/milmed/usz020.

25. Crum-Cianflone NF, Powell TM, LeardMann CA, Russell DW, Boyko EJ. Mental health and comorbidities in U.S. military members. *Mil Med*. 2016;181:537–545. doi:10.7205/MILMED-D-15-00187.

26. Dursa EK, Reinhard MJ, Barth SK, Schneiderman AI. Prevalence of a positive screen for PTSD among OEF/OIF and OEF/OIF-era veterans in a large population-based cohort. *J Trauma Stress*. 2014;27:542–549. doi:10.1002/jts.21956.

27. Head M, Goodwin L, Debell F, Greenberg N, Wessely S, Fear NT. Post-traumatic stress disorder and alcohol use: Comorbidity in UK military personnel. *Soc Psychiatry Psychiatr Epidemiol*. 2016;51:1171–1180. doi:10.1007/s00127-016-1177-8.

28. Maguen S, Cohen B, Ren L, Bosch J, Kimerling R, Seal K. Gender differences in military sexual trauma and mental health diagnoses among Iraq and Afghanistan veterans with posttraumatic stress disorder. *Womens Health Issues*. 2012;22:61–66. doi:10.1016/j.whi.2011.07.010.

29. Xue C, Ge Y, Tang B, et al. A meta-analysis of risk factors for combat-related PTSD among military personnel and veterans. *PLoS One*. 2015;10:e0120270. doi:10.1371/journal.pone.0120270.

30. Sudin J, Fear NT, Iversen A, Rona RJ, Wessely S. PTSD after deployment to Iraq: Conflicting rates, conflicting claims. *Psychol Med*. 2010;40:367–382. doi:10.1017/S0033291709990791.

31. Wisco BE, Marx BP, Miller MW, et al. A comparison of ICD-11 and DSM criteria for posttraumatic stress disorder in two national samples of U.S. military veterans. *J Affect Disord*. 2017;223:17–19. doi:10.1016/j.jad.2017.07.006.

32. Iversen AC, Fear NT, Ehlers A, et al. Risk factors for post-traumatic stress disorder among UK armed forces personnel. *Psychol Med*. 2008;38:511–522. doi:10.1017/S0033291798992778.

33. Polusny MA, Kumpula MJ, Meis LA, et al. Gender differences in the effects of deployment-related stressors and pre-deployment risk factors on the development

of PTSD symptoms in National Guard soldiers deployed to Iraq and Afghanistan. *J Psychiatr Res*. 2014;49:1–9. doi:10.1016/j.jpsychires.2013.09.016.

34. Ramchand R, Rudavsky R, Grant S, Tanielian T, Jaycox L. Prevalence of, risk factors for, and consequences of posttraumatic stress disorder and other mental health problems in military populations deployed to Iraq and Afghanistan. *Curr Psychiatry Rep*. 2015;17:37. doi:10.1007/s11920-015-0575-z.

35. Brownlow JA, Zitnik GA, McLean CP, Gehrman PR. The influence of deployment stress and life stress on post-traumatic stress disorder (PTSD) diagnosis among military personnel. *J Psychiatr Res*. 2018;103:26–32. doi:10.1016/j.jpsychires.2018.05.005.

36. Steele M, Germain A, Campbell JS. Mediation and moderation of the relationship between combat experiences and post-traumatic stress symptoms in active duty military personnel. *Mil Med*. 2017;182:e1632–e1639. doi:10.7205/MILMED-D-16-00169.

37. Arenson MB, Whooley MA, Neylan TC, Maguen S, Metzler TJ, Cohen BE. Posttraumatic stress disorder, depression, and suicidal ideation in veterans: Results from the mind your heart study. *Psychiatry Res*. 2018;265:224–230. doi:10.1016/j.psychres.2018.04.046.

38. Gilmore AK, Brignone E, Painter JM, et al. Military sexual trauma and co-occurring posttraumatic stress disorder, depressive disorders, and substance use disorders among returning Afghanistan and Iraq veterans. *Womens Health Issues*. 2016;26:546–554. doi:10.1016/j.whi.2016.07.001.

39. Norman SB, Haller M, Hamblen JL, Southwick SM, Pietrzak RH. The burden of co-occurring alcohol use disorder and PTSD in U.S. military veterans: Comorbidities, functioning, and suicidality. *Psychol Addict Behav*. 2018;32:224–229. doi:10.1037/adb0000348.

40. Stander VA, Thomsen CJ, Highfill-McRoy RM. Etiology of depression comorbidity in combat-related PTSD: A review of the literature. *Clin Psychol Rev*. 2014;34:87–98. doi:10.1016/j.cpr.2013.12.002.

41. Kulas JF, Rosenheck RA. A comparison of veterans with post-traumatic stress disorder, with mild traumatic brain injury and with both disorders: Understanding multimorbidity. *Mil Med*. 2018;183:e114–e122. doi:10.1093/milmed/usx050.

42. Bileveau PJH, Boulos D, Zamorski MA. Contribution of mental and physical disorders to disability in military personnel. *Occup Med*. 2018;68:332–339. doi:10.1093/occmed/kqy066.

43. Brignone E, Fargo JD, Blais RK, Carter ME, Samore MH, Gundlapalli AV. Non-routine discharge from military service: Mental illness, substance use disorders, and suicidality. *Am J Prev Med*. 2017;52:557–565. doi:10.1016/j.amepre.2016.11.015.

44. Buckman JE, Forbes HJ, Clayton T, et al. Early service leavers: A study of the factors associated with premature separation from the UK Armed Forces and the mental health of those who leave early. *Eur J Public Health*. 2013;23:410–415. doi:10.1093/eurpub/cks042.

45. Weeks M, Garber BG, Zamorski MA. Disability and mental disorders in the Canadian Armed Forces. *Can J Psychiatry*. 2016;61:56S–63S. doi:10.1177/0706743716628853.

46. Boscarino JA. Posttraumatic stress disorder and mortality among U.S. army veterans 30 years after military service. *Ann Epidemiol.* 2006;16:248–256. doi:10.1016/j.annepidem.2005.03.009.

47. Ramsawh HJ, Fullerton CS, Mash HB, et al. Risk for suicidal behaviors associated with PTSD, depression, and their comorbidity in the U.S. army. *J Affect Disord.* 2014;161:116–122. doi:10.1016/j.jad.2014.03.016.

48. Merskey H, Bogduk N. *Classification of Chronic Pain: Descriptions of Chronic Pain Syndromes and Definitions of Pain Terms.* Seattle, WA: IASP Press; 1994.

49. Higgins DM, Kerns RD, Brandt CA, et al. Persistent pain and comorbidity among Operation Enduring Freedom/Operation Iraqi Freedom/Operation New Dawn veterans. *Pain Med.* 2014;15:782–790. doi:10.1111/pme.12388.

50. Reif S, Adams R, Ritter G, Williams T, Larson M. Prevalence of pain diagnoses and burden of pain among active duty soldiers, FY2012. *Mil Med.* 2018;183:e330–e337. doi:10.1093/milmed/usx200.

51. Schoneboom B, Perry S, Barnhill W, Giordano N, Nicely KLW, Polomano R. Answering the call to address chronic pain in military service members and veterans: Progress in improving pain care and restoring health. *Nurs Outlook.* 2016;64:459–484. doi:10.1016/j.outlook.2016.05.010.

52. Vandenkerkhof E, VanTil L, Thompson J, et al. Pain in Canadian veterans: Analysis of data from the Survey on Transition to Civilian Life. *Pain Res Manag.* 2015;20:89–95. doi:10.1155/2015/763768.

53. US Veterans Health Administration Memorandum. *Pain as the Fifth Vital Sign.* February 1999. http://mywhatever.com/cifwriter/content/19/abcd617.html. Accessed April 9, 2020.

54. George E, Elman I, Becerra L, Berg S, Borsook D. Pain in an era of armed conflicts: Prevention and treatment for warfighters and civilian casualties. *Prog Neurobiol.* 2016;141:25–44. doi:10.1016/j.pneurobio.2016.04.002.

55. Thomas MM, Harpaz-Rotem I, Tsai J, Southwick SM, Pietrzak RH. Mental and physical health conditions in US combat veterans: Results from the National Health and Resilience in Veterans Study. *Prim Care Companion CNS Disord.* 2017;19. doi:10.4088/PCC.17m02118.

56. Cichowski SB, Rogers RG, Clark EA, Murata E, Murata A, Murata G. Military sexual trauma in female veterans is associated with chronic pain conditions. *Mil Med.* 2017;182:e1895–e1899. doi:10.7205/MILMED-D-16-00393.

57. Driscoll MA, Higgins DM, Seng EK, et al. Trauma, social support, family conflict, and chronic pain in recent service veterans: Does gender matter? *Pain Med.* 2015;16:1101–1111. doi:10.1111/pme.12744.

58. Gauntlett-Gilbert J, Wilson S. Veterans and chronic pain. *Br J Pain.* 2013;7:79–84. doi:10.1177/2049463713482082.

59. El-Gabalawy R, Thompson JM, Sweet J, et al. Comorbidity and functional correlates of anxiety and physical conditions in Canadian Veterans. *J Mil Vet Fam Health.* 2015;1:37–46. doi:10.3138/jmvfh.2014-03.

60. Seal KH, Bertenthal D, Barnes DE, et al. Traumatic brain injury and receipt of prescription opioid therapy for chronic pain in Iraq and Afghanistan veterans: Do clinical practice guidelines matter? *J Pain.* 2018;19:931–941. doi:10.1016/j.jpain.2018.03.005.

61. Booth BM, Davis TD, Cheney AM, Mengelin MA, Torner JC, Sadler AG. Physical health status of female veterans: Contributions of sex partnership and in-military rape. *Psychosom Med.* 2012;74:916–924. doi:10.1097/PSY.0b013e31827078e2.

62. Thompson JM, Pranger T, Sweet J, et al. Disability correlates in Canadian Armed Forces regular force veterans. *Disabil Rehabil.* 2015;37:884–891. doi:10.3109/ 09638288.2014.947441.

63. Stratton KJ, Clark SL, Hawn SE, Amstadter AB, Cifu DX, Walker WC. Longitudinal interactions of pain and posttraumatic stress disorder symptoms in U.S. military service members following blast exposure. *J Pain.* 2014;15:1023–1032. doi:10.1016/ j.jpain.2014.07.002.

64. Seal KH, Bertenthal D, Barnes DE, et al. Association of traumatic brain injury with chronic pain in Iraq and Afghanistan veterans: Effect of comorbid mental health conditions. *Arch Phys Med Rehabil.* 2017;98:1636–1645. doi:10.1016/ j.apmr.2017.03.026.

65. Nampiaparampil DE. Prevalence of chronic pain after traumatic brain injury: A systematic review. *JAMA.* 2008;300:711–719. doi:10.1001/jama.300.6.711.

66. Blakey SM, Wagner HR, Naylor J, et al. Chronic pain, TBI, and PTSD in military veterans: A link to suicidal ideation and violent impulses? *J Pain.* 2018;19:797–806. doi:10.1016/j.jpain.2018.02.012.

67. Elnitsky CA, Blevins C, Findlow JW, Alverio T, Weise D. Student veterans reintegrating from the military to university with traumatic injuries: How does service use relate to health status? *Arch Phys Med Rehabil.* 2018;99:S58–S64. doi:10.1016/j.apmr.2017.10.008.

68. Finley EP, Bollinger M, Noel PH., et al. A national cohort study of the association between polytrauma clinical triad and suicide-related behavior among US veterans who served in Iraq and Afghanistan. *Am J Public Health.* 2015;105:380–387. doi:10.2105/AJPH.2014.301957.

69. Lew HL, Otis JD, Tun C, Kerns RD, Clark ME, Cifu DX. Prevalence of chronic pain, posttraumatic stress disorder, and persistent postconcussive symptoms in OIF/OEF veterans: Polytrauma clinical triad. *J Rehabil Res Dev.* 2009;46:697–702.

70. Pugh MJ, Finley EP, Copeland LA, et al. Complex comorbidity clusters in OEF/OIF veterans: The polytrauma clinical triad and beyond. *Med Care.* 2014;52:172–181. doi:10.1097/MLR.0000000000000059.

71. Outcalt SD, Ang DC, Wu J, Sargent C, Yu Z, Bair MJ. Pain experience of Iraq and Afghanistan veterans with comorbid chronic pain and posttraumatic stress. *J Rehabil Res Dev.* 2014;51:559–570. doi:10.1682/JRRD.2013.06.0134.

72. Hauser W, Galek A, Erbsloh-Moller B, et al. Posttraumatic stress disorder in fibromyalgia syndrome: Prevalence, temporal relationship between posttraumatic stress and fibromyalgia symptoms, and impact on clinical outcome. *Pain.* 2013;154:1216–1223. doi:10.1016/j.pain.2013.03.034.

73. Rosenfeld JV, McFarlane AC, Bragge P, Armonda RA, Grimes JB, Ling GS. Blast-related traumatic brain injury. *Lancet Neurol.* 2013;12:882–893. doi:10.1016/ S1474-4422(13)70161-3.

74. Asmundson GJ, Coons MJ, Taylor S, Katz J. PTSD and the experience of pain: Research and clinical implications of shared vulnerability and mutual maintenance models. *Can J Psychiatry.* 2002;47:930–937. doi:10.1177/070674302047.01004.

75. Taylor S. *Anxiety Sensitivity: Theory, Research, and Treatment of the Fear of Anxiety.* Mahwah, NJ: Lawrence Erlbaum Associates; 1999.

76. Sharp TJ, Harvey AG. Chronic pain and posttraumatic stress disorder: Mutual maintenance? *Clin Psychol Rev.* 2001;21:857–877.

77. Hourani L, Council C, Hubal R, Strange L. Approaches to the primary prevention of posttraumatic stress disorder in the military: A review of the stress control literature. *Mil Med.* 2011;176:721–730. doi:10.7205/MI:MED-D-09-00227.

78. Rizzo A, Buckwalter JG, John B, et al. STRIVE: Stress Resilience in Virtual Environments: A pre-deployment VR system for training emotional coping skills and assessing chronic and acute stress responses. *Stud Health Technol Inform.* 2012;173:379–385.

79. Ilnicki S, Wiederhold BK, Maciolek J, et al. Effectiveness evaluation for short-term group pre-deployment VR computer-assisted stress inoculation training provided to Polish ISAF soldiers. *Stud Health Technol Inform.* 2012;181:113–117.

80. Holbrook TL, Galarneau MR, Dye JL, Quinn K, Dougherty AL. Morphine use after combat injury in Iraq and post-traumatic stress disorder. *N Engl J Med.* 2010;362:110–117. doi:10.1056/NEJMoa0903326.

81. Melcer T, Walker J, Sechriest VF 2nd, Lebedda M, Quinn K, Galarneau M. Glasgow coma scores, early opioids, and posttraumatic stress disorder among combat amputees. *J Trauma Stress.* 2014;27:152–159. doi:10.1002/jts.21909.

82. Reddi D, Curran N. Chronic pain after surgery: Pathophysiology, risk factors and prevention. *Postgrad Med.* 2014;90:222–227. doi:10.1136/postgradmedj-2013-132215.

83. Hicks MH. Mental health screening and coordination of care for soldiers deployed to Iraq and Afghanistan. *Am J Psychiatry.* 2011;168:341–343. doi:10.1176/appi.ajp.2011.11010074.

84. Prins A, Bovin MJ, Smolenski DJ et al. The Primary Care PTSD Screen for DSM-5 (PC-PTSD): Development and evaluation within a veteran primary care sample. *J Gen Intern Med.* 2016;31:1206–1211. doi:10.1007/s11606-016-3703-5.

85. Armed Forces Health Surveillance Branch. Surveillance snapshot: Responses to questions about back pain in post-deployment health assessment questionnaires, U.S. Armed Forces, 2005–2014. *MSMR.* 2016;23:15.

86. McCarthy MD, Thompson SJ, Knox KL. Use of the Air Force Post-Deployment Health Reassessment for the identification of depression and posttraumatic stress disorder: Public health implications for suicide prevention. *Am J Public Health.* 2012;102:S60–S65. doi:10.2105/AJPH.2011.300580.

87. Cook KF, Buckenmaier C, Gershon RC. PASTOR/PROMIS pain outcomes system: What does it mean to pain specialists? *Pain Manag.* 2014;4:277–283.

88. Veterans Affairs Canada. *Comparison to Other Countries.* Veterans Affairs Canada; 2014. https://www.veterans.gc.ca/eng/about-vac/publications-reports/reports/departmental-audit-evaluation/2009-12-nvc/4-4. Accessed April 9, 2020.

89. Bosco MA, Gallinati JL, Clark ME. Conceptualizing and treating comorbid chronic pain and PTSD. *Pain Res Treat.* 2013;2013:174728. doi:10.1155/2013/174728.

90. Otis JD, Keane TM, Kerns RD, Monson C, Scioli E. The development of an integrated treatment for veterans with comorbid chronic pain and posttraumatic stress disorder. *Pain Med.* 2009;10:1300–1311. doi:10.1111/j.1526-4673.2009.00715.x.

91. McGeary D, Moore M, Vriend CA, Peterson AL, Gatchel RJ. The evaluation and treatment of comorbid pain and PTSD in a military setting: An overview. *J Clin Psychol Med Settings*. 2011;18:155. doi:10.1007/s10880-011-9236-5.

92. Lang AJ, Schnurr PP, Jain S, et al. Evaluating transdiagnostic treatment for distress and impairment in veterans: A multi-site randomized controlled trial of Acceptance and Commitment Therapy. *Contemp Clin Trials*. 2012;33:116–123. doi:10.1016/j.cct.2011.08.007.

93. Foa EB, Hembree EA, Rothbaum BO. *Prolonged Exposure Therapy for PTSD: Emotional Processing of Traumatic Experiences, Therapist Guide*. New York, NY: Oxford University Press; 2007.

94. Monson CM, Schnurr PP, Resick PA, Friedman MJ, Young-Xu Y, Stevens SP. Cognitive processing therapy for veterans with military-related posttraumatic stress disorder. *J Consult Clin Psychol*. 2006;74:898–907. doi:10.1037/0022-006X.74.5.898.

95. Watkins LE, Sprang KR, Rothbaum BO. Treating PTSD: A review of evidence-based psychotherapy interventions. *Front Behav Neurosci*. 2018;12:258. doi:10.3389/fnbeh.2018.00258.

96. Galovski TE, Monson C, Bruce SE, Resick PA. Does cognitive-behavioral therapy for PTSD improve perceived health and sleep impairment? *J Trauma Stress*. 2009;22:197–204. doi:10.1002/jts.20418.

15

The Clinical Neuroscience of the Insomnia–Fibromyalgia Link

An Overview for Clinicians

CHRISTINA S. MCCRAE, ASHLEY F. CURTIS, AND DANIEL B. KAY ■

INTRODUCTION

The relationship between fibromyalgia (characterized by chronic widespread pain) and sleep disturbance is well established.[1] Fibromyalgia is linked to subjective sleep complaints accompanied by discomfort, fatigue, pain exacerbation,[2] and sleep architecture alterations.[3,4] Sleep disturbance is a core feature of fibromyalgia,[5] and more than 50% of fibromyalgia patients experience chronic insomnia (3 months or more of difficulty initiating and/or maintaining sleep, early-morning awakening, or nonrestorative sleep).[6] When chronic pain and chronic insomnia co-occur, treatment typically focuses on pain because insomnia is considered a symptom and is expected to improve following pain improvement. However, growing longitudinal, experimental, and trial evidence shows that sleep more reliably predicts chronic pain than vice versa[7,8] and thus may play a mechanistic role in chronic pain. Our recent work showing direct intervention for insomnia positively affects brain structure and function and improves pain in fibromyalgia supports that suggestion.

BRAIN IN FIBROMYALGIA

Sleep Architecture

Relative to healthy controls, fibromyalgia patients show subjective (diary-reported) increased sleep onset latency (SOL),[3] increased fatigue,[9] and reduced sleep quality.[9] Fibromyalgia patients also experience objective (actigraphy/polysomnography) sleep disturbance relative to controls, specifically shorter sleep duration and increased time spent awake after initial sleep onset and before final awakening (i.e., wake after sleep onset [WASO]).[10] Worse self-reported sleep quality is associated with shorter actigraphic sleep duration and increased sleep fragmentation.[9] Discrepancies between subjective and objective sleep in fibromyalgia are linked to age,[11] opioid use[12]/dosage,[11] and pain intensity.[12]

Although alpha sleep/intrusions (i.e., brain activity indicating wakefulness with eyes closed) in electroencephalography (EEG) recordings during slow-wave sleep (SWS) were originally a hallmark of fibromyalgia,[13] recent work suggests that alpha intrusions are not specific to fibromyalgia and may generally indicate non-restorative sleep.[14] Other sleep architecture metrics may better predict fibromyalgia, such as ratio of delta to alpha waves in non–rapid eye movement (NREM) sleep (lower ratios in fibromyalgia patients versus controls[14]) and altered sleep staging (more time in stage 1 "lighter" sleep and less time in SWS "deep" sleep for fibromyalgia vs. controls[15]). The sleep shift index (how many times per night sleep stages change) may be particularly important because fibromyalgia patients have higher stage shift indices than controls.[16] Studies also show that fibromyalgia patients have increased periodic leg movements.[17] Together, alpha intrusions,[18] superficial sleep, and increased muscle arousals may contribute to increased pain in fibromyalgia. Additionally, given recent work showing associations between opioids and polysomnography-assessed sleep,[19] pain medication and other factors (e.g., pain severity, body mass index) should be considered in the understanding of fibromyalgia pathophysiology.

Circadian Rhythm

The biological circadian rhythm (internal sleep–wake 24-hour "clock"), controlled by the hypothalamus and hypothalamic-pituitary-adrenal (HPA) axis, is associated with melatonin and cortisol secretion, alertness, body temperature, immune system function, and digestion and is affected by environmental factors such as light exposure.[20] In healthy adults, melatonin levels are affected by darkness/light, increasing at darkness onset, peaking near the middle of the night, and reaching minimum levels in the morning.[21] Cortisol levels are generally lowest around midnight, are highest within 30 minutes of awakening, and decrease throughout the day/evening.[22] Several studies report differences between fibromyalgia patients and controls in melatonin secretion, with one study showing decreased nighttime levels[23] and higher daytime (6:00 AM–6:00 PM) levels.[24] Greater melatonin secretion in fibromyalgia is associated with greater depression, insomnia severity, number of tender/trigger points, and with lower pain thresholds.[24] Another study found no difference in morning, afternoon, and evening serum cortisol levels between women with fibromyalgia relative to controls.[25] In this study, higher cortisol levels were observed in fibromyalgia versus controls only at midnight.[25] Other studies found no difference between fibromyalgia patients and controls in cortisol profiles (i.e., AM/PM level difference),[26] or in patterns of change over 40 hours of sleep–wake routines in three circadian rhythm makers: cortisol, melatonin, and core body temperature.[27]

Central Sensitization/Quantitative Sensory Testing

Predominant pathophysiology of fibromyalgia pain is abnormal central pain processing, or central sensitization.[7] Central sensitization leads to increased central nervous system response to both noxious and non-noxious stimuli (e.g., pressure, temperature, light, medication). Patients with fibromyalgia experience increased excitability of spinal and supraspinal neurons,[28] associated with increased sensitivity to pain (hyperalgesia) and pain in the presence of innocuous stimuli (mechanical allodynia). Central sensitization increases receptor fields of dorsal horn neurons, associated with spontaneous pain.[29,30] Quantitative sensory testing (determination of pain sensation thresholds for warm/cold stimuli) reveals that fibromyalgia patients report greater increases in pain response to repetitive noxious stimuli (e.g., heat) delivered at a constant intensity, and they experience pain increases after fewer stimulus exposures and prolonged pain aftersensations (windup) relative to pain-free controls.[28] Importantly, mechanical allodynia, enhanced windup, and prolonged aftersensations are central sensitization features that predict clinical pain.[31]

Neuroimaging

Fibromyalgia is associated with diffuse gray matter atrophy in the amygdala, cingulate, insula, medial frontal cortex, parahippocampus, and prefrontal cortex.[32-35] Early work showed a three-fold stronger association between total gray matter volume reduction and increasing age among fibromyalgia patients versus controls, suggesting that fibromyalgia might be linked to premature aging.[34] However, work from our lab revealed reductions in hippocampal volume bilaterally in patients with fibromyalgia versus controls, even after controlling for potential confounding factors such as age and depression.[36] Unlike others,[34] we did not observe an association between fibromyalgia duration and hippocampal volume difference between fibromyalgia and controls. Prior research reports decreased gray matter volume in fibromyalgia patients versus controls in left middle/rostral anterior cingulate cortex and left middle insula, and these differences were not associated with response or affective evaluation of pain.[32] Prolonged stress response (and associated disrupted HPA axis functioning and increased inflammation[37]) may lead to hippocampal volume loss.[38]

Studies examining the resting state default mode network reveal that fibromyalgia is characterized by heightened activity and connectivity patterns not typically observed in healthy persons.[39,40] Exciting pilot work from our lab shows cortical plasticity following cognitive behavioral therapy for insomnia (CBT-I). An 8-week treatment prompted reversal of cortical thinning in several brain regions.[41] This suggests that neuroplasticity in fibromyalgia may be achieved through cognitive and behavioral techniques.

Other Factors

Cognitive disturbance and altered immune response and inflammation also contribute to fibromyalgia pathophysiology. Compared with controls, fibromyalgia patients perform worse on tasks measuring mental calculations,[42] auditory concentration,[43] verbal memory,[44] visuospatial memory, working memory,[44] decision-making,[45] cognitive flexibility and planning,[46] verbal fluency,[47] and attention.[44] Regarding inflammatory processes, relative to controls, fibromyalgia patients have increased levels of peripheral blood-based[48,49] and central cerebrospinal fluid-based[50] proinflammatory cytokine interleukin-8 (IL-8). Research in human and animal fibromyalgia models show that increased IL-8 is due to increased sympathetic nervous system activation[51] and associated with increased pain intensity[48] and lower pain thresholds.[52] Figure 15.1 summarizes the proposed potential pathophysiological mechanisms underlying insomnia in fibromyalgia.

BRAIN IN INSOMNIA

Sleep Architecture

Patients with insomnia commonly report difficulty falling asleep, frequent nighttime awakenings, extended WASO, shorter sleep duration, night-to-night

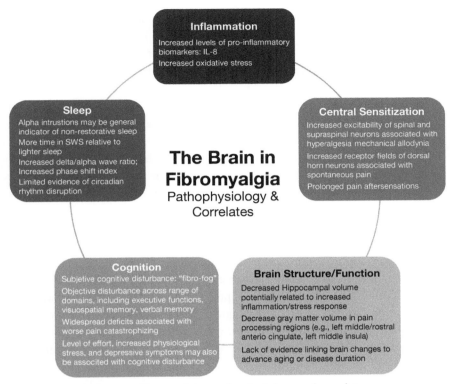

Figure 15.1. The brain in fibromyalgia—pathophysiology and correlates.

variability in sleep quality, and unrefreshing sleep. Polysomnography generally replicates self-reports but often fails to reflect the degree of sleep disturbance reported by insomnia patients.[53] One interpretation for subjective-objective discrepancy is that self-reports are more sensitive than polysomnography to sleep–wake dysfunction. More refined electrophysiological measures have detected alterations in sleep microarchitecture in insomnia, including greater high-frequency EEG activity, altered evoked potentials during sleep onset and NREM sleep, and increased cyclic alternating pattern rate.[54] These irregularities are common to many sleep and psychiatric conditions and thus are not pathognomonic of insomnia disorder but may correlate with self-reported difficulties.[53]

Neuroimaging

Insomnia is consistently associated with lower regional brain activity during active and quiet wakefulness, including greater EEG-assessed delta power[55] and lower cerebral blood flow, cerebral metabolism, or blood oxygen level–dependent signal in heteromodal regions of the neocortex, cingulate, precuneus, left medial temporal lobe, left insula, basal ganglia, thalamus, and left brainstem during either active or quiet wakefulness.[56] Increased and decreased functional connectivity is linked to insomnia during wakefulness, suggesting altered information processing. Reduced brain activity and impaired information processing, potentially due to heightened sleep drive during waking states, may underpin daytime impairments associated with insomnia.

Relative to good sleepers, insomnia patients have less NREM sleep–wake differences in relative glucose metabolism in the precuneus/posterior cingulate, left frontoparietal cortices, and lingual/fusiform areas.[57] This suggests they have less activation during wakefulness and/or less deactivation during NREM sleep. Sleep deprivation results in reduced relative cerebral glucose metabolism during recovery NREM sleep in these brain regions in good sleepers and insomnia patients, suggesting that increasing sleep drive may deactivate brain regions associated with insomnia pathophysiology.[58] During stable NREM sleep, insomnia patients have lower cerebral blood flow or relative glucose metabolism than good sleepers in the anterior cingulate, medial frontal gyrus, orbitofrontal cortex, inferior frontal gyrus, middle and posterior cingulate, precuneus, occipital lobe, superior and inferior temporal gyri, medial temporal lobe, and basal ganglia. Sleep discrepancy is linked to greater relative glucose metabolism during NREM sleep in regions associated with conscious awareness, including anterior insula, anterior cingulate, and middle/posterior cingulate.[56] Altered brain activity during NREM sleep may explain why insomnia patients report being awake during polysomnography-defined sleep. During rapid eye movement (REM) sleep, patients with insomnia have greater glucose metabolism in the dorsal anterior cingulate cortex and lower glucose metabolism in the ventromedial prefrontal cortex.[59] One hypothesis is that altered brain activity during sleep in insomnia patients reflects regionalized sleep disturbance that leads to local sleep deprivation contributing to brain region-specific impairments during wakefulness.[57]

MECHANISMS

We propose that insomnia confers vulnerability to fibromyalgia and vice versa, resulting in a "vicious, self-perpetuating cycle." Specifically, we propose that fibromyalgia alters processes involved in sleep–wake regulation (arousal, sleep drive, conscious awareness), thereby conferring insomnia risk; and insomnia symptoms result in regionalized sleep disturbance in brain areas that modulate

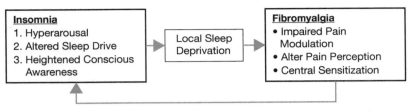

Figure 15.2. In our model, fibromyalgia alters processes involved in sleep-wake regulation (arousal, sleep drive, or conscious awareness), thereby conferring risk for insomnia. Insomnia symptoms result in localsleep deprivation in brain regions that modulate and integrate pain/sensory information, thereby conferring risk for fibromyalgia.

and integrate pain/sensory information, thereby conferring fibromyalgia risk (Figure 15.2).

Pathways: Fibromyalgia to Insomnia

As previously described, fibromyalgia is associated with central sensitization, which activates ascending arousal systems, resulting in cortical arousal. Potential evidence for heightened cortical arousal in fibromyalgia includes heightened waking state EEG beta activity, increased alpha sleep, increased NREM cyclic alternating patterns, and higher glutamate concentrations in the right posterior insula.[60] Heightened activation of brainstem arousal circuitry also blocks sleep drive expression by inhibiting hypothalamic sleep-promoting systems.[61] Heightened arousal induced by pain may explain sleep difficulties in fibromyalgia.[62]

Sleep drive alteration is another potential mechanism through which fibromyalgia confers insomnia risk. Patients with fibromyalgia spend more time inactive and napping to cope with pain.[63] These behaviors may increase daytime sleep drive expression and prevent accumulation of use-dependent sleep processes necessary to drive nocturnal sleep. Inactivity and napping may also alter circadian sleep processes in fibromyalgia[24] thereby misaligning use-dependent and circadian sleep processes. Potential markers of altered NREM sleep drive in fibromyalgia include less SWS, lower sleep spindle frequency and duration, alpha intrusions, and altered NREM delta power. However, markers of altered sleep drive are not consistently captured with global measures, necessitating brain region–specific measures of sleep drive in fibromyalgia.

Fibromyalgia may also contribute to insomnia through heightened conscious awareness during sleep. Increased pain signaling may persist during sleep, contributing to local sleep disturbance in brain regions involved in conscious awareness. Evidence that fibromyalgia patients have heightened conscious awareness during sleep include findings that they are more likely than controls to endorse being "aware of thinking all night,"[3] and they have better recall of nocturnal events (behaviorally signaled awakenings).[64] Fibromyalgia has been linked to greater sleep discrepancy, suggesting their patterns of conscious awareness may be misaligned with global sleep–wake states.[12] Several studies suggest that fibromyalgia patients experience alpha sleep. Despite some counter-evidence in patients with fibromyalgia,[65] alpha activity may reflect conscious awareness.[66] More robust measures of conscious awareness during sleep in fibromyalgia are needed.

Pathways: Insomnia to Fibromyalgia

Insomnia may impair brain functioning in regions involved in pain modulation.[67] Sleep disturbances contribute to fibromyalgia symptoms, for example, sleep loss results in reduced pain inhibition and an increase in spontaneous pain nonrestorative sleep predicting future widespread pain a core symptom of fibromyaligia.[68,69] Although earlier studies failed to find associations between alpha-sleep and post-sleep fibromyalgia symptoms,[3] one study showed that phasic alpha intrusions (but not tonic alpha activity) during NREM sleep is associated with greater morning pain in fibromyalgia,[70] Greater WASO discrepancy in patients with comorbid insomnia and fibromyalgia is associated with greater morning pain.[12] Heightened regional cortical activation associated with conscious awareness or alpha activity during NREM sleep may represent regionalized sleep disturbance that leads to local sleep deprivation in brain regions that modulate and integrate pain information.

Fibromyalgia is associated with reduced regional cerebral blood flow, glucose metabolism, and functional connectivity in several brain regions associated with pain modulation and integration during the resting state. Similar to fibromyalgia, the resting state in insomnia is associated with hypometabolism in brain regions related to pain modulation and integration, including frontal cortex; anterior, middle, and posterior cingulate; left insula; caudate; temporal lobe; parietal lobe; precuneus; occipital lobe; left hippocampus; putamen; left brainstem; and left amygdala.[56] Heightened theta activity in prefrontal and anterior cingulate cortices during the resting state is associated with daytime tenderness and tiredness in fibromyalgia.[71] Findings may suggest greater regional sleep drive in the frontal and anterior cingulate, which contributes to lower pain modulation, greater pain sensitivity, and fibromyalgia risk.

OTHER FACTORS

Other factors affecting prevalence and disease profiles of fibromyalgia and insomnia have been identified and warrant further investigation, including sex (women show higher fibromyalgia prevalence),[72] age (middle-aged and older adults at greater risk for insomnia and fibromyalgia),[72,73] race/ethnicity,[74,75] and socioeconomic status.[76]

TREATMENT

Several pharmacological and behavioral treatments are currently used to treat fibromyalgia and insomnia symptoms (Table 15.1). Generally, well-established behavioral treatments such as CBT-I and CBT for pain (CBT-P) are more promising alternatives to pharmacological interventions in terms of providing long-term sleep and pain management.

Insomnia

CBT-I, the recommended first-line treatment for chronic insomnia,[77] is an efficacious multicomponent treatment generally consisting of sleep hygiene, stimulus control, sleep restriction, and cognitive techniques. The vast majority (~70–80%) of persons treated behaviorally show sleep improvements that maintain through follow-up of up to 2 years (average, 6 months), and patients rate behavioral techniques as more acceptable than sleep medications.[78] CBT-I facilitates homeostatic sleep drive and improves sleep architecture by reducing time to delta wave peak (i.e., SWS).[79] Unlike sleep medications, behavioral approaches do not pose serious side effects and may be more effective in the long run.[80]

CONCLUSION

Pharmacological and behavioral treatments aimed at pain offer short-term symptom improvement but little benefit for long-term pain management. Mounting evidence suggests that targeting sleep and related mechanisms holds promise for improving central pain processing and long-term pain management. More research examining sleep's potential to exert positive, sustained influence on central pain mechanisms and clinical pain is needed.

Table 15.1 SUMMARY OF CURRENT TREATMENT OPTIONS FOR FIBROMYALGIA AND INSOMNIA

Treatment type	Name	Evidence
Fibromyalgia		
Pharmacological	Antidepressants	• Antidepressants such as tricyclic antidepressants (e.g., amitriptyline), which inhibit reuptake of serotonin into neuronal presynaptic terminals are associated with modest to moderate pain improvement and moderate sleep improvement in fibromyalgia.[81]
		• Adverse side effects of tricyclics (e.g., seizures, weight gain, dry mouth, gastrointestinal disturbances)[82] prompted investigations of newer antidepressants such as selective serotonin reuptake inhibitors (e.g., fluoxetine, citalopram). However, these are less effective than the former drug types for reducing symptoms.[83]
	Opioids	• Although opioids are not recommended for fibromyalgia treatment, they are commonly prescribed.[84]
		• Unfortunately, evidence showing their efficacy for long-term pain reduction is lacking.[85]
		• Additionally, long-term opioid use is associated with adverse side effects, including tolerance, immune system disturbance/suppression, and cognitive disturbance.[86,87]
		• Opioid use in fibromyalgia is also associated with disrupted sleep (i.e., longer SOL, increased lighter staged sleep, less SWS)[11,88] and sleep architecture.[19]
		• Lack of opioid efficacy in fibromyalgia may be due to reduced availability of opioid receptors in pain-processing neural regions (e.g., amygdala, dorsal anterior cingulate).[89]
Nonpharmacological	Massage therapy	• Massage therapy provides short-term relief of fibromyalgia pain.[90]
	Sulfur bath therapy	• Sulfur bath therapy improves fibromyalgia symptoms (fatigue, stiffness, physical functioning, pain severity), but pain improvement is not maintained at 3 months of follow-up.[91]
	Olive oil consumption	• Preliminary data show that daily olive oil consumption may relieve oxidative cellular stress and improve functional capacity in fibromyalgia.[92]
		• More research with larger samples is needed to further support its therapeutic efficacy.

	Pulsed ultrasound and inferential current	• Twelve sessions of pulsed ultrasound and interferential current applied at fibromyalgia tender points are associated with post-treatment reduction in number and pain threshold of tender points, as well as improvements in fatigue, SOL, and sleep depth.[93] • Interferential current is thought to reduce pain through blockage of pain potentials in dorsal horn spinal cord neurons and prevention of synaptic plastic changes that lead to features of central sensitization (i.e., hyperalgesia and allodynia).[93,94]
	Aerobic exercise	• A meta-analysis of 28 studies reports slight- to moderate-intensity aerobic exercise two to three times per week over 4 weeks leads to small post-treatment improvements in pain, fatigue, and mood.[95]
	Tai chi exercise	• Twenty-four weeks of mind-body tai chi exercise reduce fibromyalgia symptoms (global ratings on fibromyalgia impact scale) with greater treatment adherence and mood improvements after treatment relative to aerobic exercise.[96]
	CBT-I and CBT-P	• Reductions in clinically significant pain in the majority of fibromyalgia patients who underwent 8 weeks of CBT-I or CBT-P, with CBT-I (not CBT-P) showed pain reduction maintenance at 6 months of follow-up.[97] • CBT-I increased cortical thickness in brain regions associated with central sensitization (i.e., left lateral orbitofrontal cortex, left rostral middle frontal cortex), and these neural changes are associated with improved WASO.[41]
Insomnia Pharmacological	Hypnotics	• Hypnotic drugs such as benzodiazepine receptor agonists (e.g., flurazepam) and nonbenzodiazepines (e.g., zolpidem) are commonly prescribed, and they facilitate sedation by altering GABA receptors to increase affinity for the GABA inhibitory neurotransmitter.[98] • Further, benzodiazepines are associated with adverse effects such as cognitive disturbance, anxiety, physical dependence, and fall risk in older adults.[99] • While benzodiazepines improve sleep in the short-term, they are not effective for long-term management.[100] • Current guidelines only recommend hypnotics as adjunct to first-line behavioral treatments.[100]

(continued)

Table 15.1 CONTINUED

Treatment type	Name	Evidence
	Melatonin Receptor agonists	• Melatonin receptor agonists (e.g., ramelteon) are also commonly prescribed because they bind to melatonin receptors to shift the sleep–wake cycle and facilitate sleep.[101] • Melatonin receptor agonists are associated with increased fatigue and nausea.[102] Other drugs, such as antidepressants (e.g., trazodone, mirtazapine), are commonly prescribed in low doses but lack efficacy for long-term insomnia improvement.[100] • While melatonin receptor agonists improve sleep in the short-term, they are not effective for long-term management.[100]
Nonpharmacological	CBT-I	• The efficacy of CBT-I, a multicomponent treatment generally consisting of sleep hygiene, stimulus control, sleep restriction, and cognitive techniques, is well established and currently the recommended first-line treatment for insomnia.[77] • The vast majority (~70–80%) of persons treated behaviorally show sleep improvements that maintain through follow-up of up to 2 years (average, 6 months), and patients rate behavioral techniques as more acceptable than sleep medications.[78] • CBT-I facilitates homeostatic sleep drive and improves sleep architecture by reducing time to delta wave peak (i.e., reducing time to SWS).[79] • Unlike sleep medications, behavioral approaches do not pose serious side effects and may be more cost-effective in the long run.[80]

CBT-I = cognitive behavioral therapy for insomnia; CBT-P = cognitive behavioral therapy for pain; GABA = gamma-aminobutyric acid; SOL = sleep onset latency; SWS = slow-wave sleep.

REFERENCES

1. Harding SM. Sleep in fibromyalgia patients: Subjective and objective findings. *Am J Med Sci*. 1998;315(6):367–376.
2. Moldofsky H. Nonrestorative sleep and symptoms after a febrile illness in patients with fibrositis and chronic fatigue syndromes. *J Rheumatol Suppl*. 1989;19:150–153.
3. Horne JA, Shackell BS. Alpha-like EEG activity in non-REM sleep and the fibromyalgia (fibrositis) syndrome. *Electroencephalogr Clin Neurophysiol*. 1991;79(4):271–276.
4. Branco J, Atalaia A, Paiva T. Sleep cycles and alpha-delta sleep in fibromyalgia syndrome. *J Rheumatol*. 1994;21(6):1113–1117.
5. Wolfe F, Clauw DJ, Fitzcharles MA, et al. The American College of Rheumatology preliminary diagnostic criteria for fibromyalgia and measurement of symptom severity. *Arthritis Care Res*. 2010;62(5):600–610.
6. Wolfe F, Smythe HA, Yunus MB, et al. The American College of Rheumatology 1990 criteria for the classification of fibromyalgia. *Arthritis Rheum*. 1990;33(2):160–172.
7. Finan PH, Goodin BR, Smith MT. The association of sleep and pain: An update and a path forward. *J Pain*. 2013;14(12):1539–1552.
8. Smith MT, Quartana PJ, Okonkwo RM, Nasir A. Mechanisms by which sleep disturbance contributes to osteoarthritis pain: A conceptual model. *Curr Pain Headache Rep*. 2009;13(6):447–454.
9. Landis CA, Frey CA, Lentz MJ, Rothermel J, Buchwald D, Shaver JL. Self-reported sleep quality and fatigue correlates with actigraphy in midlife women with fibromyalgia. *Nurs Res*. 2003;52(3):140–147.
10. Roehrs T, Diederichs C, Gillis M, et al. Nocturnal sleep, daytime sleepiness and fatigue in fibromyalgia patients compared to rheumatoid arthritis patients and healthy controls: A preliminary study. *Sleep Med*. 2013;14(1):109–115.
11. Curtis AF, Miller MB, Boissoneault J, et al. Discrepancies in sleep diary and actigraphy assessments in adults with fibromyalgia: Associations with opioid dose and age. *J Sleep Res*. 2018:e12746.
12. Chan WS, Levsen MP, Puyat S, et al. Sleep discrepancy in patients with comorbid fibromyalgia and insomnia: Demographic, behavioral, and clinical correlates. *J Clin Sleep Med*. 2018;14(11):1911–1919.
13. Roizenblatt S, Moldofsky H, Benedito-Silva AA, Tufik S. Alpha sleep characteristics in fibromyalgia. *Arthritis Rheum*. 2001;44(1):222–230.
14. Rosenfeld VW, Rutledge DN, Stern JM. Polysomnography with quantitative EEG in patients with and without fibromyalgia. *J Clin Neurophysiol*. 2015;32(2):164–170.
15. Wu Y-L, Chang L-Y, Lee H-C, Fang S-C, Tsai P-S. Sleep disturbances in fibromyalgia: A meta-analysis of case-control studies. *J Psychosom Res*. 2017;96:89–97.
16. Burns JW, Crofford LJ, Chervin RD. Sleep stage dynamics in fibromyalgia patients and controls. *Sleep Med*. 2008;9(6):689–696.
17. González JLB, Fernández TVS, Rodríguez LA, Muñiz J, Giráldez SL. Sleep architecture in patients with fibromyalgia. *Psicothema*. 2011;23(3):368–373.
18. Moldofsky H, Lue F. The relationship of alpha and delta EEG frequencies to pain and mood in "fibrositis" patients treated with chlorpromazine and L-tryptophan. *Electroenceph Clin Neurophysiol*. 1980;50(1–2):71–80.

19. Curtis AF, Miller MB, Rathinakumar H, et al. Opioid use, pain intensity, age and sleep architecture in patients with fibromyalgia and insomnia. *Pain.* 2019;160(9):2086–2092.

20. Mahdi AA, Fatima G, Das SK, Verma NS. Abnormality of circadian rhythm of serum melatonin and other biochemical parameters in fibromyalgia syndrome. *Indian J Biochem Biophys.* 2011;48(2):82–87.

21. Brzezinski A. Melatonin in humans. *N Engl J Med.* 1997;336(3):186–195.

22. Bauer ME. Stress, glucocorticoids and ageing of the immune system. *Stress.* 2005;8(1):69–83.

23. Wikner J, Hirsch U, Wetterberg L, Röjdmark S. Fibromyalgia: A syndrome associated with decreased nocturnal melatonin secretion. *Clin Endocrinol.* 1998;49(2):179–183.

24. Caumo W, Hidalgo MP, Souza A, Torres ILS, Antunes LC. Melatonin is a biomarker of circadian dysregulation and is correlated with major depression and fibromyalgia symptom severity. *J Pain Res.* 2019;12:545–556.

25. Fatima G, Das SK, Mahdi AA, et al. Circadian rhythm of serum cortisol in female patients with fibromyalgia syndrome. *Indian J Clin Biochem.* 2013;28(2):181–184.

26. Orozco-Acosta E, Benítez-Agudelo JC, León-Jacobus A, Román NF. Serum cortisol levels and neuropsychological impairments in patients diagnosed with fibromyalgia. *Acta Esp Psiquiatr.* 2018;46(1):1–11.

27. Klerman EB, Goldenberg DL, Brown EN, Maliszewski AM, Adler GK. Circadian rhythms of women with fibromyalgia. *J Clin Endocrinol Metab.* 2001;86(3):1034–1039.

28. Staud R, Vierck CJ, Cannon RL, Mauderli AP, Price DD. Abnormal sensitization and temporal summation of second pain (wind-up) in patients with fibromyalgia syndrome. *Pain.* 2001;91(1–2):165–175.

29. Staud R. Evidence of involvement of central neural mechanisms in generating fibromyalgia pain. *Curr Rheumatol Rep.* 2002;4(4):299–305.

30. Liu H, Mantyh PW, Basbaum AI. NMDA-receptor regulation of substance P release from primary afferent nociceptors. *Nature.* 1997;386(6626):721.

31. Staud R, Robinson ME, Vierck CJ Jr, Cannon RC, Mauderli AP, Price DD. Ratings of experimental pain and pain-related negative affect predict clinical pain in patients with fibromyalgia syndrome. *Pain.* 2003;105(1–2):215–222.

32. Robinson ME, Craggs JG, Price DD, Perlstein WM, Staud R. Gray matter volumes of pain-related brain areas are decreased in fibromyalgia syndrome. *J Pain.* 2011;12(4):436–443.

33. Burgmer M, Gaubitz M, Konrad C, et al. Decreased gray matter volumes in the cingulo-frontal cortex and the amygdala in patients with fibromyalgia. *Psychosom Med.* 2009;71(5):566–573.

34. Kuchinad A, Schweinhardt P, Seminowicz DA, Wood PB, Chizh BA, Bushnell MC. Accelerated brain gray matter loss in fibromyalgia patients: Premature aging of the brain? *J Neurosci.* 2007;27(15):4004–4007.

35. Lutz J, Jäger L, de Quervain D, et al. White and gray matter abnormalities in the brain of patients with fibromyalgia: A diffusion-tensor and volumetric imaging study. *Arthritis Rheum.* 2008;58(12):3960–3969.

36. McCrae CS, O'Shea AM, Boissoneault J, et al. Fibromyalgia patients have reduced hippocampal volume compared with healthy controls. *J Pain Res.* 2015;8:47.

37. Griep EN, Boersma JW. Altered reactivity of the hypothalamic-pituitary-adrenal axis in the primary fibromyalgia syndrome. *J Rheumatol.* 1993;20(3):469–474.
38. McEwen BS, Magarinos AM. Stress and hippocampal plasticity: Implications for the pathophysiology of affective disorders. *Hum Psychopharmacol.* 2001;16(S1):S7–S19.
39. Cifre I, Sitges C, Fraiman D, et al. Disrupted functional connectivity of the pain network in fibromyalgia. *Psychosom Med.* 2012;74(1):55–62.
40. Napadow V, LaCount L, Park K, As-Sanie S, Clauw DJ, Harris RE. Intrinsic brain connectivity in fibromyalgia is associated with chronic pain intensity. *Arthritis Rheum.* 2010;62(8):2545–2555.
41. McCrae CS, Mundt JM, Curtis AF, et al. Gray matter changes following cognitive behavioral therapy for patients with comorbid fibromyalgia and insomnia: A pilot study. *J Clin Sleep Med.* 2018;14(09):1595–1603.
42. Reyes del Paso GA, Pulgar A, Duschek S, Garrido S. Cognitive impairment in fibromyalgia syndrome: The impact of cardiovascular regulation, pain, emotional disorders and medication. *Eur J Pain.* 2012;16(3):421–429.
43. Grace GM, Nielson WR, Hopkins M, Berg MA. Concentration and memory deficits in patients with fibromyalgia syndrome. *J Clin Exp Neuropsychol.* 1999;21(4):477–487.
44. Dick BD, Verrier MJ, Harker KT, Rashiq S. Disruption of cognitive function in fibromyalgia syndrome. *Pain.* 2008;139(3):610–616.
45. Hess LE, Haimovici A, Muñoz MA, Montoya P. Beyond pain: Modeling decision-making deficits in chronic pain. *Front Behav Neurosci.* 2014;8:263.
46. Galvez-Sánchez CM, Reyes del Paso GA, Duschek S. Cognitive impairments in fibromyalgia syndrome: Associations with positive and negative affect, alexithymia, pain catastrophizing and self-esteem. *Front Psychol.* 2018;9:377.
47. Park DC, Glass JM, Minear M, Crofford LJ. Cognitive function in fibromyalgia patients. *Arthritis Rheum.* 2001;44(9):2125–2133.
48. Gur A, Karakoc M, Erdogan S, Nas K, Cevik R, Sarac A. Regional cerebral blood flow and cytokines in young females with fibromyalgia. *Clinical and experimental rheumatology.* 2002;20(6):753–760.
49. Wang H, Moser M, Schiltenwolf M, Buchner M. Circulating cytokine levels compared to pain in patients with fibromyalgia: A prospective longitudinal study over 6 months. *J Rheumatol.* 2008;35(7):1366–1370.
50. Kadetoff D, Lampa J, Westman M, Andersson M, Kosek E. Evidence of central inflammation in fibromyalgia: Increased cerebrospinal fluid interleukin-8 levels. *J Neuroimmunol.* 2012;242(1–2):33–38.
51. Black PH. Stress and the inflammatory response: A review of neurogenic inflammation. *Brain Behav Immunity.* 2002;16(6):622–653.
52. Yamamoto J, Nishiyori A, Takami S, Ohtani Y, Minami M, Satoh M. A hyperalgesic effect of intracerebroventricular cytokine-induced neutrophil chemoattractant-1 in the rat paw pressure test. *Eur J Pharmacol.* 1998;363(2–3):131–133.
53. Maes J, Verbraecken J, Willemen M, et al. Sleep misperception, EEG characteristics and autonomic nervous system activity in primary insomnia: A retrospective study on polysomnographic data. *Int J Psychophysiology.* 2014;91(3):163–171.
54. Feige B, Baglioni C, Spiegelhalder K, Hirscher V, Nissen C, Riemann D. The microstructure of sleep in primary insomnia: An overview and extension. *Int J Psychophysiol.* 2013;89(2):171–180.

55. Freedman RR. EEG power spectra in sleep-onset insomnia. *Electroencephalogr Clin Neurophysiol.* 1986;63(5):408–413.
56. Kay DB, Buysse DJ. Hyperarousal and beyond: New insights to the pathophysiology of insomnia disorder through functional neuroimaging studies. *Brain Sci.* 2017;7(3):pii: 23.
57. Kay DB, Karim HT, Soehner AM, et al. Sleep-wake differences in relative regional cerebral metabolic rate for glucose among patients with insomnia compared with good sleepers. *Sleep.* 2016;39(10):1779–1794.
58. Kay DB, Karim HT, Hasler BP, et al. Impact of acute sleep restriction on cerebral glucose metabolism during recovery non-rapid eye movement sleep among individuals with primary insomnia and good sleeper controls. *Sleep Med.* 2019;55:81–91.
59. Pace-Schott EF, Germain A, Milad MR. Sleep and REM sleep disturbance in the pathophysiology of PTSD: The role of extinction memory. *Biol Mood Anxiety Disord.* 2015;5:3.
60. Harris RE, Sundgren PC, Craig AD, et al. Elevated insular glutamate in fibromyalgia is associated with experimental pain. *Arthritis Rheum.* 2009;60(10):3146–3152.
61. Saper CB, Fuller PM, Pedersen NP, Lu J, Scammell TE. Sleep state switching. *Neuron.* 2010;68(6):1023–1042.
62. Rizzi M, Sarzi-Puttini P, Atzeni F, et al. Cyclic alternating pattern: A new marker of sleep alteration in patients with fibromyalgia? *J Rheumatol.* 2004;31(6):1193–1199.
63. Morin CM, Kowatch RA, Wade JB. Behavioral management of sleep disturbances secondary to chronic pain. *J Behav Ther Exp Psychiatry.* 1989;20(4):295–302.
64. Anch AM, Lue FA, MacLean AW, Moldofsky H. Sleep physiology and psychological aspects of the fibrositis (fibromyalgia) syndrome. *Can J Psychol.* 1991;45(2):179–184.
65. Perlis ML, Giles DE, Bootzin RR, et al. Alpha sleep and information processing, perception of sleep, pain, and arousability in fibromyalgia. *Int J Neurosci.* 1997;89(3–4):265–280.
66. Simon CW, Emmons WH. EEG, consciousness, and sleep. *Science.* 1956;124(3231):1066–1069.
67. Krause AJ, Prather AA, Wager TD, Lindquist MA, Walker MP. The pain of sleep loss: A brain characterization in humans. *J Neurosci.* 2019;39(12):2291–2300.
68. McBeth J, Lacey RJ, Wilkie R. Predictors of new-onset widespread pain in older adults: Results from a population-based prospective cohort study in the UK. *Arthritis Rheum.* 2014;66(3):757–767.
69. Smith MT, Edwards RR, McCann UD, Haythornthwaite JA. The effects of sleep deprivation on pain inhibition and spontaneous pain in women. *Sleep.* 2007;30(4):494–505.
70. Roizenblatt S, Moldofsky H, Benedito-Silva AA, Tufik S. Alpha sleep characteristics in fibromyalgia. *Arthritis Rheum.* 2001;44(1):222–230.
71. Fallon N, Chiu Y, Nurmikko T, Stancak A. Altered theta oscillations in resting EEG of fibromyalgia syndrome patients. *Eur J Pain.* 2018;22(1):49–57.
72. Queiroz LP. Worldwide epidemiology of fibromyalgia. *Curr Pain Headache Rep.* 2013;17(8):356.
73. Jaussent I, Dauvilliers Y, Ancelin M-L, et al. Insomnia symptoms in older adults: Associated factors and gender differences. *Am J Geriatr Psychiatry.* 2011;19(1):88–97.

74. Clark P, Paiva ES, Ginovker A, Salomón PA. A patient and physician survey of fibromyalgia across Latin America and Europe. *BMC Musculoskel Disord.* 2013;14(1):188.
75. Roberts RE, Roberts CR, Chan W. Ethnic differences in symptoms of insomnia among adolescents. *Sleep.* 2006;29(3):359–365.
76. Gellis LA, Lichstein KL, Scarinci IC, et al. Socioeconomic status and insomnia. *J Abnorm Psychol.* 2005;114(1):111.
77. Morin CM, Bootzin RR, Buysse DJ, Edinger JD, Espie CA, Lichstein KL. Psychological and behavioral treatment of insomnia: Update of the recent evidence (1998–2004). *Sleep.* 2006;29(11):1398–1414.
78. Morin CM, Hauri PJ, Espie CA, Spielman AJ, Buysse DJ, Bootzin RR. Nonpharmacologic treatment of chronic insomnia. *Sleep.* 1999;22(8):1134–1156.
79. Cervena K, Dauvilliers Y, Espa F, et al. Effect of cognitive behavioural therapy for insomnia on sleep architecture and sleep EEG power spectra in psychophysiological insomnia. *J Sleep Res.* 2004;13(4):385–393.
80. Morin CM, Colecchi C, Stone J, Sood R, Brink D. Behavioral and pharmacological therapies for late-life insomnia: A randomized controlled trial. *JAMA.* 1999;281(11):991–999.
81. Arnold LM, Keck PE, Welge JA. Antidepressant treatment of fibromyalgia: A meta-analysis and review. *Psychosomatics.* 2000;41(2):104–113.
82. Wang S-M, Han C, Bahk W-M, et al. Addressing the side effects of contemporary antidepressant drugs: A comprehensive review. *Chonnam Med J.* 2018;54(2):101–112.
83. Staud R. Pharmacological treatment of fibromyalgia syndrome. *Drugs.* 2010;70(1):1–14.
84. Goldenberg DL, Clauw DJ, Palmer RE, Clair AG. Opioid use in fibromyalgia: A cautionary tale. Paper presented at: Mayo Clinic Proceedings; 2016.
85. Chou R, Turner JA, Devine EB, et al. The effectiveness and risks of long-term opioid therapy for chronic pain: A systematic review for a National Institutes of Health Pathways to Prevention Workshop. *Ann Intern Med.* 2015;162(4):276–286.
86. Eriksen J, Sjøgren P, Bruera E, Ekholm O, Rasmussen NK. Critical issues on opioids in chronic non-cancer pain: An epidemiological study. *Pain.* 2006;125(1–2):172–179.
87. Vallejo R, de Leon-Casasola O, Benyamin R. Opioid therapy and immunosuppression: A review. *Am J Therapeut.* 2004;11(5):354–365.
88. Miller MB, Chan WS, Curtis AF, et al. Pain intensity as a moderator of the association between opioid use and insomnia symptoms among adults with chronic pain. *Sleep Med.* 2018;52:98–102.
89. Harris RE, Clauw DJ, Scott DJ, McLean SA, Gracely RH, Zubieta J-K. Decreased central μ-opioid receptor availability in fibromyalgia. *J Neurosci.* 2007;27(37):10000–10006.
90. Brattberg G. Connective tissue massage in the treatment of fibromyalgia. *Eur J Pain.* 1999;3(3):235–244.
91. Buskila D, Abu-Shakra M, Neumann L, et al. Balneotherapy for fibromyalgia at the Dead Sea. *Rheumatol Int.* 2001;20(3):105–108.
92. Rus A, Molina F, Ramos MM, Martínez-Ramírez MJ, del Moral ML. Extra virgin olive oil improves oxidative stress, functional capacity, and health-related psychological status in patients with fibromyalgia: A preliminary study. *Biol Res Nurs.* 2017;19(1):106–115.

93. Almeida TF, Roizenblatt S, Benedito-Silva AA, Tufik S. The effect of combined therapy (ultrasound and interferential current) on pain and sleep in fibromyalgia. *Pain*. 2003;104(3):665–672.

94. Sarnoch H, Adler F, Scholz OB. Relevance of muscular sensitivity, muscular activity, and cognitive variables for pain reduction associated with EMG biofeedback in fibromyalgia. *Percept Motor Skills*. 1997;84(3):1043–1050.

95. Häuser W, Klose P, Langhorst J, et al. Efficacy of different types of aerobic exercise in fibromyalgia syndrome: A systematic review and meta-analysis of randomised controlled trials. *Arthritis Res Ther*. 2010;12(3):R79.

96. Wang C, Schmid CH, Fielding RA, et al. Effect of tai chi versus aerobic exercise for fibromyalgia: Comparative effectiveness randomized controlled trial. *BMJ*. 2018;360:k851.

97. McCrae CS, Williams J, Roditi D, et al. Cognitive behavioral treatments for insomnia and pain in adults with comorbid chronic insomnia and fibromyalgia: Clinical outcomes from the SPIN randomized controlled trial. *Sleep*. 2018;42(3):zsy234.

98. Gottesmann C. GABA mechanisms and sleep. *Neuroscience*. 2002;111(2):231–239.

99. Longo LP, Johnson B. Addiction: Part I. Benzodiazepines: Side effects, abuse risk and alternatives. *Am Fam Physician*. 2000;61(7):2121–2128.

100. Buysse DJ, Rush AJ, Reynolds CF. Clinical management of insomnia disorder. *JAMA*. 2017;318(20):1973–1974.

101. Emens JS, Burgess HJ. Effect of light and melatonin and other melatonin receptor agonists on human circadian physiology. *Sleep Med Clin*. 2015;10(4):435–453.

102. Arendt J, Rajaratnam SM. Melatonin and its agonists: An update. *Br J Psychiatry*. 2008;193(4):267–269.

16

Alcohol and Chronic Pain

Shared Neural Circuits and Clinical Features

TESSA M. FROHE, BENJAMIN L. BEREY, KATIE WITKIEWITZ,
ELIZABETH A. MCCALLION, AND KEVIN E. VOWLES ■

INTRODUCTION

Globally, the prevalence of current and lifetime rates of alcohol use disorder (AUD) are estimated to be 16% and 32%, respectively.[1] As such, it is important to identify correlates and predictors of AUDs. Chronic pain is estimated to affect 20% of adults worldwide.[2] While few studies have estimated the prevalence of AUD and chronic pain concurrently, there is growing evidence of significant comorbidity between these conditions.[3–5] This chapter will discuss the interactions between alcohol use and chronic pain, highlight the prevalence and clinical characteristics of the two, and provide an overview of neural mechanisms associated with each disorder. Finally, behavioral and pharmacological interventions will be discussed and future directions considered.

CHRONIC PAIN

Acute pain is normal and necessary for survival because it alerts humans to retreat from harmful factors and to inhibit action to promote healing.[6]

Conversely, chronic pain is prevalent, is complex, has no added value to survival, and often relates to significant levels of distress and disability.[2] Specifically, one in five adults report experiencing chronic pain in their lifetime.[7] Despite the pervasiveness of chronic pain and the costs associated with treatment, it has been relatively understudied as a contributing factor to the global disease burden. Further, definitions of chronic pain vary in the current literature, with fluctuating timeframes for a chronic pain diagnosis (i.e., >1 month, >3 months, >6 months), various medical etiologies, and pain locations.

Pain lasting longer than 3 months is a widely used definition for chronic pain; however, this is not accepted universally as a standard timeframe.[8] Other timeframes include past-year persistent, daily pain lasting 6 months or more.[9] Moreover, the American College of Rheumatology (ACR) utilizes the 3-month timeframe; however, the ACR definition of where the pain must be present covers the entire body and is defined as a chronic widespread pain (i.e., left and right side of the body, above and below the waist, plus axial skeletal pain). Chronic pain is commonly diagnosed without a biomedical marker present, and the amount of pain experienced is sometimes disproportional to the amount of tissue damage that has occurred.[6] For example, 85% of back pain is considered nonspecific, making diagnoses diverse and complex.

Chronic pain is one of the primary reasons adults seek medical care,[9] costing the United States $635 billion per annum.[10] Importantly, interpretation of pain may predict functioning better than pain intensity alone, and pain severity increases when fear of pain is higher and persistent pain-avoidant behavior occurs.[11,12] Additionally, chronic pain relates to poorer interpersonal social resources, both physical and psychological health,[2,9] as well as economic well-being.[13] Because chronic pain is reliably associated with poorer functioning, chronic pain–based psychosocial interventions often prioritize overall functioning as a key treatment target.[12]

ALCOHOL USE

Like pain, AUD is prevalent and costly. An AUD diagnosis is defined by meeting criteria for at least two symptoms in the *Diagnostic and Statistical Manual of Mental Disorders,* fifth edition (DSM-5) within the past year.[14] The progression from alcohol use to AUD is often characterized by three stages: compulsive alcohol consumption, an inability to control alcohol consumption, and withdrawal when access to alcohol is limited.[14] As recently as 2012, the National Epidemiological Survey on Alcohol and Related Conditions (NESARC) found that current and lifetime rates of AUD were 13.9% and 29.1%, respectively,[15] and approximately 14% of individuals with an AUD ever received treatment from 2001 to 2002.[16]

AUD is associated with significant years of life lost due primarily to disability and premature mortality. Moreover, total volume of alcohol consumed and heavy drinking predict negative health outcomes, including poorer HIV/AIDS outcomes and several types of cancer, while heavy drinking is associated with ischemic heart disease.[17] In 2010, heavy drinking and AUD accounted for more than 80% of the overall costs in lost productivity and health. From a developmental perspective, adolescence and early adulthood (i.e., 18–29 years of age) are high-risk periods for AUDs.[15] Other established risk factors for AUD are being male, having a family history of alcohol problems, and having heightened negative affect.[18]

COMORBIDITY OF CHRONIC PAIN AND SUBSTANCE USE DISORDERS

People with chronic pain are 33% more likely to use substances,[19] and persistent pain significantly increases the risk for subsequent substance use following detoxification.[3] This may be due to alcohol's analgesic effects, given that up to 25% of people use alcohol to reduce their pain.[4] Individuals with an AUD are more likely to treat pain with alcohol,[20] and alcohol use after treatment is positively associated with pain.[5] Further, alcohol is often used to self-manage chronic pain,[4] and heavy drinking is related to pain severity and pain-management strategies.[20] Greater pain frequency, depression, being unmarried, and having higher levels of education are also associated with using alcohol to manage chronic pain.[4] Similarly, pain is common during alcohol detoxification, and among those in treatment, persistent pain increases the odds of a substance use lapse longitudinally.[3] Thus, it is important to understand the neurobiological interactions between pain and alcohol, including how interventions can reduce chronic pain and/or alcohol use.

NEURAL CIRCUITRY OF CHRONIC PAIN

Recently, our understanding of pain has evolved to show that chronic pain relates to various brain changes.[21] Nociceptors encompass biological (physical and psychological) pain, which are afferent neurons that converge at the spinal cord's dorsal root ganglia leading to spinal and brainstem pathways and projections to the brain regions that include the thalamus, nucleus accumbens (NAc), and amygdala (i.e. the "pain pathway").[6] The "pain pathway" links the sensory inflow of tactile information with the cortex to make a conscious perception of painful sensations.

Before interpretation by the primary and secondary somatosensory cortices, pain arising from the stimulation of nerve cell (nociceptive) signals may be inhibited or amplified.[22] Internal body and/or environmental cues can cause this effect at the posterior column by way of the descending modulation system. Chronic pain is understood as the development and maintenance of pain through the central nervous system (i.e., brain and nerves of the spinal cord), called *central sensitization*. Central sensitization occurs gradually, where stimuli impair brain functions by inhibiting brain orchestrated mechanisms[23] and overactivate both the ascending and descending pathways.[24] This means that central sensitization sustains chronic pain without any resolution, and any injuries that occur subsequently can aggravate or further sustain the nociceptive input, which can cause more pain overall. This process, which both inhibits pain and facilitates higher sensitization to pain, will also alter the sensory processing that occurs in the brain.[24] Chronic pain is commonly understood to be a sensory abnormality or a disorder of reward function.[6] Studies suggest that chronic pain alters brain structures, such that individuals with chronic pain have highly active regions within the prefrontal/limbic networks compared with individuals with acute pain.[25]

The NAc and dorsal striatum are two important subregions of the basal ganglia located deep in the brain.[26] The NAc controls the hedonic, pleasurable sensations, and the dorsal striatum is responsible for habit formation. Further, the prefrontal cortex (PFC) is associated with, but not limited to, the suppression of pain.[27] The PFC contains several interrelated regions, including the anterior cingulate cortex (ACC), which receives information that is partially responsible for drug-seeking behavior.[28] Vos and colleagues found that ongoing pain can alter the thalamus's somatotopic map responsible for sense of touch.[29] Others found less brain metabolites, suggesting more distorted brain circuits, among individuals with, rather than without, chronic pain.[30] Findings indicate that chronic pain is interconnected with limbic properties and helps explain negative affective states. Pain may also be due to lesions in the thalamus, the midbrain, or the cortex; and the perception of pain may be related to lesions close to the neospinothalamic tract, which could reduce the inhibitory mechanisms on nearby conducting pathways. However, those with chronic pain rarely have recognizable nociceptive input and can be affected in many different domains, ranging from biological to psychological to social.

NEURAL CIRCUITRY OF ALCOHOL USE DISORDERS

Three main regions are consistently linked with aspects of addiction, namely the extended amygdala, and similar to chronic pain, the basal ganglia and PFC.[26]

The extended amygdala is located beneath the basal ganglia. It is responsible for the "fight or flight" response and controls behavioral aspects, including negative affect and anxiety.[31] In addition to the aforementioned role of the PFC, it is also responsible for higher order executive functions, including emotion regulation, working memory, and decision-making (among others).[27] Addiction can be viewed cyclically and in three stages: binge/intoxication, withdrawal/negative affect, and preoccupation/anticipation.[32] The first stage consists of experiencing hedonic effects of a substance following use (i.e., alcohol intoxication); the second stage exists during an absence of the substance, which causes negative emotional states (i.e., alcohol withdrawal); and the third stage consists of drug-seeking following abstinence.[32] While these stages are intricately interconnected, each stage pertains to one of the three brain regions discussed previously.

The limbic system consists of a complex system throughout the brain near the edge of the cortex and is known for being a major part of the reward system. The limbic system includes the striatum and basil ganglia, which controls the basic emotions (e.g., fear) and drives (e.g., hunger, sex). The basal ganglia and its subregions are greatly involved during the binge/intoxication stage. For instance, during alcohol consumption, the activation of the NAc produces positive, pleasurable feelings, which helps to positively reinforce the behavior that may lead to repetitive alcohol use in animals[33] and humans.[34] These rewarding effects include the activation of the dopamine and opioid signaling systems.[26] Further, neuroimaging studies have found alcohol to activate dopamine neurotransmitters. This may engender changes in the dorsal striatum[35] and can help to explain why alcohol-seeking and consumption habits are strengthened over time. While the brain reward system produces pleasurable feelings during alcohol consumption, it also elicits differential responses to substance-related cues (e.g., drug paraphernalia). As people learn to associate a substance with internal or external stimuli, exposure to those stimuli can produce similar activation of the dopamine system that produces powerful cravings for the substance.[26] Thus, even the exposure to alcohol cues can trigger cravings and alcohol use.

The duration before experiencing withdrawal symptoms can vary from hours or days and consists of physical withdrawal symptoms and negative emotional states during abstinence. These adverse feelings are believed to come from dampened dopamine release, also located in the basal ganglia, and greater activation of the brain stress systems located in the extended amygdala. During withdrawal, several stress neurotransmitters, such as corticotropin-releasing factor (CRF), norepinephrine, and dynorphin, are activated in the extended amygdala. As such, these neurotransmitters are associated with withdrawal and subsequent substance use due to increased stress. It is possible that individuals experiencing withdrawal are motivated to use substances to stifle activated brain stress systems that are responsible for negative, aversive feelings (i.e., preoccupation/anticipation stage).

NEURAL CIRCUITRY OF CHRONIC PAIN AND ALCOHOL USE DISORDERS

Physical and emotional pain during drug and alcohol withdrawal is common, and many addiction models are characterized by impaired hedonic capacity, which pain significantly impedes.[6,36] Moreover, the processes of alcohol and pain share several commonalities in neural circuitry. Both physical and psychological pain have overlapping neurobiological mechanisms, and alcohol may be a means of escaping one's pain.[37] Heightened activation serves as a greater risk factor for individuals who have AUDs and chronic pain already, and similarities in the neural circuitry have been found to underlie both.[6,28] Reward circuits (i.e., medial prefrontal cortex [mPFC], amygdala, and NAc) play a key role in heightened activation among individuals with chronic pain and/or AUDs, which is distinct from the general population.[37] Both pain and AUD underlie reward and memory processes. Specifically, activity in the mPFC is involved in substance use and chronic pain. One study found that the interactions between the mPFC and NAc were causal factors facilitating pain chronification.[38] These findings supported previous work suggesting that the reward pathway, or mesocorticolimbic circuitry, is influenced by the interaction of brain valuation circuitry. This interaction can affect motivational values,[39] implying that addiction circuitry, such as AUDs, may be linked with chronic pain. Further, the basal ganglia relate to hedonic and addictive behaviors, which increase the likelihood of chronic pain and AUD.

During adolescence, several brain structures undergo dynamic changes that may render the brain vulnerable to myriad unhealthy or risky environmental influences. Specifically, abnormalities of the PFC may contribute to overall executive control and information processing[40] and are believed to relate to risky behaviors. The PFC consists of several interrelated regions, including the ACC, which receives information that is partially responsible for drug-seeking behavior.[28] Brumback and colleagues[41] conducted a longitudinal functional magnetic resonance imaging (fMRI) study examining substance-naïve adolescent brain structures and found that thinner PFC areas in early adolescence predicted negative alcohol outcomes in late adolescence. Further, a transactional relation exists between drinking and stress levels that account for both behavioral and neurological associations. Puberty is a peak period of vulnerability to complex structures such as the hypothalamic-pituitary-adrenocortical axis, which is made up of the hypothalamus, the pituitary gland, and suprarenal glands.[42] Studies show that increased levels of cortisol affect several brain structures that influence chronic pain.[42] Further, the rate of chronic pain reported in adolescence increases dramatically from earlier stages of childhood[42] and can predispose to the development of adult chronic pain.[43] Adolescent alcohol use and chronic pain may alter brain function and confer risk for comorbid chronic pain and AUD later in life by potentially reorganizing limbic circuitries.[38,41,42]

Overall, the central nucleus of the amygdala accomplishes a major output function of the amygdala in pain processing (nociceptive amygdala), fear, and anxiety. Its impaired function may translate in persistent, uncontrolled emotional-affective symptoms in pain and alcohol use.[26] This evidence highlights the associations between brain regions that are crucial to functional brain networks with both chronic pain and substance use behaviors at earlier developmental stages. Addressing ways to modify stress responses in adolescent development may offer protective strategies to control affective states that may otherwise be accounted for by potential development of chronic pain or AUDs.

TREATMENTS FOR CHRONIC PAIN AND ALCOHOL USE DISORDERS

Given the neurobiological similarities between AUD and chronic pain, pharmacotherapy and behavioral treatments aimed at one condition may be beneficial to the other. Of clinical relevance, greater levels of pain predicted time to first heavy drinking lapse and time to first lapse during or following AUD treatment.[5] Relative to veterans with a substance use disorder (SUD) diagnosis and intermittent or no pain, veterans with an SUD diagnosis and persistent pain were more likely to drop out of treatment and were less likely to abstain from alcohol or drugs through 1 year of follow-up.[19] Thus, pain is an important factor that negatively influences treatment outcomes.

Cognitive behavioral therapy (CBT) is an effective treatment for SUDs,[26] including AUD,[44] and chronic pain.[45] CBT is a relatively short-term treatment approach (typically 8 to 24 sessions)[26] that emphasizes techniques to modify maladaptive behaviors and improve coping skills through identifying and adjusting dysfunctional thinking. Similarly, acceptance and commitment therapy (ACT)[46] and mindfulness-based stress reduction (MBSR)[47] can be utilized for both pain and AUDs.[48–50] Both have shown increases in psychological plasticity through acceptance and mindfulness of one's own life experiences.[46]

Despite myriad behavioral interventions aimed at increasing overall health by reducing alcohol use, few pharmacotherapies have been developed for, and approved by, the US Food and Drug Administration (FDA) for treating AUD.[26]

One is naltrexone, an opioid antagonist, that reduces craving and rewarding alcohol effects.[26] Naltrexone has been shown to decrease the percentage of heavy drinking days and increase the percentage of days abstinent in some alcohol-dependent individuals, particularly individuals with a family history of AUD.[51] This is important because the desire to eliminate negative physical and emotional states during withdrawal is a salient motivator for continued substance use. These results are especially promising considering two small studies also found that low-dose naltrexone is an effective treatment for pain reduction in patients with fibromyalgia.[52] Perhaps naltrexone, which acts as an opioid antagonist, also has anti-inflammatory effects, which helps to reduce pain symptoms. Future studies would benefit from examining the effects of naltrexone on pain intensity, pain interference, and AUD outcomes simultaneously.

To help individuals remain abstinent following withdrawal symptoms (e.g., epigastric pain, trembling), acamprosate has been shown to be a safe and effective treatment for individuals with AUD.[53] It appears that acamprosate may interact with the neurotransmitter systems, such as N-methyl-D-aspartate (NMDA) receptors (i.e., ionotropic glutamate receptor) and calcium channels, that have been changed because of alcohol abuse, thus returning them from a hyperactive to a normal state. Recently, a meta-analysis found acamprosate to be most efficacious in increasing the length of alcohol abstinence.[54] This may be due to findings showing that acamprosate reduces withdrawal symptoms (e.g., pain), thereby reducing the likelihood of future lapses. Acamprosate does not have any significant drug interactions; therefore, it may be an appropriate treatment for individuals with multiple medical problems that take multiple medications. Specifically, this may be especially beneficial to individuals with comorbid chronic pain and AUD.

Although the evidence is slim, effective treatments for chronic pain and AUD separately are established, whereas effective treatments for comorbid chronic pain *and* AUD have been far less studied. However, recent findings suggest that an integrated CBT intervention for chronic pain and SUD improved pain interference, reduced cravings for alcohol, and decreased past-month alcohol use.[55] Given preliminary data in support of mindfulness-oriented recovery enhancement (MORE) as a combined intervention for chronic pain and opioid misuse among patients with chronic pain, it may be possible that behavioral interventions such as integrated CBT and mindfulness-based interventions could be used to treat concurrent pain and AUD. Further, pharmacotherapies such as naltrexone and topiramate appear to decrease craving and the subjective effects of alcohol[56] while also acting as anti-inflammatory agents that decrease pain. Thus, examining treatments aimed at reducing chronic pain and alcohol use has great benefit and should be explored in future efficacy trials.

FUTURE DIRECTIONS

In general, better assessment and treatment of chronic pain patients may be associated with improvements in alcohol use outcomes. Multidisciplinary interventions that incorporate elements of physical and emotional components have produced successful outcomes.[57] Therefore, future research on comorbid chronic pain and AUD should focus on accurate means of measuring appropriate outcomes in order to determine whether these treatments are successful. For example, research suggests that desire for control over pain, rather than pain intensity, may be the most accurate measurement of individual levels of pain.[58] Additionally, clinicians should assess their patient's alcohol use for pain management and be aware of any psychosocial impairment in order to make proper referrals and/or any adjustments to treatment that may be necessary. Further, it is important to monitor patient functioning and quality of life in chronic pain because this may offer further insight into alcohol use as well as pain-related functioning.[59] Preliminary findings suggest that assessing pain interference and intensity as potential triggers for alcohol relapse may be an important component of relapse prevention interventions for AUD.[5] It is important to examine an individual's interpretation of pain, including psychological components (i.e., effects on pain interference or effects on returning to work), which may have positive short- and long-term effects on pain interference. Clinicians should remain attentive to older pain patients with fewer social resources, especially men, in order to monitor potential hazardous drinking problems.

By remaining focused on multiple characteristics, clinicians may be better able to offer preventative care to pain patients who fit this profile. Similarly, recognizing pain as a potential clinical target in behavioral interventions for AUD may result in better overall treatment outcomes. Based on the positive outcomes naltrexone has had for patients with chronic pain and alcohol, pharmacological treatments may provide added benefit in the treatment of both chronic pain and AUD. Pairing pharmaceuticals with behavioral interventions may offer higher treatment success rates than either on their own. Examining the utility of pharmacological treatments with other behavioral interventions, such as ACT or mindfulness-based relapse prevention,[46] may offer insight into the efficacy of multidisciplinary treatments for individuals who have both chronic pain and AUDs. Research on chronic pain and AUD continues to develop and enrich each discipline separately; however, it remains important to examine both together in order to enhance our understanding of these complex, comorbid disorders. Enriching the two disciplines together holds great opportunity for improvement in both fields and, most important, to the treatments for patients who are affected by both daily.

REFERENCES

1. World Health Organization. *Global Status Report on Alcohol and Health 2014.* Geneva: Author; 2014.

2. Breivik H, Collett B, Ventafridda V, Cohen R, Gallacher D. Survey of chronic pain in Europe: Prevalence, impact on daily life, and treatment. *Eur J Pain.* 2006;10(4):287–333.

3. Larson MJ, Paasche-Orlow M, Cheng DM, Lloyd-Travaglini C, Saitz R, Samet JH. Persistent pain is associated with substance use after detoxification: A prospective cohort analysis. *Addiction.* 2007;102(5):752–760.

4. Riley JL, King C. Self-report of alcohol use for pain in a multi-ethnic community sample. *J Pain.* 2009;10(9):944–952.

5. Witkiewitz K, Vowles KE, McCallion E, Frohe T, Kirouac M, Maisto SA. Pain as a predictor of heavy drinking and any drinking lapses in the COMBINE study and the UK Alcohol Treatment Trial. *Addiction.* 2015;110(8):1262–1271.

6. Elman I, Borsook D. Common brain mechanisms of chronic pain and addiction. *Neuron.* 2016;89(1):11–36.

7. van Hecke O, Torrance N, Smith BH. Chronic pain epidemiology: Where do lifestyle factors fit in? *Br J Pain.* 2013;7(4):209–217.

8. Harstall C, Ospina M. How prevalent is chronic pain. *Pain Clin Updates.* 2003;11(2):1–4.

9. Gureje O, Von Korff M, Simon GE, Gater R. Persistent pain and well-being: A World Health Organization study in primary care. *JAMA.* 1998;280(2):147–151.

10. Gaskin DJ, Richard P. The economic costs of pain in the United States. *J Pain.* 2012;13(8):715–724.

11. Vowles KE, McCracken LM, Eccleston C. Patient functioning and catastrophizing in chronic pain: The mediating effects of acceptance. *Health Psychol.* 2008;27(2S):S136.

12. Gatchel RJ, Peng YB, Peters ML, Fuchs PN, Turk DC. The biopsychosocial approach to chronic pain: Scientific advances and future directions. *Psychol Bull.* 2007;133(4):581.

13. Latham J, Davis B. The socioeconomic impact of chronic pain. *Disabil Rehabil.* 1994;16(1):39–44.

14. American Psychiatric Association. *Diagnostic and Statistical Manual of Mental Disorders.* 5th ed. American Psychiatric Publishing; 2013.

15. Grant BF, Goldstein RB, Saha TD, et al. Epidemiology of DSM-5 alcohol use disorder: Results from the National Epidemiologic Survey on Alcohol and Related Conditions III. *JAMA Psychiatry.* 2015;72(8):757–766.

16. Cohen E, Feinn R, Arias A, Kranzler HR. Alcohol treatment utilization: Findings from the National Epidemiologic Survey on Alcohol and Related Conditions. *Drug and Alcohol Dependence.* 2007;86(2):214–221.

17. Rehm J, Baliunas D, Borges GL, et al. The relation between different dimensions of alcohol consumption and burden of disease: An overview. *Addiction.* 2010;105(5):817–843.

18. Witkiewitz K, McCallion E, Vowles KE, et al. Association between physical pain and alcohol treatment outcomes: The mediating role of negative affect. *J Consult Clin Psychol.* 2015;83(6):1044.

19. Caldeiro RM, Malte CA, Calsyn DA, et al. The association of persistent pain with out-patient addiction treatment outcomes and service utilization. *Addiction*. 2008;103(12):1996–2005.

20. Brennan PL, Schutte KK, Moos RH. Pain and use of alcohol to manage pain: Prevalence and 3-year outcomes among older problem and non-problem drinkers. *Addiction*. 2005;100(6):777–786.

21. Tracey I, Bushnell MC. How neuroimaging studies have challenged us to rethink: Is chronic pain a disease? *J Pain*. 2009;10(11):1113–1120.

22. Eippert F, Finsterbusch J, Bingel U, Büchel C. Direct evidence for spinal cord involvement in placebo analgesia. *Science*. 2009;326(5951):404.

23. Nijs J, Van Houdenhove B, Oostendorp RA. Recognition of central sensitization in patients with musculoskeletal pain: Application of pain neurophysiology in manual therapy practice. *Man Ther*. 2010;15(2):135–141.

24. Staud R, Craggs JG, Robinson ME, Perlstein WM, Price DD. Brain activity related to temporal summation of C-fiber evoked pain. *Pain*. 2007;129(1–2):130–142.

25. Apkarian AV, Krauss BR, Fredrickson BE, Szeverenyi NM. Imaging the pain of low back pain: Functional magnetic resonance imaging in combination with monitoring subjective pain perception allows the study of clinical pain states. *Neurosci Lett*. 2001;299(1):57–60.

26. Office of the Surgeon General. *Facing Addiction in America: The Surgeon General's Report on Alcohol, Drugs, and Health*. Washington, DC: US Department of Health and Human Services;2016.

27. Kane MJ, Engle RW. The role of prefrontal cortex in working-memory capacity, executive attention, and general fluid intelligence: An individual-differences perspective. *Psychonom Bull Rev*. 2002;9(4):637–671.

28. Egli M, Koob GF, Edwards S. Alcohol dependence as a chronic pain disorder. *Neurosci Biobehav Rev*. 2012;36(10):2179–2192.

29. Vos BP, Strassman AM. Fos expression in the medullary dorsal horn of the rat after chronic constriction injury to the infraorbital nerve. *J Compar Neurol*. 1995;357(3):362–375.

30. Grachev ID, Fredrickson BE, Apkarian AV. Abnormal brain chemistry in chronic back pain: An in vivo proton magnetic resonance spectroscopy study. *Pain*. 2000;89(1):7–18.

31. Davis M, Walker DL, Miles L, Grillon C. Phasic vs sustained fear in rats and humans: Role of the extended amygdala in fear vs anxiety. *Neuropsychopharmacology*. 2010;35(1):105–135.

32. Koob GF, Le Moal M. Drug abuse: Hedonic homeostatic dysregulation. *Science*. 1997;278(5335):52–58.

33. Yoshimoto K, McBride W, Lumeng L, Li T-K. Alcohol stimulates the release of dopamine and serotonin in the nucleus accumbens. *Alcohol*. 1992;9(1):17–22.

34. Boileau I, Assaad JM, Pihl RO, et al. Alcohol promotes dopamine release in the human nucleus accumbens. *Synapse*. 2003;49(4):226–231.

35. Yin HH, Knowlton BJ. The role of the basal ganglia in habit formation. *Nat Rev Neurosci*. 2006;7(6):464–476.

36. Shurman J, Koob GF, Gutstein HB. Opioids, pain, the brain, and hyperkatifeia: A framework for the rational use of opioids for pain. *Pain Med*. 2010;11(7):1092–1098.

37. Apkarian AV, Neugebauer V, Koob G, et al. Neural mechanisms of pain and alcohol dependence. *Pharmacol Biochem Behav*. 2013;112:34–41.

38. Baliki MN, Petre B, Torbey S, et al. Corticostriatal functional connectivity predicts transition to chronic back pain. *Nat Neurosci*. 2012;15(8):1117–1119.

39. Pessiglione M, Lebreton M. From the reward circuit to the valuation system: How the brain motivates behavior. In: Gendolla GHE, Tops M, Koole SL, eds. *Handbook of Biobehavioral Approaches to Self-Regulation*. New York, NY: Springer; 2015:157–173.

40. Shimamura AP. The role of the prefrontal cortex in dynamic filtering. *Psychobiology*. 2000;28(2):207–218.

41. Brumback T, Worley M, Nguyen-Louie TT, Squeglia LM, Jacobus J, Tapert SF. Neural predictors of alcohol use and psychopathology symptoms in adolescents. *Dev Psychopathol*. 2016;28(4 part 1):1209–1216.

42. Walco GA, Krane EJ, Schmader KE, Weiner DK. Applying a lifespan developmental perspective to chronic pain: Pediatrics to geriatrics. *J Pain*. 2016;17(9):T108–T117.

43. Walker LS, Dengler-Crish CM, Rippel S, Bruehl S. Functional abdominal pain in childhood and adolescence increases risk for chronic pain in adulthood. *Pain*. 2010;150(3):568–572.

44. Magill M, Ray LA. Cognitive-behavioral treatment with adult alcohol and illicit drug users: A meta-analysis of randomized controlled trials. *J Stud Alcohol Drugs*. 2009;70(4):516–527.

45. Wetherell JL, Afari N, Rutledge T, et al. A randomized, controlled trial of acceptance and commitment therapy and cognitive-behavioral therapy for chronic pain. *Pain*. 2011;152(9):2098–2107.

46. Hayes S, Strosahl K, Wilson K. Acceptance and commitment therapy: The process and practice of mindful change, 2nd ed. *Psychother Psychosom*. 2012;81(4):263.

47. Kabat-Zinn J, Lipworth L, Burney R. The clinical use of mindfulness meditation for the self-regulation of chronic pain. *J Behav Med*. 1985;8(2):163–190.

48. Vowles KE, Thompson M. Acceptance and commitment therapy for chronic pain. In: McCracken LM, ed. *Mindfulness and Acceptance in Behavioral Medicine: Current Theory and Practice*. Oakland, CA: Context Press/New Harbinger Publications; 2011:31–60.

49. Thekiso TB, Murphy P, Milnes J, Lambe K, Curtin A, Farren CK. Acceptance and commitment therapy in the treatment of alcohol use disorder and comorbid affective disorder: A pilot matched control trial. *Behav Ther*. 2015;46(6):717–728.

50. Bowen S, Witkiewitz K, Clifasefi SL, et al. Relative efficacy of mindfulness-based relapse prevention, standard relapse prevention, and treatment as usual for substance use disorders: A randomized clinical trial. *JAMA Psychiatry*. 2014;71(5):547–556.

51. Garbutt JC, Greenblatt AM, West SL, et al. Clinical and biological moderators of response to naltrexone in alcohol dependence: A systematic review of the evidence. *Addiction*. 2014;109(8):1274–1284.

52. Younger J, Mackey S. Fibromyalgia symptoms are reduced by low-dose naltrexone: A pilot study. *Pain Med*. 2009;10(4):663–672.

53. Rösner S, Hackl-Herrwerth A, Leucht S, Lehert P, Vecchi S, Soyka M. Acamprosate for alcohol dependence. *Cochrane Database Syst Rev*. 2010;(9):CD004332.

54. Maisel NC, Blodgett JC, Wilbourne PL, Humphreys K, Finney JW. Meta-analysis of naltrexone and acamprosate for treating alcohol use disorders: When are these medications most helpful? *Addiction.* 2013;108(2):275–293.

55. Morasco BJ, Greaves DW, Lovejoy TI, Turk DC, Dobscha SK, Hauser P. Development and preliminary evaluation of an integrated cognitive-behavior treatment for chronic pain and substance use disorder in patients with the hepatitis C virus. *Pain Med.* 2016;17(12):2280–2290.

56. Drobes DJ, Anton RF, Thomas SE, Voronin K. Effects of naltrexone and nalmefene on subjective response to alcohol among non-treatment-seeking alcoholics and social drinkers. *Alcoholism.* 2004;28(9):1362–1370.

57. McCracken L, Gross R, Eccleston C. Multimethod assessment of treatment process in chronic low back pain: Comparison of reported pain-related anxiety with directly measured physical capacity. *Behav Res Ther.* 2002;40(5):585–594.

58. Fordyce WE. Pain and suffering: A reappraisal. *Am Psychologist.* 1988;43(4):276.

59. Vowles KE, Witkiewitz K, Levell J, Sowden G, Ashworth J. Are reductions in pain intensity and pain-related distress necessary? An analysis of within treatment change trajectories in relation to improved functioning following interdisciplinary acceptance and commitment therapy for adults with chronic pain. *J Consult Clin Psychol.* 2017;85(2):87–98.

17

Catastrophizing in Comorbid Chronic Pain and Mental Illness

A Primer for Clinicians

CYNTHIA O. TOWNSEND AND DONALD R. TOWNSEND ■

In the wake of the opioid overdose epidemic, there has been a reinvigoration of efforts to critically explore how psychological variables, such as catastrophizing, contribute to either worsening or mitigating one's vulnerability to chronic pain and mental health disorders. The National Pain Strategy[1] has emphasized an imperative for clinical practice to align with empirical research, which favors multimodal therapies encompassing a "social-psycho-bio" conceptualization[2] of chronic pain. Catastrophizing, a mental health variable viewed dynamically as a contributor, mediator, and result of chronic pain suffering, remains important in the psychological and pain medicine literature.[3] Pain catastrophizing, defined as "an exaggerated negative mental set brought to bear during actual or anticipated painful experience,"[4,5] has been a mainstay of psychological constructs in the treatment of chronic pain.

The evolution, theoretical models, and significance of catastrophizing have been thoroughly reviewed.[4,6–13] Key components of the construct include a maladaptive cognitive coping style characterized by irrational ideas that cause psychological distress from engaging a negative forecast of future events, exaggerating struggles, perceiving experiences are worse than reality, exaggeration of the frequency of danger, and judgment that there is nothing one can do about the impending situation.[6]

MEASURING CATASTROPHIZING

Assessment of pain-related catastrophizing was advanced through the development of the Pain Catastrophizing Scale (PCS).[8] The PCS comprises three domains, including (a) rumination about one's pain (inability to inhibit thinking about one's current or anticipated pain); (b) magnification of pain (exaggerating one's pain); and (c) helplessness (holding the belief that one's pain will never get better).[7,8,14] The PCS short form, a seven-item abbreviated version of the PCS, has been used to screen for individuals at high risk for worrisome catastrophizing.[15] Derived from the PCS, the Symptom Catastrophizing Scale (SCS)[13] was recently developed to assess catastrophic thinking related to health or mental health conditions, rather than pain. The SCS has demonstrated ability to detect change following interventions targeting catastrophizing. The Pain Appraisal Scale (PAS) is a similar scale to assess pain-related self-efficacy and pain catastrophizing[16] but was named to decrease stigma associated with the term *pain catastrophizing*.

CATASTROPHIZING AND NEUROPLASTICITY OF PAIN

Exciting advancements in neuroimaging studies investigating cortical structural alterations in chronic pain and changes in pain-related hemodynamic responses have revealed possible neural correlates of pain catastrophizing. A systematic review of structural and functional magnetic resonance imaging (fMRI) studies[17] confirmed a connection between pain catastrophizing and brain areas associated with pain perception, the sensory-discriminative and affective components of processing of noxious stimuli, and modulation of conscious pain experience. The review noted a correlation between pain catastrophizing and a decrease in gray matter volume. Additionally, results suggested that increased activity of brain areas involved in pain processing and increased functional connectivity between them were associated with higher pain catastrophizing scores.[17] Galambos et al.[17] suggested that pain catastrophizing might be associated with the affective and intensity-related components of pain. Catastrophizing may modulate top-down attentional processes and weaken adaptive pain modulation, therefore allowing painful stimuli to become subjectively more salient and intense.[17] Another systematic review investigating cortical changes and pain-related cognitive and emotional factors[18] similarly concluded that pain catastrophizing is associated with alterations in gray matter morphology, resting-state functional connectivity, and task-related brain activation in brain areas linked to pain processing, attention to pain, emotion and motor activity, and reduced top-down pain inhibition. Atrophy of gray matter in these brain regions could indicate a decrease of activity of the orbitofrontal region leading to loss of top-down inhibition, greater level of perceived pain, more negative perceptions, and greater catastrophizing overall.[18]

A complementary line of research demonstrated that patients with idiopathic chronic pain and greater catastrophizing also had increased pain sensitivity supporting the theory that negative affective and cognitive factors in response to pain may serve as a mechanism in central pain sensitization.[19] Amygdala reactivity is also believed to play a role in the promotion of dysfunctional cognitive/emotional reactions to pain and development of internalizing symptoms.[20] In a highly selective community sample, individuals with chronic pain without mental health diagnoses or medication use were found to have exaggerated and abnormal amygdala connectivity with the central executive network (CEN), which was most exaggerated in patients with the greatest pain catastrophizing.[20] Pain catastrophizing helplessness and rumination were found to explain the relationship between catastrophizing and exaggerated amygdala–CEN connectivity. This network is believed to exert cognitive control through selective attention and working memory maintenance.

The alignment of cognitive behavioral pain management therapies with reversal of cortical structural alterations in response to treatment is cause for much excitement. Seminowicz et al.[21] demonstrated evidence of structural neuroplasticity in response to cognitive behavioral therapy (CBT). Improvement in pain catastrophizing after intervention was the only clinical measure that significantly correlated with structural changes in multiple regions and is thought to reflect greater top-down mechanisms of pain control and cognitive reappraisal of pain, and alterations in the perception of noxious signals. In a longitudinal randomized controlled trial study of the effects of CBT on brain connectivity in pain-processing areas[22] for patients characterized as high catastrophizers, resting-state fMRI scans revealed that patients in the CBT group showed a substantial reduction in resting-state connectivity in primary pain-processing areas, with concurrent and persisting reductions in pain and catastrophizing.[22]

Clinical Implications

The past decade of pain neuroscience research has noted an important shift toward exploring neuroplasticity and the central sensitization process, which contribute to the chronification of pain.[23] Research has enriched our understanding of the complex relationship between central sensitization and chronic pain, as well as the complexities of the overlapping sensory, emotional, cognitive, and behavioral responses to pain mediated in cortical and subcortical regions. This expanded knowledge propagates opportunities to increase educational interventions aimed at changing patients' understanding of the biological process of pain as a mechanism to reduce pain itself.[24,25] Mental health clinicians not familiar with the neuroscience of chronic pain should become well-informed about research in the neurophysiology and neurobiology of pain.[26,27]

CATASTROPHIZING AND PAIN-RELATED OUTCOMES

As a cognitive coping strategy affecting pain perception and clinical outcomes, catastrophizing is regarded as vital to improving decision-making and optimizing chronic pain treatment outcomes when engaging a multidisciplinary team approach to pain management.[6,28] It is recognized as a powerful psychological determinant of pain-related disability.[11,29,30] Several reviews in the past 5 years have examined catastrophizing as a prognostic factor for pain-related outcomes (i.e., pain sensitivity, physical disability, delayed recovery, treatment response). Wertli et al.[31] offered one of the first systematic reviews of catastrophizing as a predictive factor in patients with low back pain. The authors concluded that two-thirds of studies reviewed found that greater catastrophizing was associated with greater pain, disability, and delayed recovery. Catastrophizing was also found to be predictive of poor pain outcomes, such as the risk for restricted functioning, development of persistent symptoms, poorer expectations of relief, pain interference, and prolonged bed rest at 1 year.[31] More recently, Martinez-Calderon et al.[30] found that even after controlling for multiple covariates, higher levels of pain catastrophizing were significantly associated with higher pain intensity and more disability over time across a variety of pain conditions.

Research on the effects of catastrophizing on pain intervention efficacy reveals the complexities of catastrophizing. A systematic review of psychological interventions for chronic musculoskeletal pain[32] concluded that catastrophizing mediated treatment effects in all the studies examined. Despite the volume of research regarding the role of pain catastrophizing as a mediator of pain-related disability, many questions remain. Lee et al.[33] underscored the need to improve flawed research methodologies, including underpowered studies, heterogeneous pain populations, inefficient statistical methods, poor control of potential confounds, and reliance on cross-sectional designs.

Longitudinal studies are necessary to examine pain-specific psychosocial factors, such as pain-related catastrophizing, mediating the transition from acute to chronic pain conditions and the role that early intervention plays.[11] A population-based study[34] found that pain catastrophizing was a predictor of future chronic pain for individuals with and without chronic pain at baseline. Longitudinal studies of individuals experiencing work-related injury,[35] post-trauma whiplash injury,[36] severe trauma,[37] and postsurgical interventions[38-41] have examined pain catastrophizing as a mediator of pain chronicity, disability, functional outcomes, recovery expectations, work limitations, and postoperative morphine consumption,[38] finding that pain catastrophizing accounted for significant overall variance in outcomes.

Clinical Implications

Pain catastrophizing has a significant and unique, predictive influence on pain intensity, pain-related physical disability, return to work status, risk for prescription opioid misuse, suicidal ideation, health care utilization, and delayed surgical recovery.[11] Catastrophizing is believed to also interact with social environmental factors (e.g., spouse catastrophizing, health care provider communication) and behavioral responses (e.g., isolation, sedentary activity, excessive medical information seeking). Besen et al.[35] offered practical recommendations for addressing pain catastrophizing, including a focus on interpretation of the pain instead of pain relief, as well as proactive communication with support systems. The complexities of chronic pain suggest that CBT techniques aimed at addressing misinterpretations of pain and catastrophic views of health outcomes should ideally be embedded in a comprehensive pain management approach.[42,43] Catastrophizing is modifiable and is a mediator of treatment outcomes for both multidisciplinary and stand-alone pain management treatment approaches.[44]

CATASTROPHIZING, CHRONIC PAIN, AND DEPRESSION

Pain and depression are highly comorbid conditions of the most critical public health issues facing health care providers.[45] Beyond the bidirectional relationship between pain and depression is an unexpected but persistent finding that pain does not have a direct relationship with depression.[46-48] Instead, it is believed that several cognitive variables, including catastrophizing, have a mediating effect on pain and depression.[45] Research suggests that treatments for chronic pain necessitate targeting pain-related catastrophic thought processes to reduce pain levels and depression and to improve patients' quality of life.[45,48-51]

Individuals endorsing pain catastrophizing report a greater likelihood of depression.[45,52] Catastrophizing has an indirect effect on depression through increased feelings of helplessness and hopelessness.[47] Withdrawal from valued activities because of fear of pain may further lead to rumination about not being physically able to engage in such activities and thus can lead to depression.[53,54] Additionally, preexisting or coexisting depression symptoms can result in greater activity reduction, focus on negative personal health information, and tendency to interpret ambiguous information as being more threatening,[55] thus perpetuating a vicious cycle of pain, depression, catastrophizing, and even increased risk for suicide.[50,56-58]

The transdiagnostic approach to pain and emotion focuses on the shared underlying mechanism driving the pain, depression, and catastrophizing triad.[59,60] This conceptualization approaches catastrophizing as a mechanism in emotion regulation in response to significant emotional stress caused by recurring pain and depression.[60] In this model, pain flares trigger catastrophic worry, which, in turn, strains individuals' emotion regulation systems, resulting in a downward spiral of negative affect and increased pain,[60] potentially due to activation of the hypothalamic-pituitary-adrenal (HPA) axis, the primary regulator of the stress response system underlying centralized pain disorder syndromes.[61]

Clinical Implications

As a result of attentional biases, both individuals with depression and high catastrophizers are more attuned to their pain, ruminate on daily struggles, and fail to successfully regulate the extent to which their suffering dominates their thought processes.[50,62] The underlying catastrophic dysfunctional belief schema implicated in depression is considered parallel to cognitive distortions contributing to maladaptive responses to debilitating chronic pain.[63] Maladaptive ruminative thought patterns contributing to greater depression, suicide risk, and catastrophizing are critical to target in multimodal treatments.[56] Clinicians should enhance adaptive strategies for emotion regulation through expression (not thought suppression) and modification of dysfunctional cognitive pain responses.[47,60,64] Emerging evidence suggests that metacognitive therapy (MCT) and other CBT approaches (e.g., acceptance and commitment therapy [ACT], mindfulness-based cognitive therapy) are beneficial to target repetitive negative thinking in order to regain attentional flexibility.[65-67]

CATASTROPHIZING, CHRONIC PAIN, AND INSOMNIA

Difficulty falling asleep, difficulty staying asleep, and feeling tired contribute to poor quality of life for individuals with chronic pain.[68,69] A review[70] examining the bidirectional relationship between sleep and pain determined that sleep impairment reliably predicts new episodes and exacerbations in chronic pain. Pain catastrophizing may be predictive of insomnia in patients with debilitating pain,[71] and the content of presleep cognitions may contribute to sleep disturbance independent from depression and pain severity. Pain symptoms contributing to insomnia are often cited by patients, while negative cognitive processes (sleep catastrophizing) are often overlooked.[70,72]

Sleep catastrophizing entails the magnification and rumination of negative thoughts related to the perceived worst possible outcomes of poor sleep.[73] Similar to pain-related hypervigilance,[74] the same mechanism is considered to be responsible for catastrophic sleep-related thoughts contributing to insomnia.[73] The cognitive model of insomnia[75] suggests that sleep catastrophizing develops when persons suffering from insomnia tend to worry about sleep and consequences of sleep loss, which triggers autonomic and emotional arousal, altering attention toward sleep-related threat cues.[75] Harvey and Greenall[73] found that sleep-related catastrophizing is more common in persons with insomnia. Persons with insomnia have more negative thoughts regarding the impact of sleep loss and judge those outcomes to be more probable.

Addressing maladaptive thoughts about sleep has been a common component of cognitive behavior therapy for insomnia (CBT-I).[76,77] The cognitive portion of CBT-I targets erroneous beliefs, expectations, and excessive worry.[78] One of the primary targets for intervention is the exaggerated consequences of sleep loss following a night of insomnia.[79] CBT-I has also been effective for patients with diverse pain conditions.[80–83] Morin, Blais, and Svard[84] targeted maladaptive thoughts in individuals with chronic pain and found that sleep efficiency and changes in maladaptive thinking were associated with maintenance of treatment gains. Patients with chronic pain and insomnia reported a significant and longitudinal reduction in pain-related beliefs and attitudes about sleep, insomnia, and pain interference after receiving hybrid CBT intervention for pain and insomnia.[81,85,86]

Clinical Implications

Insomnia is no longer considered a symptom of either chronic pain or chronic depression, but rather is a co-occurring disorder warranting treatment consideration.[70,87] Potential contributors to insomnia within chronic pain, including maladaptive thought patterns related to sleep, should be assessed and targeted as part of an effective CBT-I intervention. Compared with the highly manualized aspects of CBT-I (i.e., sleep restriction and stimulus control), cognitive-specific interventions in CBT-I targeting maladaptive beliefs about sleep and sleep–pain consequences have neither been consistently utilized, adequately standardized in treatment protocols, nor effectively replicated. The largest area of variable treatment application is in assessment and application of cognitive interventions for insomnia treatment. Mental health providers should simultaneously assess and treat catastrophizing thought patterns related to both sleep and pain to improve self-management of both syndromes. Engaging a systematic approach to assessing and treating sleep catastrophizing is important in determining whether treatment strategies to address dysfunctional sleep cognitions have added significant value to overall cognitive behavioral insomnia interventions.

FUTURE OF PAIN CATASTROPHIZING MANAGEMENT

Interventions for modifying pain catastrophizing have primarily included CBT, ACT, mindfulness meditation and exercise, as well as a combination of these within multidisciplinary and interdisciplinary treatment programs. In a meta-analysis of interventions to address pain catastrophizing in adults with chronic pain, Schutze et al.[9] found that CBT, multimodal treatment (usually combined CBT and exercise), and ACT showed the most efficacy at post-test evaluation. Skill acquisition and cognitive, emotional, and behavior changes were implied as the mechanism to achieve treatment benefits and were also noted to demonstrate significant improvements in reducing pain catastrophizing.[9] Effective through additive effects on cognitive, behavioral, and emotional processes, as well as modulation of descending inhibitory pain pathways, multidimensional pain treatment programs provide a comprehensive management plan, with interventions designed to improve functioning in multiple domains.[9,12,88–90]

Mental health providers should be attuned to both assessment and treatment strategies targeting pain catastrophizing to achieve personalized treatment plans and optimal outcomes for persons with chronic pain conditions.[9,44,91] Individuals who engage in pain symptom magnification may benefit from neuroscience pain education and CBT cognitive restructuring skills training to decrease behavioral inhibition and activity avoidance that contribute to deconditioning, isolation, and possibility depression.[9] Additionally, interventions such as ACT and mindfulness meditation that target negative thought patterns and rumination are likely to address underlying catastrophizing. Enhanced emotional awareness strategies[92,93] and cognitive behavioral analysis can add benefit to treatment planning through analysis of themes in pain catastrophizing to optimize treatment interventions.[9]

Future research and clinical training on the development of treatment interventions targeting catastrophizing should continue to examine the reliability of existing psychological approaches and relapse-prevention strategies.[30] There is also continued need to explore and assess additional psychological constructs, such as psychological inflexibility, and interventional opportunities to mitigate how cognitive error patterns may lead to further deleterious effects of rumination, magnification, and helplessness in response to pain.[94] Prospective research and clinical interventions should reverse neglect of presurgical psychological distress factors, such as catastrophizing, and opportunities to maximize the success of multimodal prehabilitation efforts to improve healing and pain surgical outcomes.[95,96]

Given the devastating effects of chronic pain and necessity of research to more fully understand its nature, the future direction for the construct of pain catastrophizing has been laid. With more accurate assessment, statistical measurement, and clinical interventions to reduce pain catastrophizing, this important work promises to reduce its detrimental effects on the individual and psychiatric comorbidities.[3,97] Because of the mediating impact of catastrophizing on nearly every area of chronic pain and comorbid psychiatric disorders, pain catastrophizing should be a major target of assessment and intervention for mental health clinicians dedicated to decreasing the suffering in individuals with chronic pain.

REFERENCES

1. Interagency Pain Research Coordinating Committee (IPRCC). National pain strategy: A comprehensive population health-level strategy for pain. 2016. https://www.iprcc.nih.gov/National-Pain-Strategy/Overview. Accessed 5/25/2020.
2. Carr DB, Bradshaw YS. Time to flip the pain curriculum? *Anesthesiology.* 2014;120(1):12–14.
3. Gatchel RJ. Introduction to the "special issue on pain catastrophizing." *J Appl Biobehav Res.* 2017;22(1).
4. Sullivan MJL, Thorn B, Haythornthwaite JA, et al. Theoretical perspectives on the relation between catastrophizing and pain. *Clin J Pain.* 2001;17(1):52–64.
5. Sullivan MJ, D'Eon JL. Relation between catastrophizing and depression in chronic pain patients. *J Abnorm Psychol.* 1990;99(3):260–263.
6. Neblett R. Pain catastrophizing: An historical perspective. *J Appl Biobehav Res.* 2017;22(1):e12086.
7. Miller MM, Meints SM, Hirsh AT. Catastrophizing, pain, and functional outcomes for children with chronic pain: A meta-analytic review. *Pain.* 2018;159(12):2442–2460.

8. Flaskerud JH. Pain and culture: The catastrophizing construct and measurement. *Issues Ment Health Nurs.* 2015;36(2):152–155.

9. Schutze R, Rees C, Smith A, Slater H, Campbell JM, O'Sullivan P. How can we best reduce pain catastrophizing in adults with chronic noncancer pain? A systematic review and meta-analysis. *J Pain.* 2018;19(3):233–256.

10. Schütze R. Re-thinking over-thinking pain: What can metacognition add to our understanding of pain catastrophising? *Clin Psychologist.* 2016;20(3):147–153.

11. Edwards RR, Dworkin RH, Sullivan MD, Turk DC, Wasan AD. The role of psychosocial processes in the development and maintenance of chronic pain. *J Pain.* 2016;17(9 suppl):T70–T92.

12. Quartana PJ, Campbell CM, Edwards RR. Pain catastrophizing: A critical review. *Expert Rev Neurother.* 2009;9(5):745–758.

13. Moore E, Adams H, Ellis T, Thibault P, Sullivan MJL. Assessing catastrophic thinking associated with debilitating mental health conditions. *Disabil Rehabil.* 2018;40(3):317–322.

14. Sullivan MJL, Bishop SR, Pivik J. The Pain Catastrophizing Scale: Development and validation. *Psychol Assess.* 1995;7(4):524–532.

15. Cheng ST, Chen PP, Chow YF, et al. The Pain Catastrophizing Scale—short form: Psychometric properties and threshold for identifying high-risk individuals. *Int Psychogeriatr.* 2019;31(11):1665–1674.

16. Amtmann D, Liljenquist K, Bamer A, et al. Measuring pain catastrophizing and pain-related self-efficacy: Expert panels, focus groups, and cognitive interviews. *Patient.* 2018;11(1):107–117.

17. Galambos A, Szabo E, Nagy Z, et al. A systematic review of structural and functional MRI studies on pain catastrophizing. *J Pain Res.* 2019;12:1155–1178.

18. Malfliet A, Coppieters I, Van Wilgen P, et al. Brain changes associated with cognitive and emotional factors in chronic pain: A systematic review. *Eur J Pain.* 2017;21(5):769–786.

19. Meints SM, Mawla I, Napadow V, et al. The relationship between catastrophizing and altered pain sensitivity in patients with chronic low-back pain. *Pain.* 2019;160(4):833–843.

20. Jiang Y, Oathes D, Hush J, et al. Perturbed connectivity of the amygdala and its subregions with the central executive and default mode networks in chronic pain. *Pain.* 2016;157(9):1970–1978.

21. Seminowicz DA, Shpaner M, Keaser ML, et al. Cognitive-behavioral therapy increases prefrontal cortex gray matter in patients with chronic pain. *J Pain.* 2013;14(12):1573–1584.

22. Lazaridou A, Kim J, Cahalan CM, et al. Effects of cognitive-behavioral therapy (CBT) on brain connectivity supporting catastrophizing in fibromyalgia. *Clin J Pain.* 2017;33(3):215–221.

23. Pelletier R, Higgins J, Bourbonnais D. Is neuroplasticity in the central nervous system the missing link to our understanding of chronic musculoskeletal disorders? *BMC Musculoskelet Disord.* 2015;16(25):25.

24. Nijs J, Meeus M, Cagnie B, et al. A modern neuroscience approach to chronic spinal pain: Combining pain neuroscience education with cognition-targeted motor control training. *Phys Ther.* 2014;94(5):730–738.

25. Moseley GL, Butler DS. Fifteen years of explaining pain: The past, present, and future. *J Pain*. 2015;16(9):807–813.

26. Louw A, Zimney K, Puentedura EJ, Diener I. The efficacy of pain neuroscience education on musculoskeletal pain: A systematic review of the literature. *Physiother Theory Pract*. 2016;32(5):332–355.

27. Malfliet A, Kregel J, Coppieters I, De Pauw R, Meeus M, Roussel N. Effect of pain neuroscience education combined with cognition-targeted motor control training on chronic spinal pain: A randomized clinical trial. *JAMA Neurol*. 2018;75(7):808–817.

28. Rigoard P, Gatzinsky K, Deneuville JP, et al. Optimizing the management and outcomes of failed back surgery syndrome: A consensus statement on definition and outlines for patient assessment. *Pain Res Manag*. 2019;2019:3126464.

29. Flink IL, Boersma K, Linton SJ. Pain catastrophizing as repetitive negative thinking: A development of the conceptualization. *Cogn Behav Ther*. 2013;42(3):2015–2223.

30. Martinez-Calderon J, Jensen MP, Morales-Asencio JM, Luque-Suarez A. Pain catastrophizing and function in individuals with chronic musculoskeletal pain: A systematic review and meta-analysis. *Clin J Pain*. 2019;35(3):279–293.

31. Wertli MM, Eugster R, Held U, Steurer J, Kofmehl R, Weiser S. Catastrophizing: A prognostic factor for outcome in patients with low back pain. A systematic review. *Spine J*. 2014;14(11):2639–2657.

32. Mansell G, Kamper SJ, Kent P. Why and how back pain interventions work: What can we do to find out? *Best Pract Res Clin Rheumatol*. 2013;27(5):685–697.

33. Lee H, Hubscher M, Moseley GL, et al. How does pain lead to disability? A systematic review and meta-analysis of mediation studies in people with back and neck pain. *Pain*. 2015;156(6):988–997.

34. Landmark T, Dale O, Romundstad P, Woodhouse A, Kaasa S, Borchgrevink PC. Development and course of chronic pain over 4 years in the general population: The HUNT pain study. *Eur J Pain*. 2018;22(9):1606–1616.

35. Besen E, Gaines B, Linton SJ, Shaw WS. The role of pain catastrophizing as a mediator in the work disability process following acute low back pain. *J Appl Biobehav Res*. 2017;22(1).

36. Andersen TE, Karstoft KI, Brink O, Elklit A. Pain-catastrophizing and fear-avoidance beliefs as mediators between post-traumatic stress symptoms and pain following whiplash injury: A prospective cohort study. *Eur J Pain*. 2016;20(8):1241–1252.

37. Archer KR, Abraham CM, Song Y, Obremskey WT. Cognitive-behavioral determinants of pain and disability two years after traumatic injury: A cross-sectional survey study. *J Trauma Acute Care Surg*. 2012;72(2):473–479.

38. Tuna T, Boz S, Van Obbergh L, Lubansu A, Engelman E. Comparison of the pain sensitivity questionnaire and the pain catastrophizing scale in predicting postoperative pain and pain chronicization after spine surgery. *Clin Spine Surg*. 2018;31(9):E432–E440.

39. Burns LC, Ritvo SE, Ferguson MK, Clarke H, Seltzer Z, Katz J. Pain catastrophizing as a risk factor for chronic pain after total knee arthroplasty: A systematic review. *J Pain Res*. 2015;8:21–32.

40. Forsythe ME, Dunbar MJ, Hennigar AW, Sullivan MJL, Gross M. Prospective relation between catastrophizing and residual pain following knee arthroplasty: Two-year follow-up. *Pain Res Manage*. 2008;13(4):335–341.

41. Edwards RR, Haythornthwaite JA, Smith MT, Klick B, Katz JN. Catastrophizing and depressive symptoms as prospective predictors of outcomes following total knee replacement. *Pain Res Manage*. 2009;14(4):307–311.
42. Gatchel RJ, McGeary DD, McGeary CA, Lippe B. Interdisciplinary chronic pain management: Past, present, and future. *Am Psychol*. 2014;69(2):119–130.
43. Gatchel RJ, Okifuji A. Evidence-based scientific data documenting the treatment and cost-effectiveness of comprehensive pain programs for chronic nonmalignant pain. *J Pain*. 2006;7(11):779–793.
44. Gilliam WP, Craner JR, Morrison EJ, Sperry JA. The mediating effects of the different dimensions of pain catastrophizing on outcomes in an interdisciplinary pain rehabilitation program. *Clin J Pain*. 2017;33(5):443–451.
45. Goesling J, Clauw DJ, Hassett AL. Pain and depression: An integrative review of neurobiological and psychological factors. *Curr Psychiatry Rep*. 2013;15(12):421.
46. Tran P, Sturgeon JA, Nilakantan A, Foote A, Mackey S, Johnson K. Pain catastrophizing mediates the relationship between trait happiness and depressive symptoms in individuals with current pain. *J Appl Biobehav Res*. 2017;22(4).
47. Hulsebusch J, Hasenbring MI, Rusu AC. Understanding pain and depression in back pain: The role of catastrophizing, help-/hopelessness, and thought suppression as potential mediators. *Int J Behav Med*. 2016;23(3):251–259.
48. Ramirez-Maestre C, Esteve R, Ruiz-Parraga G, Gomez-Perez L, Lopez-Martinez AE. The key role of pain catastrophizing in the disability of patients with acute back pain. *Int J Behav Med*. 2017;24(2):239–248.
49. Edwards RR, Smith MT, Kudel I, Haythornthwaite J. Pain-related catastrophizing as a risk factor for suicidal ideation in chronic pain. *Pain*. 2006;126(1–3):272–279.
50. Noyman-Veksler G, Lerman SF, Joiner TE, et al. Role of pain-based catastrophizing in pain, disability, distress, and suicidal ideation. *Psychiatry*. 2017;80(2):155–170.
51. Nicholas MK, Asghari A, Blyth FM, et al. Self-management intervention for chronic pain in older adults: A randomised controlled trial. *Pain*. 2013;154(6):824–835.
52. McWilliams LA, Asmundson GJ. The relationship of adult attachment dimensions to pain-related fear, hypervigilance, and catastrophizing. *Pain*. 2007;127(1–2):27–34.
53. Brecht DM, Gatchel RJ. An overview of a biopsychosocial model of epigenetics and pain catastrophizing. *J Appl Biobehav Res*. 2019;24(3):e12171.
54. Marshall PWM, Schabrun S, Knox MF. Physical activity and the mediating effect of fear, depression, anxiety, and catastrophizing on pain related disability in people with chronic low back pain. *PLoS One*. 2017;12(7):e0180788.
55. Pincus T, Smeets RJ, Simmonds MJ, Sullivan MJ. The fear avoidance model disentangled: Improving the clinical utility of the fear avoidance model. *Clin J Pain*. 2010;26(9):739–746.
56. Edwards RR, Cahalan C, Mensing G, Smith M, Haythornthwaite JA. Pain, catastrophizing, and depression in the rheumatic diseases. *Nat Rev Rheumatol*. 2011;7(4):216–224.
57. Ilgen MA, Zivin K, McCammon RJ, Valenstein M. Pain and suicidal thoughts, plans and attempts in the United States. *Gen Hosp Psychiatry*. 2008;30(6):521–527.
58. Racine M. Chronic pain and suicide risk: A comprehensive review. *Prog Neuropsychopharmacol Biol Psychiatry*. 2018;87(part B):269–280.

59. Linton SJ. A transdiagnostic approach to pain and emotion. *J Appl Biobehav Res.* 2013;18(2):82–103.

60. Linton SJ, Bergbom S. Understanding the link between depression and pain. *Scand J Pain.* 2011;2(2).

61. Eller-Smith OC, Nicol AL, Christianson JA. Potential mechanisms underlying centralized pain and emerging therapeutic interventions. *Front Cell Neurosci.* 2018;12(35):35.

62. Eccleston C, Crombez G. Pain demands attention: A cognitive–affective model of the interruptive function of pain. *Psychol Bull.* 1999;125(3):356–366.

63. Gellatly R, Beck AT. Catastrophic thinking: A transdiagnostic process across psychiatric disorders. *Cogn Ther Res.* 2016;40(4):441–452.

64. Lumley MA, Cohen JL, Borszcz GS, et al. Pain and emotion: A biopsychosocial review of recent research. *J Clin Psychol.* 2011;67(9):942–968.

65. Schutze R, Rees C, Slater H, Smith A, O'Sullivan P. "I call it stinkin' thinkin'": A qualitative analysis of metacognition in people with chronic low back pain and elevated catastrophizing. *Br J Health Psychol.* 2017;22(3):463–480.

66. Ziadni MS, Sturgeon JA, Darnall BD. The relationship between negative metacognitive thoughts, pain catastrophizing and adjustment to chronic pain. *Eur J Pain.* 2018;22(4):756–762.

67. Normann N, Morina N. The efficacy of metacognitive therapy: A systematic review and meta-analysis. *Front Psychol.* 2018;9:2211.

68. Turk DC, Dworkin RH, Revicki D, et al. Identifying important outcome domains for chronic pain clinical trials: An IMMPACT survey of people with pain. *Pain.* 2008;137(2):276–285.

69. Ohayon MM. Relationship between chronic painful physical condition and insomnia. *J Psychiatr Res.* 2005;39(2):151–159.

70. Finan PH, Goodin BR, Smith MT. The association of sleep and pain: An update and a path forward. *J Pain.* 2013;14(12):1539–1552.

71. Yun SY, Kim DH, Do HY, Kim SH. Clinical insomnia and associated factors in failed back surgery syndrome: A retrospective cross-sectional study. *Int J Med Sci.* 2017;14(6):536–542.

72. Smith MT, Perlis ML, Carmody TP, Smith MS, Giles DE. Presleep cognitions in patients with insomnia secondary to chronic pain. *J Behav Med.* 2001;24(1):93–114.

73. Harvey AG, Greenall E. Catastrophic worry in primary insomnia. *J Behav Ther Exp Psychiatry.* 2003;34(1):11–23.

74. Picavet HS, Vlaeyen JW, Schouten JS. Pain catastrophizing and kinesiophobia: Predictors of chronic low back pain. *Am J Epidemiol.* 2002;156(11):1028–1034.

75. Harvey AG. A cognitive model of insomnia. *Behav Res Ther.* 2002;40(8):869–893.

76. Brasure M, Fuchs E, MacDonald R, et al. Psychological and behavioral interventions for managing insomnia disorder: An evidence report for a clinical practice guideline by the American College of Physicians. *Ann Intern Med.* 2016;165(2):113–124.

77. Cheatle MD, Foster S, Pinkett A, Lesneski M, Qu D, Dhingra L. Assessing and managing sleep disturbance in patients with chronic pain. *Sleep Med Clin.* 2016;11(4):531–541.

78. Belanger L, Savard J, Morin CM. Clinical management of insomnia using cognitive therapy. *Behav Sleep Med.* 2006;4(3):179–198.

79. Harvey AG, Sharpley AL, Ree MJ, Stinson K, Clark DM. An open trial of cognitive therapy for chronic insomnia. *Behav Res Ther.* 2007;45(10):2491–2501.

80. Bohra MH, Espie CA. Is cognitive behavioural therapy for insomnia effective in treating insomnia and pain in individuals with chronic non-malignant pain? *Br J Pain.* 2013;7(3):138–151.

81. Tang NK, Goodchild CE, Salkovskis PM. Hybrid cognitive-behaviour therapy for individuals with insomnia and chronic pain: A pilot randomised controlled trial. *Behav Res Ther.* 2012;50(12):814–821.

82. Finan PH, Carroll CP, Moscou-Jackson G, et al. Daily opioid use fluctuates as a function of pain, catastrophizing, and affect in patients with sickle cell disease: An electronic daily diary analysis. *J Pain.* 2018;19(1):46–56.

83. Finan PH, Buenaver LF, Coryell VT, Smith MT. Cognitive-behavioral therapy for comorbid insomnia and chronic pain. *Sleep Med Clin.* 2014;9(2):261–274.

84. Morin CM, Blais F, Savard J. Are changes in beliefs and attitudes about sleep related to sleep improvements in the treatment of insomnia? *Behav Res Ther.* 2002;40(7):741–752.

85. Tang NK, Goodchild CE, Hester J, Salkovskis PM. Pain-related insomnia versus primary insomnia: A comparison study of sleep pattern, psychological characteristics, and cognitive-behavioral processes. *Clin J Pain.* 2012;28(5):428–436.

86. Afolalu EF, Moore C, Ramlee F, Goodchild CE, Tang NK. Development of the Pain-Related Beliefs and Attitudes about Sleep (PBAS) scale for the assessment and treatment of insomnia comorbid with chronic pain. *J Clin Sleep Med.* 2016;12(9):1269–1277.

87. Asih S, Neblett R, Mayer TG, Brede E, Gatchel RJ. Insomnia in a chronic musculoskeletal pain with disability population is independent of pain and depression. *Spine J.* 2014;14(9):2000–2007.

88. Bujak BK, Regan E, Beattie PF, Harrington S. The effectiveness of interdisciplinary intensive outpatient programs in a population with diverse chronic pain conditions: A systematic review and meta-analysis. *Pain Manag.* 2019;9(4):417–429.

89. Wachter K, Schultz R, Gatchel RJ. Three approaches found effective for pain catastrophizing. *Pract Pain Manage.* 2018;18(2).

90. Townsend CO, Kerkvliet JL, Bruce BK, et al. A longitudinal study of the efficacy of a comprehensive pain rehabilitation program with opioid withdrawal: Comparison of treatment outcomes based on opioid use status at admission. *Pain.* 2008;140(1):177–189.

91. Craner JR, Gilliam WP, Sperry JA. Rumination, magnification, and helplessness: How do different aspects of pain catastrophizing relate to pain severity and functioning? *Clin J Pain.* 2016;32(12):1028–1035.

92. Lumley MA, Schubiner H. Psychological therapy for centralized pain: An integrative assessment and treatment model. *Psychosom Med.* 2019;81(2):114–124.

93. Lumley MA, Schubiner H. Emotional awareness and expression therapy for chronic pain: Rationale, principles and techniques, evidence, and critical review. *Curr Rheumatol Rep.* 2019;21(7):30.

94. Talaei-Khoei M, Fischerauer SF, Lee SG, Ring D, Vranceanu AM. Pain catastrophizing mediates the effect of psychological inflexibility on pain intensity and upper extremity physical function in patients with upper extremity illness. *Pain Pract*. 2017;17(1):129–140.

95. Levett DZH, Grimmett C. Psychological factors, prehabilitation and surgical outcomes: Evidence and future directions. *Anaesthesia*. 2019;74(suppl 1):36–42.

96. Scheede-Bergdahl C, Minnella EM, Carli F. Multi-modal prehabilitation: Addressing the why, when, what, how, who and where next? *Anaesthesia*. 2019;74(suppl 1):20–26.

97. Flink IL, Boersma K, Linton SJ. Pain catastrophizing as repetitive negative thinking: A development of the conceptualization. *Cogn Behav Ther*. 2013;42(3):215–223.

18

Untangling Comorbid Irritable Bowel Syndrome and Psychiatric Disorders

MIHAELA FADGYAS STANCULETE
AND DAN L. DUMITRASCU ■

CLINICAL VIGNETTE

A. M. is a 37-year-old female schoolteacher. She was healthy until 18 months ago, when she started to report heartburn of mild intensity, not necessitating therapy. After a few weeks, heartburn increased in severity and disturbed her sleep. She began thinking about cancer and read on the Internet about esophageal cancer. She started therapy with proton pomp inhibitor (PPI) and was referred for upper digestive endoscopy, which showed mild esophagitis. After 2 months of well-being, she started complaining of abdominal pain and diarrhea. Hematological and biochemical tests were normal, and fecal calprotectin levels were also normal. She started therapy with antispasmodic drugs and rifaximin, with mild improvement. Nine months later, the pain worsened and started to obsess the patient. She reported pain of severe intensity several days per week, preventing her from working in good conditions. The pain was not related to eating and somewhat improved after defecation. Intensity was variable from discomfort to unbearable, requiring emergency department visits. Bowel movements were less than three per week and occasionally diarrheic. Appetite was preserved, as was body weight. Colonoscopy was normal. Irritable bowel syndrome (IBS) diagnosis was established. She continued therapy with antispasmodic drugs, no PPIs. Antidepressant drugs were recommended, but she refused to take them. She was alexithymic, oncophobic, and depressive. Cognitive behavioral therapy (CBT) was started, but she declined to continue. Finally, she accepted buspirone but rejected this therapy after few days, claiming adverse effects. She said, "Please send me to a surgeon to take out the bad from me." Despite several sessions of CBT and relaxation therapy, she still has the same symptoms.

IRRITABLE BOWEL SYNDROME: A SOMATIC OR A PSYCHIATRIC CONDITION?

IBS is the prototype of functional gastrointestinal disorders (FGIDs).[1] The Rome Foundation is an independent nonprofit organization that provides an evidence-based approach to the diagnosis of FGIDs. With the advent of the papers of the Rome IV committees, changes of paradigm in the approach of including IBS have been accepted.[2] Thus, FGIDs are no longer considered idiopathic but rather are self-constituted entities with specific features caused by disorders of the gut–brain interaction.[3] Among them, functional bowel disorders are the most frequent, and among them, IBS, the galleon figure of FGIDs.[4] IBS itself has gone through some changes in respect to definition and characterization. According to the new Rome IV criteria, it should now be defined as an FGID of the bowels characterized by abdominal pain (not discomfort) and defecation changes.[1,5]

The main pathogenic factors of IBS are displayed in Table 18.1. They include genetic, environmental, and physiological factors.[1,6–12]

Table 18.2 displays the most common psychosocial factors encountered in IBS.[13–18]

In severe forms, the psychological factors are predominant, while in mild forms, the psychological factors are almost nonexistent (Figure 18.1).

Thus, individual entities, characterized by abdominal symptoms and emotional disorders, in the absence of organic or biochemical conditions able to explain these complaints, may be referred either to a gastroenterologist (when gastrointestinal symptoms are prevalent, i.e., mainly in less severe cases) or to a psychiatrist (when emotional symptoms are frequent, i.e., in severe cases), or to both of these specialists (when both categories of symptoms have similar severity, i.e., in moderate and severe cases).

Table 18.1 PATHOGENIC FACTORS IN IRRITABLE BOWEL SYNDROME

Genetic	Environmental	Physiological
Familial	Infection	Motility
Twins	Stress	Visceral hypersensitivity
KDEL endoplasmic reticulum protein retention receptor 2 (KDELR2)	Diet	Abnormal input processing: central and peripheral
Glutamate receptor, ionotropic, delta 2 (GRID2) interacting protein		Autonomic dysfunction
Single-nucleotide polymorphisms (SNPs)		Hypothalamic-pituitary-adrenal (HPA) axis dysfunction
Serotonin transporter–linked polymorphic region (5-HTTLPR)		Immune dysfunction
		Intestinal microbiota
		Intestinal permeability

Psychiatric symptoms are highly prevalent in IBS. Some years ago, we could consider IBS a somatoform disorder of the gastrointestinal tract.[19] Now, with the advent of the *Diagnostic and Statistical Manual of Mental Disorders,* fifth edition (DSM-V),[20] we might contemplate seeing an IBS case as a psychiatric case of somatic symptom disorder. But even this term shows that the somatician (i.e., the gastroenterologist) has priority over the psychiatrist in managing the patient.[21] Analyzing the conceptual change of somatization through all five editions of the DSM, one can find a persistent trend to consider IBS patients less "psychological" and more "somatic."[22]

Table 18.2 PSYCHOSOCIAL FACTORS IN IRRITABLE BOWEL SYNDROME

Psychological factors	Social factors
• Anger	• Adverse life events (sexual, emotional, physical abuse)
• Anxiety	
• Depression	• Chronic life stress
• Cognitive and affective processes:	• Parental beliefs and behaviors
(a) Alexithymia	• Learning illness behavior through positive reinforcement or reward
(b) Anxiety	
(c) Catastrophizing	• Modeling
(d) Coping mechanisms	• Illness behavior
	• Social support
	• Beliefs and norms

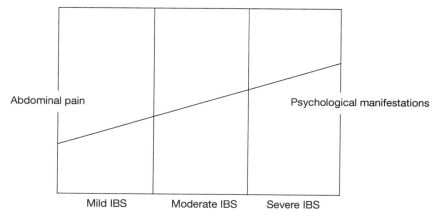

Figure 18.1. Relationship between the severity of abdominal and psychological manifestations in irritable bowel syndrome (IBS).

SQUEEZING THE PSYCHOLOGICAL FROM THE BIOPSYCHOSOCIAL MODEL

In an attempt to explain the pathogenic mechanisms of IBS, Drossman has suggested a model based on the biopsychosocial model of Engel[23] that can be applied to IBS and in large part to all FGIDs.[24] This model was refined by the groups of Fukudo and Drossman.[25] These models emphasize the role of psychosocial factors in association with genetic and physiological factors. This model was adopted by clinical physicians, psychiatrists, and psychosomaticians and has been re-evaluated several times.[26,27]

Stress is also an important factor involved in IBS. Starting with the pioneer studies of the effect of stress on colonic motility in IBS, it came out that stress and post-traumatic stress disorder can affect psychological health and lead to biological changes in the patient.

Of course, not everybody was satisfied with the explanatory model, and these were mainly the psychiatrists. They formulated more or less pertinent criticism: lack of philosophical coherence,[28] lack of importance given to subjective meanings and needs of the patient,[29] or even the incapacity to explain the "unexplained symptoms."[30]

FGIDs become a psychiatric condition when symptoms are intense or have a frequent incidence, causing disability. Therefore, it is crucial that the gastroenterologist or the general practitioner correctly identify the expression form of IBS.[31] But these severe forms of IBS are encountered in patients in whom the feelings and cognitions fall in the field of mental pathology.[32]

For a comprehensive covering of FGID patients, gastroenterologists associated with the Rome IV working committee have recently developed a Multidimensional Clinical Profile (MDCP).[33] According to this operative model, the functional patient has to be evaluated for the following aspects: (a) categorical diagnosis, (b) clinical modifiers, (c) impact on daily activity, (d) psychosocial modifiers, and (e) physiological features and biomarkers.[32] This way of thinking leaves a lot of room for the intervention of the psychiatrist, and point (d) may require the advice of a psychiatrist.

WHAT REMAINS FOR THE PSYCHIATRIST?

Of course, the psychiatrist should contribute to the care of the patient with severe forms of IBS and with psychiatric comorbidities. Reasons for psychiatric consultation include the following:

- Current anxiety or depression symptoms
- Personal history of psychiatric conditions
- Prior/current suicidal ideation or self-harm behavior
- Family history of major mental disorders

Pain and Irritable Bowel Syndrome

Abdominal pain is a cardinal symptom in patients with IBS and is mediated by nociceptors in the intestinal wall (visceral hypersensitivity). Visceral pain is less defined and often poorly localized clinically.

Chronic pain involves both central nervous system (CNS) reorganization and dysregulation of the brain–gut axis. Several brain regions are involved in the central processing of the pain. The most important are considered: the insular cortex, prefrontal cortex (PFC), anterior cingulate cortex (ACC), amygdala, and hippocampus.

Recent research demonstrated that patients with IBS have a greater engagement of regions associated with emotional arousal and endogenous pain modulation.[34] Also, a similar activation of regions involved in the processing of visceral afferent information was observed. The afferent visceral stimulation can be experienced as painful both as a result of peripheral intensity and as a result of central processing. Chronic pain can lead to modified brain circuitry, change in motility and permeability in the gastrointestinal tract, and interact with gut microbiota; all result in an intensified visceral pain perception.

Studies using functional imaging demonstrated that IBS patients show lesser activation of the ACC (which is responsible for descending pain inhibition) and greater activation of the midcingulate cortex (MCC). Thus, it was hypothesized that in IBS, the adaptive inhibitory response to painful visceral stimuli is replaced with a maladaptive response.

A growing body of data suggests that psychological factors strongly influence IBS pain.[35-37] On the other hand, pain has been recognized as a significant symptom with implications for mental health. Many studies pointed out that IBS patients pay greater attention to pain and tend to catastrophize the symptoms. Other researchers have confirmed that symptom catastrophizing (magnifying the threat or the seriousness of pain and feeling helpless to do anything about it) negatively affects subjective pain reporting and daily functioning.

Comorbidities of Irritable Bowel Syndrome in Psychiatry

Several comorbidities have been described in IBS because functional disorders, like IBS, are always at the frontier between physical disease and mental disorder. Accumulating evidence supports that many patients with IBS have psychiatric comorbidity, and the most common conditions are depressive and anxiety disorders.[38-42] Studies suggest that multiple factors are involved in the determination of this comorbidity. The relationship between IBS and psychiatric illnesses is bidirectional between the gastrointestinal tract and the brain, through neural, neuroimmune, and neuroendocrine pathways. The model of comorbidity is illustrated in Figure 18.2.

Understanding the relationship between the neurobiology, psychiatric symptoms, and psychosocial factors can guide comprehensive interventions. The care of IBS patients benefits from collaboration with mental health professionals. With special training and experience in the use of psychotropic medications and various psychotherapies, psychiatrists are a significant part of the multidisciplinary team.

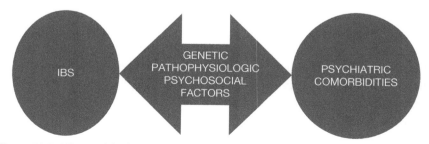

Figure 18.2. The model of psychiatric comorbidities in irritable bowel syndrome (IBS).

The hypothesis linking emotional and cognitive areas in the CNS with the autonomic nervous system (ANS) and the enteric nervous system (ENS) made a lasting contribution to the understanding of psychiatric comorbidities.

One of the latest disease models of IBS comprises the overlap of brain circuits involved in emotion regulation, autonomic responses, and pain modulation as one of the most important features. Descending neural modulatory circuits from the brain can inhibit or facilitate ascending nociceptive transmission. Chronic pain from IBS appears to be associated with a dysregulation in descending pain modulation (DPM). Those circuits are also known to be influenced by cognitive processes and mood. Stress and emotional dysregulation (anxiety and depression) can cause efferent stimulation and amplify the pain signal. Evaluation of pain also appears to be modified in IBS. Those postulations are confirmed by functional and possibly structural brain changes involving prefrontal and cingulate regions.[43,44] Moreover, brain–gut dysregulation predisposes patients with chronic IBS pain to anxiety and depression. Table 18.3 presents the psychiatric comorbidities reported in IBS.

The simultaneous presence of mental illness and IBS increases the costs of dealing with both of them, worsens the prognosis, has a substantial negative impact on quality of life and self-care.

Psychiatric comorbidities appear to play significant roles, including the following:

- Moderation of symptom severity
- Involvement in symptom persistence

Table 18.3 PSYCHIATRIC COMORBIDITIES REPORTED IN IRRITABLE BOWEL SYNDROME

Anxiety disorders	Generalized anxiety disorder (GAD)
	Panic disorder (PD)
	Post-traumatic stress disorder (PTSD)
	Obsessive-compulsive disorder (OCD)
	Agoraphobia
	Social phobia
Affective disorders	Major depression disorder (MDD)
	Bipolar disorder
	Dysthymia
Sleep disorders	Poor sleep quality
	Increased daytime sleepiness
	Prolonged sleep latency
	Sleep fragmentation
Somatoform and related disorders	
Schizophrenia	

- Participation in decisions-making and consent to treatment
- Moderation of response to treatment

Psychiatric symptoms in IBS patients are highly prevalent but are often unrecognized and undertreated. A population-based study reported a lifetime prevalence of anxiety and depressive disorder of 50.5%.[45] The incidence of psychiatric comorbidity is even higher in patients with IBS receiving care in tertiary gastroenterology centers. These comorbidities should be systematically checked and treated.[46]

One significant problem arises if the patient is suicidal. IBS is frequently considered as a minor, non–life-threatening condition. One study conducted in a tertiary care facility found that 38% of patients reported suicidal ideation as a result of their hopelessness.[47] The main risk factors are represented by concurrent depression, hopelessness, anxiety, inefficient coping mechanisms, and inadequate treatment options. Guthrie et al. conducted a study that suggests that suicidal ideations and episodes of self-harm may be relatively frequent in patients with high levels of health care utilization rates and multiple psychosocial risk factors.[39] It seems important to ask about suicidal ideation and behaviors at the initial evaluation and in the follow-up visits.

Genetic Factors of Psychiatric Disorders in Irritable Bowel Syndrome

Several studies have reported that there is a link between IBS and psychiatric disorders, including in families.[48,49] Table 18.4 presents nine potential target genes associated with psychiatric disorders that were also investigated in IBS but with inconclusive results.

Psychiatric Therapy in Irritable Bowel Syndrome

A biopsychosocial treatment of psychiatric comorbidities is probably the most appropriate involving pharmacotherapy, psychotherapy, and education.[50] It is noteworthy to remember that many patients with IBS and psychiatric comorbidities do not receive effective treatment for their psychiatric comorbidities. This situation is the result of many factors, especially the gastroenterologists, who often do not pay sufficient attention to the presence of psychiatric disorders in their patients.

Table 18.4 GENES INVOLVED IN IRRITABLE BOWEL SYNDROME
AND PSYCHIATRIC DISORDERS

Gene	Psychiatric condition
SLC6A4 (solute carrier family 6 member 4)	Obsessive-compulsive disorder
	Depression
Gene encoding FK506 binding protein 51 (FKBP5)	Post-traumatic stress disorder
Catechol-O-methyltransferase (COMT) gene: COMT Val 158Met	Obsessive-compulsive disorder
	Panic disorder
	Cognitive impairment
Brain-derived neurotrophic factor (BDNF) gene	Schizophrenia
	Anorexia and bulimia nervosa
BDNF Val166Met	Post-traumatic stress disorder
	Mood disorders
Opioid receptor mu 1(OPRM1) gene	Opioid dependence
OPRM1 118AG variant	Pain sensitivity
	Social sensitivity
NPY (neuropeptide Y)	Stress response
Ankyrin repeat and kinase domain containing 1 (ANKK1) gene	Impulse control disorders
	Alexithymia
Dopamine receptor D2 (DRD2) gene	Cocaine dependence
DRD2 Taq1A	Schizophrenia
Fatty acid amide hydrolase (FAAH) gene	Substance dependence

PHARMACOLOGICAL THERAPY: ANTIDEPRESSANTS

Several studies have emphasized that psychotropic drugs can play a major role in the treatment of IBS patients. Treatment of anxiety and depression in IBS is similar to the treatment of idiopathic depression.[51,52]

Antidepressants are used to treat both depression and IBS symptoms. Until now it was demonstrated that two types of antidepressants could help IBS symptoms: tricyclic antidepressants and selective serotonin reuptake inhibitors. The antidepressants represent a treatment option in patients with moderate and severe symptoms. Antidepressants are often chosen for their side-effect profile to help moderate symptoms like constipation or diarrhea.

The beneficial effects of antidepressants could be the result of the increase in central pain threshold. Other mechanisms of action are represented by the anticholinergic effects (influence on gastrointestinal motility and secretion) and their reduction of the pain sensitivity of peripheral nerves.[53] The most commonly used antidepressants are illustrated in Table 18.5

The psychiatrist will choose a particular antidepressant based on many factors, including the following:

Table 18.5 ANTIDEPRESSANTS USED IN IRRITABLE BOWEL SYNDROME TREATMENT

Medication class	Generic names	Side effects	Special consideration
Tricyclic antidepressants (TCAs)	Amitriptyline Imipramine Desipramine Nortriptyline	Sedation Dry mouth Blurred vision Difficulty urinating Constipation Drowsiness	Avoid TCAs in constipation-predominant irritable bowel syndrome
Selective serotonin reuptake inhibitors (SSRIs)	Citalopram Escitalopram Paroxetine Sertraline Fluoxetine	Nervousness Vivid dreams Sleep disturbances Sexual difficulties Diarrhea	Start cautiously and discuss transient worsening of bowel symptoms
Serotonin-norepinephrine reuptake inhibitors (SNRIs)	Venlafaxine Duloxetine Desvenlafaxine Milnacipran	Nausea Headaches	Usefulness is limited by gastrointestinal side effects. There is a lack of evidence for their effectiveness.

- Symptom pattern (diarrhea or constipation)
- Severity
- Associated emotional symptoms (anxiety, depression)
- General medical health
- Possible side effects

Evidence to support general use of antidepressants for IBS patients to minimize the risk for psychiatric comorbidities is lacking at this time. In some countries, antidepressants are not approved for the treatment of IBS, so they only can be used off-label. Because of the side effects (loss of appetite, nausea, sexual impairments), antidepressants in the treatment of IBS without psychiatric comorbidities are considered only if other treatments have not proved successful. The use of psychotropic medication is cautioned in elderly patients because of anticholinergic side effects. Nonpharmacological approaches, including psychotherapy, relaxation, and stress management, could be considered as alternatives.

PSYCHOTHERAPY IN IRRITABLE BOWEL SYNDROME
Psychotherapy has demonstrated effectiveness relieving both gastrointestinal and mood disturbances. Data suggest that patients with severe IBS that has not responded to usual treatment may benefit from psychological treatment.

Psychological therapies such as counseling, relaxation, hypnotherapy, and psychotherapy can be very effective.[54] Cognitive behavioral therapy (CBT), brief psychodynamic interpersonal therapy, group therapy, and hypnotherapy have all been demonstrated to improve overall well-being and IBS symptoms. The psychotherapy might help the patients cope with their symptoms better than previously.

CBT seems to produce a significant improvement in daily functioning, larger than that produced by relaxation therapy.[55]

Hypnotherapy is an effective treatment alternative for patients with refractory IBS and aims to teach patients the necessary hypnotic skills to control and help normalize gut function. The beneficial effects of gut-directed hypnotherapy are durable, making it a highly valuable therapeutic option.[56]

CONCLUSION

According to the biopsychosocial model of disease, the modern approach to the chronic pain patient is to address not only the mental or somatic disease but also the interaction between these two intricate components of the human body. In the case of FGIDs, mainly in the case of IBS, the pathogenesis of symptoms and their expression are indeed caused by mental and somatic factors. Their preponderance is variable from case to case, but it is well accepted that, usually, the severe cases of IBS present with psychiatric disorders. On the other hand, the psychiatrist should never minimize the somatic origin of the pain in some of the patients. Comorbidity with pain and psychiatric disturbances increases the IBS burden, which is reflected in greater severity of the symptoms, longer duration of disease, and worse outcomes. Thus, it is essential to treat both pain and psychiatric disorders when they coexist to achieve optimal therapeutic success.

REFERENCES

1. Lacy BE, Mearin F, Chang L, et al. Bowel disorders. *Gastroenterology*. 2016;150(6): 1393–1407.
2. Drossman DA, Dumitrascu DL, Rome III. New standard for functional gastrointestinal disorders. *J Gastrointest Liver Dis*. 2006;15(3):237–41.
3. Drossman DA, Hassler WL. Rome IV: Functional GI disorders of gut brain interaction. *Gastroenterology*. 2016;150(6):1257–1261.
4. Dumitrascu DL. Making a positive diagnosis of irritable bowel syndrome. *J Clin Gastroenterol*. 2011;45(suppl):S82–S85.
5. Bai T, Xia J, Jiang Y, et al. Comparison of the Rome IV and Rome III criteria for IBS diagnosis: A cross-sectional survey. *J Gastroenterol Hepatol*. 2016;32(5):1018–1025.

6. Ek WE, Reznichenko A, Ripke S, et al. Exploring the genetics of irritable bowel syndrome: A GWA study in the general population and replication in multinational case-control cohorts. *Gut.* 201;64(11):1774–1782.

7. Niesler B, Kapeller J, Fell C, et al. 5-HTTLPR and STin2 polymorphisms in the serotonin transporter gene and irritable bowel syndrome: Effect of bowel habit and sex. *Eur J Gastroenterol Hepatol.* 2010;22(7):856–861.

8. Camilleri M, Katzka DA. Irritable bowel syndrome: Methods, mechanisms, and pathophysiology: Genetic epidemiology and pharmacogenetics in irritable bowel syndrome. *Am J Physiol Gastrointest Liver Physiol.* 2012;302(10):G1075–G1084.

9. Hotoleanu C, Popp R, Trifa AP, Nedelcu L, Dumitrascu DL. Genetic determination of irritable bowel syndrome. *World J Gastroenterol.* 2008;14(43):6636–6640.

10. Drossman DA, Leserman J, Nachman G, et al. Sexual and physical abuse in women with functional or organic gastrointestinal disorders. *Ann Intern Med.* 1990;113(11):828–833.

11. Galati JS, McKee DP, Quigley EM. Response to intraluminal gas in irritable bowel syndrome: Motility versus perception. *Dig Dis Sci.* 1995;40(6):1381–1387.

12. Naliboff BD, Munakata J, Fullerton S, et al. Evidence for two distinct perceptual alterations in irritable bowel syndrome. *Gut.* 1997;41(4):505–512.

13. Drossman DA, Chang L, Bellamy N, et al. Severity in irritable bowel syndrome: A Rome Foundation Working Team report. *Am J Gastroenterol.* 2011;106(10):1749–1759.

14. Van Oudenhove L, Levy RL, Crowell MD, et al. Biopsychosocial aspects of functional gastrointestinal disorders. *Gastroenterology.* 2016;150(6):1355–1367.

15. Surdea-Blaga T, Băban A, Dumitrascu DL. Psychosocial determinants of irritable bowel syndrome. *World J Gastroenterol.* 2012;18(7):616–626.

16. Crowell MD, Harris L, Jones MP, Chang L. New insights into the pathophysiology of irritable bowel syndrome: Implications for future treatments. *Curr Gastroenterol Rep.* 2005;7(4):272–279.

17. Fadgyas Stanculete M. Psychiatric comorbidities in irritable bowel syndrome (IBS). In: Choban V, ed. *Irritable Bowel Syndrome—Novel Concepts for Research and Treatment.* Rijeka: InTechOpen; 2016:7–24.

18. Gerson CD, Gerson MJ, Chang L, et al. A cross-cultural investigation of attachment style, catastrophizing, negative pain beliefs, and symptom severity in irritable bowel syndrome. *Neurogastroenterol Motil.* 2015;27(4):490–500.

19. American Psychiatric Association. *Diagnostic and Statistical Manual of Mental Disorders,* fourth edition, text revision. Arlington, VA: American Psychiatric Publishing; 2000.

20. American Psychiatric Association. *Diagnostic and Statistical Manual of Mental Disorders,* fifth edition. Arlington, VA: American Psychiatric Publishing; 2013.

21. Basilisco G, Coletta M, Arsiè E, Cesana BM. Study of somatization in IBS. *Neurogastroenterol Motil.* 2015;27(5):741.

22. Moldovan R, Radu M, Băban A, Dumitraşcu DL. Evolution of psychosomatic diagnosis in DSM: Historical perspectives and new development for internists. *Rom J Intern Med.* 2015;53(1):25–30.

23. Engel GL. From biomedical to biopsychosocial: Being scientific in the human domain. *Psychosomatics.* 1997;38(6):521–528.

24. Gaynes BN, Drossman DA. The role of psychosocial factors in irritable bowel syndrome. *Baillieres Best Pract Res Clin Gastroenterol.* 1999;13(3):437–452.
25. Tanaka Y, Kanazawa M, Fukudo S, Drossman DA. Biopsychosocial model of irritable bowel syndrome. *J Neurogastroenterol Motil.* 2011;2:131–139.
26. Fava GA, Sonino N. The biopsychosocial model thirty years later. *Psychother Psychosom.* 2008;77(1):1–2.
27. Adler RH. Engel's biopsychosocial model is still relevant today. *J Psychosom Res.* 2009;67(6):607–611.
28. Benning TB. Limitations of the biopsychosocial model in psychiatry. *Adv Med Educ Pract.* 2015;6:347–352.
29. Ghaemi N. The rise and fall of the bio-psychosocial model. *Br J Psychiatry.* 2009;195:3–4.
30. Butler CC, Evans M, Greaves D, Simpson S. Medically unexplained symptoms: The biopsychosocial model found wanting. *J R Soc Med.* 2004;97:219–222.
31. Boeckxstaens GE, Drug V, Dumitrascu D, et al. COST Action BM1106 GENIEUR members. Phenotyping of subjects for large scale studies on patients with IBS. *Neurogastroenterol Motil.* 2016;28(8):1134–1147.
32. Fadgyas-Stanculete M, Buga AM, Popa-Wagner A, Dumitrascu DL. The relationship between irritable bowel syndrome and psychiatric disorders: From molecular changes to clinical manifestations. *J Mol Psychiatry.* 2014;2(1):4.
33. Garakani A, Win T, Virk S, Gupta S, et al. Comorbidity of irritable bowel syndrome in psychiatric patients: A review. *Am J Ther.* 2003;10(1):61–67.
34. Tillisch K, Mayer EA, Labus JS. Quantitative meta-analysis identifies brain regions activated during rectal distension in irritable bowel syndrome. *Gastroenterology.* 2011;31;140(1):91–100.
35. Edebol-Carlman H, Ljótsson B, Linton SJ, et al. Face-to-face cognitive-behavioral therapy for irritable bowel syndrome: The effects on gastrointestinal and psychiatric symptoms. *Gastroenterol Res Pract.* 2017;2017:8915872.
36. Deiteren A, de Wit A, van der Linden L, De Man JG, Pelckmans PA, De Winter BY. Irritable bowel syndrome and visceral hypersensitivity: Risk factors and pathophysiological mechanisms. *Acta Gastroenterol Bel.* 2015;79(1):29–38.
37. Moloney RD, Johnson AC, O'Mahony SM, Dinan TG, Meerveld GV, Cryan JF. Stress and the microbiota–gut–brain axis in visceral pain: Relevance to irritable bowel syndrome. *CNS Neurosci Ther.* 2016;22(2):102–117.
38. Fond G, Loundou A, Hamdani N, et al. Anxiety and depression comorbidities in irritable bowel syndrome (IBS): A systematic review and meta-analysis. *Eur Arch Psychiatry Clin Neurosci.* 2014;264(8):651–660.
39. Guthrie E, Barlow J, Fernandes L, et al. Changes in tolerance to rectal distension correlate with changes in psychological state in patients with severe irritable bowel syndrome. *Psychosom Med.* 2004;66(4):578–582.
40. Spiegel BM. The burden of IBS: Looking at metrics. *Curr Gastroenterol Report.* 2009;11(4):265–269.
41. Hausteiner-Wiehle C, Henningsen P. Irritable bowel syndrome: Relations with functional, mental, and somatoform disorders. *World J Gastroenterol.* 2014;20(20):6024–6030.

42. Wouters MM, Boeckxstaens GE. Is there a causal link between psychological disorders and functional gastrointestinal disorders? *Expert Rev Gastroenterol Hepatol.* 2016;10(1):5–8.

43. Elsenbruch S. Abdominal pain in irritable bowel syndrome: A review of putative psychological, neural and neuro-immune mechanisms. *Brain Behav Immun.* 2011;25(3):386–394.

44. Chakiath RJ, Siddall PJ, Kellow JE, et al. Descending pain modulation in irritable bowel syndrome (IBS): A systematic review and meta-analysis. *Syst Rev.* 2015;4(1):175.

45. Mykletun A, Jacka F, Williams L, Pasco J, et al. Prevalence of mood and anxiety disorder in self-reported irritable bowel syndrome (IBS): An epidemiological population based study of women. *BMC Gastroenterol.* 2010;10(1):88.

46. Koloski NA, Jones M, Kalantar J, Weltman M, Zaguirre J, Talley NJ. The brain-gut pathway in functional gastrointestinal disorders is bidirectional: A 12-year prospective population-based study. *Gut.* 2012;61(9):1284–1290.

47. Miller V, Hopkins L, Whorwell P. Suicidal ideation in patients with irritable bowel syndrome. *Clin Gastroenterol Hepatol.* 2004;2(12):1064–1068.

48. Saito YA. The role of genetics in IBS. *Gastroenterol Clin North Am.* 2011;40(1):45–67.

49. Henström M, D'Amato M. Genetics of irritable bowel syndrome. *Mol Cell Pediatr.* 2016;3(1):1.

50. Sinagra E, Romano C, Cottone M. Psychopharmacological treatment and psychological interventions in irritable bowel syndrome. *Gastroenterol Res Pract.* 2012;2012:486067.

51. Ruepert L, Quartero AO, de Wit NJ, van der Heijden GJ, Rubin G, Muris JW. Bulking agents, antispasmodics and antidepressants for the treatment of irritable bowel syndrome. *Cochrane Database Syst Rev.* 2011;(8):CD003460.

52. Halland M, Talley NJ. New treatments for IBS. *Nat Rev Gastroenterol Hepatol.* 2013;10(1):13–23.

53. Macedo D, Chaves Filho AJM, de Sousa CNS, et al. Antidepressants, antimicrobials or both? Gut microbiota dysbiosis in depression and possible implications of the antimicrobial effects of antidepressant drugs for antidepressant effectiveness. *J Affect Disord.* 2017;208:22–32.

54. Lackner JM, Brasel AM, Quigley BM, et al. The ties that bind: Perceived social support, stress, and IBS in severely affected patients. *Neurogastroenterol Motil.* 2010;22(8):893–900.

55. Laird KT, Tanner-Smith EE, Russell AC, Hollon SD, Walker LS. Comparative efficacy of psychological treatments for improving mental health and daily functioning in irritable bowel syndrome: A systematic review and meta-analysis. *Clin Psychol Review.* 2017;51:142–152.

56. Lindfors P, Unge P, Arvidsson P, Nyhlin H, et al. Effects of gut-directed hypnotherapy on IBS in different clinical settings: Results from two randomized, controlled trials. *Am J Gastroenterol.* 2012;107(2):276–285.

19

The Many Faces of Chronic Urogenital Pain

Vulvodynia and Psychiatric Comorbidities

BERNARD L. HARLOW, MIRIAM J. HAVILAND, AND SOPHIE BERGERON ■

INTRODUCTION

Vulvodynia is a condition in which women experience chronic vulvar pain. Although it is a highly prevalent disorder of reproductive age and can cause serious physical and psychological distress, the biological and psychological causes of vulvodynia remain poorly understood. Psychological morbidity is highly prevalent among women with vulvodynia, and thus it is important for both medical and psychological care providers to understand the association between these two conditions. In this chapter, we will discuss the definition, distribution, pathophysiology, and psychosocial risk factors associated with vulvodynia, as well as current treatment options for vulvodynia and associated psychiatric comorbidities.

OVERVIEW OF VULVODYNIA

Definition

Vulvodynia is chronic vulvar pain for which there is no known clinical pathology.[1,2] The pain must be present for at least 3 months, although the onset of pain can be either acute or gradual and then constant or intermittent. Vulvodynia is diagnosed after other explanations for vulvar pain, such as inflammatory vaginitis, candidiasis, sexually transmitted infections, dermatoses, or other pelvic pain disorders, are ruled out.[3]

Phenotypic Patterns

Vulvodynia can be classified by symptom onset or site of pain. There are two subgroups of vulvodynia based on the timing of symptom onset: primary and secondary. Women with primary vulvodynia experience pain at the time of first sexual intercourse, first use of tampons, or first pelvic examination. Generally these women are younger and have never been pregnant.[4] In contrast, women with secondary onset of vulvodynia develop their symptoms after having had pain-free sexual intercourse or other pain-free introital events.[5] Vulvodynia can also be classified into subgroups based on site of pain. Localized vulvodynia is pain that is consistently located at a particular location within the vulvar vestibule. It may represent a single location, multiple specific locations, or a particular region of the vestibule. Localized vulvar pain can be either provoked by physical contact, unprovoked, or mixed (a combination of provoked and unprovoked).

The diagnosis of localized vulvodynia has two components: self-report and clinical assessment. Women with localized vulvodynia report contact pain and pain with any vaginal touch or entry (such as the insertion of a tampon) for more than 3 months. The diagnosis is then made when pain is elicited with pressure from a cotton-tipped swab applied sequentially around the vulvar vestibule with no other identifiable cause.[6] Localized vulvodynia is likely caused by neuroinflammatory pain from nociceptors in the vulvar vestibule that have been sensitized by inflammation or trauma.[7] Generalized vulvodynia is episodic stinging, burning, aching, stabbing, or rawness anywhere in the vulva. Generalized vulvar pain can be either provoked by physical contact, unprovoked, or mixed (a combination of provoked and unprovoked). Women with generalized vulvodynia typically have pain-free periods and may not experience dyspareunia. This may represent neuropathic pain from damage to the pudendal nerve.[8,9]

Prevalence

Data on the prevalence of vulvodynia are limited. Until recently, the only method of assessing prevalence was through women seeking clinical care.

Recent research, however, has shown that a large proportion of women choose not to seek care and even when they do so, often receive incorrect diagnoses.[10] Thus, prevalence assessments done in clinical settings will dramatically underestimate the true prevalence. Recent US-based cross-sectional studies of women from the general population have found that vulvodynia affects women of all ages and race/ethnicities. The annual prevalence is reported to be as high as 3 to 7%.[11] A community-based study found that as many as 16% of women may experience vulvodynia over the course of their lives,[10] and by age 40 years, 7 to 8% of women may experience symptoms consistent with vulvodynia. The incidence of vulvodynia is highest among younger women, with 4% of women experiencing their first episode of vulvodynia before age 25 years. The incidence decreases among women in their late 20s and 30s, and then increases again as women enter their 40s.[12] Women of all ethnicities experience vulvodynia, but one study which compared the prevalence of vulvodynia among women of different ethnic groups found that among the 19,101 women surveyed, Hispanic women were 1.4 times more likely to develop vulvar pain symptoms (95% confidence interval [CI] = 1.1–1.8) compared with white women.[12] There is, however, as of yet no explanation for this difference.

Pathogenesis and Comorbid Conditions

The pathogenesis of vulvodynia is unknown, but many have speculated that it is the result of an altered immune-inflammatory response mechanism. Although it is unclear to what extent factors that occur in the genital tract influence the pathogenesis of vulvodynia, one of the innate properties of the genital tract is selective expression of cytokines and bactericidal peptides. Stress, chronic disease, or local chemical irritation may cause pro-inflammatory mediators to overpower the endogenous inhibitors, changing the inflammatory reaction from protective to destructive.[13] A histopathology study conducted by Chadha et al. found that all of the patients with vulvodynia from whom they collected punch biopsies had chronic inflammatory infiltrates—particularly T lymphocytes—whereas their controls did not.[14] Other studies have shown that women with vulvodynia have higher average levels of interleukin-1β and tumor necrosis factor-α in their perineal tissue.[15,16] These alterations may be caused by a variety of factors, including hormonal and environmental exposures, infection, and psychiatric morbidities.[17-20] It is unclear whether these immune-inflammatory processes directly cause vulvodynia or serve as an intermediate step on the causal pathway.

Women with vulvodynia are more likely to experience a variety of comorbid functional somatic syndromes than women with no history of vulvodynia.

Examples include chronic fatigue syndrome, fibromyalgia, irritable bowel syndrome, and interstitial cystitis. The temporal relationship between these conditions and vulvodynia is not well understood, and it is possible that these conditions may have similar etiologies.[11]

RELATIONSHIP BETWEEN VULVODYNIA AND PSYCHOLOGICAL CONDITIONS

Psychobiological Underpinnings

Neuroscience research has found that a variety of factors such as genetic and psychosocial risk factors, infectious triggers, and personality traits can contribute to mind–body–brain interactions, which affect how the brain perceives, processes, and manages pain. This research, combined with the absence of identifiable pathology for vulvodynia, historically led to the view that vulvodynia may be caused solely by psychological factors. This view is likely erroneous.[21] Researchers currently believe that the interaction between psychosocial risk factors and physiological changes can both cause and mediate vulvodynia symptoms.[22-24] Physiologically, women with vulvodynia have increased density of superficial nerve endings, increased immunoreactivity, and nociceptor sensitivity.[16,25,26] These physiological alterations, combined with the high prevalence of psychosocial risk factors among women with vulvodynia,[23,27] suggests that there is an interaction between psychiatric morbidities and physiological causes of vulvodynia.[21]

Psychological stress, both acute and chronic, has been shown to cause changes in innate and adaptive immune responses, predominantly by impacting neuroendocrine mediators from the hypothalamic-pituitary-adrenal (HPA) axis and the sympathetic-adrenal axis.[28] The HPA axis is responsible for regulating the body's cortisol levels and mediates and controls the immune and inflammatory response of cytokines. Chronic stresses can dysregulate the HPA axis, which can cause inflammation.[22] As discussed earlier in this chapter, women with vulvodynia have been shown to have higher levels of cytokines in their perianal tissue, which may be caused by the dysregulation of the HPA axis.

The interaction between psychosocial risk factors and physiological changes can occur at different levels of functional complexity. Research using positron emission tomography scans found that there was a relationship between perceived pain intensity and the activation of a diverse group of brain regions, including those involved in the processing of negative emotions.[29] Vulvodynia also causes increased sensitization of the peripheral and central nervous systems. This sensitization leads to (a) decreased thresholds for nociceptor stimulation, (b) an increased field of nociceptor reception, and (c) nociceptor responsiveness to allodynia, increased intensity of response, and the occurrence of spontaneous pain.[30,31]

Direct and Indirect Effects of Childhood Maltreatment

A covariate highly related to psychiatric sequelae is childhood maltreatment, which in and of itself has been shown to be associated with vulvodynia. A community-based study of 125 women with vulvodynia and 125 age-matched controls showed that women with vulvodynia were twice as likely to report never or rarely receiving family support as a child compared with women without vulvodynia (odds ratio [OR] = 2.6; 95% CI = 1.3–5.1). The same study also found that women with vulvodynia were significantly more likely to report feeling in danger at home, in their neighborhood, or at school a few times or more compared with women without vulvodynia.[32] A second study found that women with vulvodynia were significantly more likely to report that they suffered severe physical (OR = 2.4; 95% CI = 1.3–4.4) or sexual (OR = 9.7; 95% CI = 1.2–79.1) abuse as children compared with women without vulvodynia. Among the subset of women who suffered severe abuse as children (physical and/or sexual), women with vulvodynia were significantly more likely to have lived in fear of abuse than women without vulvodynia.[20] This suggests that it may not be the abuse itself that causes vulvodynia, but rather the constant stress of living in fear of abuse.

Direct Psychological/Psychiatric Associations and Issues of Temporality

Psychiatric conditions such as mood and anxiety disorders have been shown to increase a woman's risk for developing vulvodynia. A study published in 2011 by Khandker et al. assessed the temporal relationship between psychological distress and adult-onset vulvodynia. The authors administered the Structured Clinical Interview for DSM-IV Axis I Disorders (SCID) to 240 case-control pairs of women with and without vulvodynia to establish the age of onset of diagnosed mood and anxiety disorders. This information was then used to determine whether the first episode of the mood anxiety disorder was antecedent to subsequent onset of vulvodynia symptoms. The authors found that women with antecedent mood or anxiety disorders were four times as likely to develop vulvodynia compared with those without.[27] In another study looking at the role of chronic childhood stressors and the development of vulvodynia, Khandker et al. found that in a subset of participants who had not experienced abuse as a child, women with a history of mood disorder had a six-fold increase of developing vulvodynia compared with women with no history of mood disorders.[20] This finding suggests that adult-onset mood disorders may be significant risk factors for vulvodynia independent of childhood abuse.

Multiple studies have demonstrated that compared with women without vulvodynia, those with vulvodynia are more likely to be psychologically distressed.[11,33,34] Arnold et al. conducted a nested case-control study of 100 women with vulvodynia and 325 matched controls and found that women with vulvodynia were significantly more likely to report symptoms of anxiety or depression than controls (OR = 1.93; 95% CI = 1.08–3.46).[11] In a population-based study of 1795 women, Iglesias-Rios et al. found that women who screened positive for depression were 50% more likely to have vulvodynia (Prevalence Ratio [PR] = 1.53; 95% CI = 1.12–2.10) than women who did not screen positive for depression. The authors also found that women who screened positive for post-traumatic stress disorder were twice as likely to have vulvodynia (PR = 2.37; 95% CI = 1.07–5.25.[35] These studies, however, failed to assess the temporal relationship between psychological distress and onset of vulvodynia. Given the biological link between these two conditions, it is plausible that vulvodynia could be associated with psychological distress.

As discussed earlier in this chapter, women with antecedent mood disorders are significantly more likely to develop vulvodynia. In a subgroup analysis of 62 women with vulvodynia and 82 age-matched controls, Khandker et al. found that vulvodynia cases had six times the odds of antecedent mood disorders.[20] Women with vulvodynia are also more likely to develop new-onset depression and anxiety. In a different study of 240 case-control pairs, Khandker et al. found that women with vulvodynia were more likely to develop new or recurrent mood and anxiety disorders even after adjusting for antecedent history of mood disorders (Hazard Ratio [HR] = 1.7; 95% CI = 1.1–2.6).[27]

Vulvodynia can also cause new or recurrent onset of psychological symptoms. The interaction between vulvodynia and psychological distress might also increase the severity of vulvodynia symptoms. Masheb et al. found that among the 53 women surveyed with a vulvodynia diagnosis, those with current major depressive disorder (MDD) were significantly more likely to report greater pain severity and worse quality of life than women without current MDD.[23] Boerner and Rosen found a significant inverse correlation between pain acceptance and depression and anxiety among women with vulvodynia.[36] This may be because increased pain acceptance decreases women's avoidance and catastrophizing about pain, two factors that have been shown to increase intensity of pain in women with vulvodynia.[37]

Methodological Weakness of Past Research

Research on the association between vulvodynia and psychological conditions has several limitations. One example is that investigation into this association has been primarily cross-sectional and therefore has failed to establish the temporal relationship between these two conditions. Although many studies have utilized validated screening instruments such as the Patient Health Questionnaire Depression Scale (PHQ-8)[38] and the SCID,[39] these instruments may only capture current mood disorders or, when history of mood disorders are captured, may not accurately reflect timing of depression over the life course.

Additional limitations of this research stem from the fact that childhood abuse and psychological conditions assessed as risk factors for vulvodynia have all been largely retrospectively assessed, and thus may suffer from recall bias, because women with vulvodynia may be more likely to recall experiencing these risk factors, the severity of these factors, and the timing of these factors than women with no history of vulvar pain. However, use of structured clinical interviews such as the SCID has been shown to contribute less recall bias than unstructured interviews or self-reported measures.[40] Outcome misclassification may also occur unless vulvodynia cases are clinically confirmed. It is common for women with vulvovaginal pain symptoms from another cause to be misclassified as having vulvodynia.

CLINICAL ISSUES TREATING CO-OCCURRING VULVODYNIA AND PSYCHIATRIC DISORDERS

Assessment

Women with vulvodynia typically consult several health care professionals for their pain, often without success.[12] As a result, they often feel stigmatized and misunderstood, which can add to their psychological burden and complicate their clinical presentation.[41] Hence, the assessment of both the biomedical and psychosocial dimensions of vulvodynia, as either causal or maintenance factors, is crucial. Three medical procedures are required for a proper diagnosis: (a) a gynecological history, (b) a cotton-swab palpation of the vestibular area with the woman rating her pain at various locations, and (c) vaginal and cervical cultures. In addition to the clinical examination, it is highly recommended to make a psychosocial assessment with both the woman and her partner.

Psychosocial assessment recommendations include the following:

1. **Pain.** Pain quality, location, duration, onset, elicitors, and intensity should first be queried. We use a 0 to 10 scale with 0 representing *no pain at all* and 10 representing *the worst pain ever* as a tool throughout assessment and treatment. An immediate focus on the pain validates the patient's suffering and demonstrates an understanding of the problem and its impacts, which is central to establishing the therapeutic alliance. Many women with vulvodynia are skeptical of psychological approaches to pain management, and any hint that the pain might be caused by psychological issues will hamper the treatment process, sometimes even leading to discontinuation of therapy.

2. **Sexuality.** Given that vulvodynia has a major negative impact on sexuality,[34] including reduced sexual desire, arousal, satisfaction, and frequency of sexual activity, this needs to be carefully assessed. Despite the pain, most women continue to engage in sexual intercourse with their partner, sometimes inadvertently worsening the problem.

3. **Cognition.** Two types of cognitions may lead to the maintenance of vulvodynia. One has to do with thoughts concerning the overall pain condition, for example, "I will be stuck with this problem for life." Women with vulvodynia who believe that their pain is affecting all aspects of their life report lower relationship satisfaction, as well as more sexual dysfunction and psychological distress.[42] A second type of cognition involves the thoughts preceding, during, and following the pain experience. Higher levels of pain catastrophizing before entering psychological treatment have been shown to predict worse outcomes following treatment.[43]

4. **Affective dimension.** The affective component of vulvodynia can also take on a general form (e.g., an elevated degree of anxiety concerning the overall condition) and a more situational one (e.g., fear of pain during sexual activity). Fear of engaging in pain-generating activities is common among chronic pain sufferers and can lead to avoidance.[44] Women who report higher levels of fear of pain, anxiety, and avoidance have worse treatment outcomes.[43] Assessing the extent of pain-related fear and anxiety early on in treatment is thus essential. It is up to the clinician to determine whether levels of anxiety reach a clinical threshold or not. Independent of level of anxiety, its reduction is always a therapeutic target given it is such a strong modulator of pain intensity. The same is true of depressive symptoms. Although many women presenting with vulvodynia do not score within the clinical

range on depression measures such as the Beck Depression Inventory, many will exhibit modest levels of symptomatology requiring clinical attention. A focus on depressive symptoms is usually embedded in psychological approaches to pain management, with a view to reducing pain. Focusing on depression and anxiety in assessment and treatment is most successful when presenting this work as a means for further pain reduction and improved quality of life, as opposed to inferring causality relationships, which only increases patient resistance to psychological treatment. A full-blown mood disorder may require medication, depending on the severity of the presentation.

5. **Interpersonal dimension.** Relationship factors must be considered because these may affect the pain and sexual adjustment of the couple. These include partner responses to the pain, or how the partner reacts when the women experiences pain during sexual activity, intimacy, sexual communication, and emotion regulation patterns. Because more and more research is showing that relationship factors modulate the pain and associated sexual dysfunction and psychological distress, we now emphasize including the partner in assessment and treatment.[45]

6. **Medications.** Finally, assessment of use of current pain, psychotropic, or other medication, in addition to drug and alcohol consumption, is a prerequisite to the establishment of any treatment plan.

Treatment

Treatment generally begins with noninvasive approaches (e.g., cognitive behavioral therapy [CBT], physical therapy) and may progress to oral or topical medical management options (e.g., gabapentin, topical hormones). If these treatments fail, vestibulectomy (for provoked vestibulodynia only) may be recommended.[46] A multimodal approach to treatment should be adopted to target the multiple, often interdependent dimensions of vulvodynia.

Psychological interventions focus on reducing pain, improving sexual function and satisfaction, reducing psychological distress, and strengthening the romantic relationship by targeting the thoughts, emotions, behaviors, and couple interactions associated with vulvodynia.[47] Such interventions can be delivered in individual, couple, or group formats. CBT is the most common and most studied psychological treatment.

The efficacy of group and individual CBT was examined in three different randomized clinical trials (RCTs). The first study compared vestibulectomy, biofeedback, and CBT. Participants who received CBT reported significant improvements in pain at a 6-month follow-up.[48] At a 2.5-year follow-up, their ratings of pain during intercourse were equivalent to those of women having undergone a vestibulectomy.[49] In a second RCT involving a mixed group of 50 women with vulvodynia, Masheb et al. found that individual CBT yielded significantly greater improvements in pain and sexual function than supportive psychotherapy, with gains maintained at 1-year follow-up.[50] A third RCT compared a corticosteroid cream to group CBT for a 13-week treatment period. Intent-to-treat multilevel analyses showed that the CBT group reported significantly more pain reduction at 6-month follow-up. At post-treatment, women in the CBT condition displayed significantly less pain catastrophizing, and at 6-month follow-up, they reported significantly better global improvements in pain and sexual functioning as well as better treatment satisfaction.[51] In summary, CBT constitutes an empirically validated and noninvasive treatment for vulvodynia, which has the added benefit of addressing sexual dysfunction and psychological distress.

Treatment in the Presence of Psychiatric Morbidity

When psychological distress reaches clinical levels, this aspect of the patient's presentation will become more central. At this point, mental health professionals may need to move beyond pain and sexuality-focused CBT. Reasons for elevated psychological distress can range from a history of childhood maltreatment to significant relationship conflict, including domestic violence. Childhood maltreatment can become the focus of treatment if briefer CBT interventions are ineffective and the woman is ready to attend to this aspect of her past more directly. Two lines of caution are warranted: (a) the mental health professional needs to have sufficient experience and training in trauma-informed psychotherapy, and (b) childhood maltreatment must never be presented as the sole cause of vulvodynia, given that chronic pain is a complex, multifactorial phenomenon requiring a multimodal treatment approach. Namely, focusing on childhood maltreatment to the exclusion of other potential exacerbating factors could prolong treatment unnecessarily and be less helpful. We recommend that work on childhood maltreatment be included within a cognitive behavioral framework also involving strategies to reduce pain and immediate distress.

Significant relationship difficulties should be addressed in couple therapy, especially since that may interfere with ongoing treatment, for example, if a partner sabotages the woman's efforts at improving her condition or exhibits angry and critical remarks on a regular basis. Women with a preexisting mood or anxiety disorder could be in need of more intensive psychotherapy to cope with the added burden of vulvodynia. Finally, women who have tried multiple treatments with no success, or women who have experienced many negative side effects or complications from treatments such as surgery, may be at an increased risk for developing a psychiatric disorder. They may require additional psychological support and/or psychotherapy targeting their mood or anxiety disorder directly, such as empirically validated CBT, or antidepressant and/or anxiolytic medication.

In an ideal world, mental health professionals treating women with vulvodynia have some knowledge of trauma, psychiatric disorders, pain, couple relationships, and sexuality. When this is not the case, referrals are key, and clinicians should consider working within a multidisciplinary team in order to provide optimal health care to women with vulvodynia.

PUBLIC HEALTH IMPACT AND FUTURE RESEARCH

Vulvodynia is a serious, debilitating, chronic condition that is highly prevalent among women of reproductive age. Because the pathophysiology of vulvodynia is not well understood, women with vulvodynia and their providers are often frustrated by the lack of clear etiology and thus treatment options for the condition.[52] Given the high prevalence of adverse psychosocial factors and psychiatric morbidity among women with vulvodynia, holistic treatment that encompasses CBT and biomedical interventions may represent the best approach for treatment. Furthermore, given that childhood maltreatment and other antecedent psychosocial risk factors have been shown to be associated with vulvodynia,[20,32,53] clinicians and public health practitioners may wish to adapt a life-course approach to treating these conditions because this may either prevent vulvodynia from occurring altogether or lessen the severity of symptoms among women who are already suffering from the condition.

Continued research on vulvodynia is essential to improve prevention of, and treatment for, vulvodynia. A better understanding of the pathophysiology of vulvodynia could lead to the development of more effective treatment options. With such a strong biological link between vulvodynia and psychosocial risk factors, it may not be possible to effectively treat vulvodynia without also addressing a woman's psychiatric comorbidities.

REFERENCES

1. Bornstein J, Goldstein AT, Stockdale CK, et al. 2015 ISSVD, ISSWSH, and IPPS consensus terminology and classification of persistent vulvar pain and vulvodynia. *J Low Genit Tract Dis.* 2016;20(2):126–130.

2. Bachmann GA, Rosen R, Pinn VW, et al. Vulvodynia: A state-of-the-art consensus on definitions, diagnosis and management. *J Reprod Med*. 2006;51:447–456.
3. Lynch PJ, Moyal-Barracco M, Scurry J, Stockdale C. 2011 ISSVD terminology and classification of vulvar dermatological disorders. *J Low Genit Tract Dis*. 2012;16:339–344.
4. Witkin SS, Gerber S, Ledger WJ. Differential characterization of women with vulvar vestibulitis syndrome. *Am J Obstet Gynecol*. 2002;187:589–594.
5. Jantos M, Burns NR. Vulvodynia: Development of a psychosexual profile. *J Reprod Med*. 2007;52:63–71.
6. Stockdale CK, Lawson HW. 2013 Vulvodynia guideline update. *J Low Genit Tract Dis*. 2014;18:93–100.
7. Bohm-Starke N, Hilliges M, Brodda-Jansen G, Rylander E, Torebjörk E. Psychophysical evidence of nociceptor sensitization in vulvar vestibulitis syndrome. *Pain* 2001;94:177–183.
8. Turner ML, Marinoff SC. Pudendal neuralgia. *Am J Obstet Gynecol*. 1991;165:1233–1236.
9. De Andres J, Sanchis-Lopez N, Asensio-Samper JM, et al. Vulvodynia: An evidence-based literature review and proposed treatment algorithm. *Pain Pract*. 2016;16:204–236.
10. Harlow BL, Stewart EG. A population-based assessment of chronic unexplained vulvar pain: Have we underestimated the prevalence of vulvodynia? *J Am Med Womens Assoc*. 2003;58:82–88.
11. Arnold LD, Bachmann GA, Rosen R, Rhoads GG. Assessment of vulvodynia symptoms in a sample of US women: A prevalence survey with a nested case control study. *Am J Obstet Gynecol*. 2007;196:128.e1–e6.
12. Harlow BL, Kunitz CG, Nguyen RH, et al. Prevalence of symptoms consistent with a diagnosis of vulvodynia: Population-based estimates from 2 geographic regions. *Am J Obstet Gynecol*. 2014;210:40.e1–e8.
13. Fichorova RN, Tucker LD, Anderson DJ. The molecular basis of nonoxynol-9-induced vaginal inflammation and its possible relevance to human immunodeficiency virus type 1 transmission. *J Infect Dis*. 2001;184:418–428.
14. Chadha S, Gianotten WL, Drogendijk AC, et al. Histopathologic features of vulvar vestibulitis. *Int J Gynecol Pathol*. 1998;17:7–11.
15. Seckin-Alac E, Akhant SE, Bastu E, Tuzlalik S, Yavuz E. Elevated tissue levels of tumor necrosis factor-α in vulvar vestibulitis syndrome. *Clin Exp Obstet Gynecol*. 2014;41:691–693.
16. Foster DC, Hasday JD. Elevated tissue levels of interleukin-1 beta and tumor necrosis factor-alpha in vulvar vestibulitis. *Obstet Gynecol*. 1997;89:291–296.
17. Harlow BL, He W, Nguyen RHN. Allergic reactions and risk of vulvodynia. *Ann. Epidemiol*. 2009;19:771–777.
18. Fichorova RN. Guiding the vaginal microbicide trials with biomarkers of inflammation. *J Acquir Immune Defic Syndr*. 2004;37(suppl 3):S184–S193.
19. Fichorova RN, Trifonova RT, Gilbert RO, et al. Trichomonas vaginalis lipophosphoglycan triggers a selective upregulation of cytokines by human female reproductive tract epithelial cells. *Infect Immun*. 2006;74:5773–5779.

20. Khandker M, Brady S, Stewart E, Harlow B. Is chronic stress during childhood associated with adult-onset vulvodynia? *J Womens Heal.* 2014;23:649–656.
21. Jantos M. Vulvodynia: A psychophysiological profile based on electromyographic assessment. *Appl Psychophysiol Biofeedback.* 2008;33:29–38.
22. Basson R. The recurrent pain and sexual sequelae of provoked vestibulodynia: A perpetuating cycle. *J Sex Med.* 2012;9:2077–2092.
23. Masheb RM, Wang E, Lozano C, Kerns RD. Prevalence and correlates of depression in treatment-seeking women with vulvodynia. *J Obstet Gynaecol.* 2005;25:786–791.
24. Granot M, Friedman M, Yarnitsky D, Zimmer EZ. Enhancement of the perception of systemic pain in women with vulvar vestibulitis. *BJOG* 2001;109:863–866.
25. Bohm-Starke N. Medical and physical predictors of localized provoked vulvodynia. *Acta Obstet Gynecol Scand.* 2010;89:1504–1510.
26. Bohm-Starke N, Hilliges M, Falconer C, Rylander E. Increased intraepithelial innervation in women with vulvar vestibulitis syndrome. *Gynecol Obste. Invest.* 1998;46:256–260.
27. Khandker M, Brady SS, Vitonis AF, et al. the influence of depression and anxiety on risk of adult onset vulvodynia. *J Womens Heal.* 2011;20:1445–1451.
28. Kemeny ME, Schedlowski M. Understanding the interaction between psychosocial stress and immune-related diseases: A stepwise progression. *Brain Behav Immun.* 2007;21:1009–1018.
29. Coghill RC, Sang CN, Maisog JM, Iadarola MJ. Pain intensity processing within the human brain: A bilateral, distributed mechanism. *J Neurophysiol.* 1999;82:1934–1943.
30. Hawthorn J, Redmond K. *Pain: Causes and Management.* Oxford, UK: Blackwell Science; 1998:7–28.
31. Lowenstein L, Vardi Y, Deutsch M, et al. Vulvar vestibulitis severity: Assessment by sensory and pain testing modalities. *Pain.* 2004;107:47–53.
32. Harlow BL, Stewart EG. Adult-onset vulvodynia in relation to childhood violence victimization. *Am J Epidemiol.* 2005;161:871–880.
33. Wylie K, Hallam-Jones R, Harrington C. Psychological difficulties within a group of patients with vulvodynia. *J Psychosom Obstet Gynaecol.* 2004;25:257–265.
34. Desrochers G, Bergeron S, Landry T, Jodoin M. Do psychosexual factors play a role in the etiology of provoked vestibulodynia? A critical review. *J Sex Marital Ther.* 2008;34:198–226.
35. Iglesias-Rios L, Harlow SD, Reed BD. Depression and posttraumatic stress disorder among women with vulvodynia: Evidence from the Population-Based Woman to Woman Health Study. *J Women's Heal.* 2015;**00**:150507121748004.
36. Boerner KE, Rosen NO. Acceptance of vulvovaginal pain in women with provoked vestibulodynia and their partners: Associations with pain, psychological, and sexual adjustment. *J Sex Med.* 2015;12:1450–1462.
37. Desrochers G, Bergeron S, Khalifé S, Dupuis M-J, Jodoin M. Fear avoidance and self-efficacy in relation to pain and sexual impairment in women with provoked vestibulodynia. *Clin J Pain.* 2009;25:520–527.
38. Kroenke K, Strine TW, Spitzer RL, Williams JB, Berry JT, Mokdad AH. The PHQ-8 as a measure of current depression in the general population. *J Affect Disord.* 2009;114:163–173.

39. First MB, Spitzer RL, Gibbon M, Williams JB. *Structured Clinical Interview for DSM-IV-TR Axis I Disorders*. New York State Psychiatric Institute; 2002. http://www.scid4.org/revisions/november_2001_02.htm.
40. Sanchez-Villegas A, Schlatter J, Ortuno F, et al. Validity of a self-reported diagnosis of depression among participants in a cohort study using the Structured Clinical Interview for DSM-IV (SCID-I). *BMC Psychiatry.* 2008;8:43.
41. Nguyen RHN, Turner RM, Rydell SA, Maclehose RF, Harlow BL. Perceived stereotyping and seeking care for chronic vulvar pain. *Pain Med.* 2013;14:1461–1467.
42. Jodoin M, Bergeron S, Khalifé S, Dupuis M-J, Desrochers G, Leclerc B. Attributions about pain as predictors of psychological symptomatology, sexual function, and dyadic adjustment in women with vestibulodynia. *Arch Sex Behav.* 2011;40:87–97.
43. Desrochers G, Bergeron S, Khalifé S, Dupuis M-J, Jodoin M. Provoked vestibulodynia: Psychological predictors of topical and cognitive-behavioral treatment outcome. *Behav Res Ther.* 2010;48:106–115.
44. Linton SJ, Melin L, Götestam KG. Behavioral analysis of chronic pain and its management. *Prog Behav Modif.* 1984;18:1–42.
45. Rosen NO, Rancourt K, Corsini-Munt S, Bergeron S. Beyond a "woman's problem": The role of relationship processes in female genital pain. *Curr Sex Health Rep.* 2014;6:1–10.
46. Goldstein AT, Pukall CF, Brown C, Bergeron S, Stein A, Kellogg-Spadt S. Vulvodynia: Assessment and treatment. *J Sex Med.* 2016;13:572–590.
47. Bergeron S, Rosen NO, Pukall CR. Genital pain in women and men: It can hurt more than your sex life. In: Binik YM, Hall K, eds. *Principles and Practice of Sex Therapy, 5th edition*. New York, NY: Guilford Press; 159–176.
48. Bergeron S, Binik YM, Khalifé S, et al. A randomized comparison of group cognitive-behavioral therapy, surface electromyographic biofeedback, and vestibulectomy in the treatment of dyspareunia resulting from vulvar vestibulitis. *Pain.* 2001;91:297–306.
49. Bergeron S, Khalifé S, Glazer HI, Binik YM. Surgical and behavioral treatments for vestibulodynia: Two-and-one-half year follow-up and predictors of outcome. *Obstet Gynecol.* 2008;111:159–166.
50. Masheb RM, Kerns RD, Lozano C, Minkin MJ, Richman S. A randomized clinical trial for women with vulvodynia: Cognitive-behavioral therapy vs. supportive psychotherapy. *Pain.* 2009;141:31–40.
51. Bergeron S, Khalifé S, Dupuis M-J, McDuff P. A randomized clinical trial comparing group cognitive-behavioral therapy and a topical steroid for women with dyspareunia. *J Consult Clin Psychol.* 2016;84:259–268.
52. Gunter J. Vulvodynia: New thoughts on a devastating condition. *Obstet Gynecol Surv.* 2007;62:812–819.
53. Khandker M, Brady SS, Vitonis AF, et al. The influence of depression and anxiety on risk of adult onset vulvodynia. *J Womens Health.* 2011;20:1445–1451.

20

Understanding and Managing Personality Disorders in Chronic Pain

JAMES N. WEISBERG, CHANNING TWYNER, AND CHRISTOPHER PAUL ■

INTRODUCTION

As previously discussed in this text, chronic pain is a significant health care issue at epidemic proportions in the United States,[1] and there is a high incidence of both clinical psychiatric disorders[2,3] and personality disorders (PDs) in the chronic pain population.[4,5] Furthermore, the incidence of opioid use disorders both in the general population[6] and in the chronic pain population is on the rise in the United States.[5] Opioid overdose deaths have increased from 2.1 per 100,000 in 1999 to 9.3 per 100,000 in 2015.[7] Individuals with psychiatric disorders, including PDs, are also at higher risk for opioid abuse.[5] Given that PDs are more common both in those with opioid use disorders and in those with chronic pain, the importance of understanding, recognizing, and addressing PDs is crucial when working with chronic pain patients. It is incumbent on the pain clinician to understand the basic PDs in order to identify and mitigate potential risk factors that may interfere with treatment outcomes and increase the likelihood of comorbid substance use disorders.

While some attention is given to the history of the study of personality in chronic pain, this chapter is mostly limited to a discussion of PDs rather than "nonpathological" personality traits or characteristics. For a more extensive review of nonpathological and pathological personality characteristics in chronic pain, the reader is referred to a recent review article.[8]

BRIEF HISTORY OF PERSONALITY AND PAIN

The relationship between personality and pain can easily be traced to ancient Greece. Hippocrates posited that physical pain was caused by an imbalance in the four humors (blood, black bile, yellow bile, and phlegm) and that these humors were the basis of personality temperaments. Plato and his student Aristotle viewed pain as arising from a combination of both physical stimulation and emotions.[9] In the late 19th century, psychodynamic theorists discussed the connection between emotional factors and the experience of chronic pain.[10] Freud theorized that such individuals might "convert" their emotional distress into physical symptoms, including pain, through the mechanism of hysteria and that the body part associated with the pain was often symbolic of the emotional trauma.[10] Later theorists followed in the early psychodynamic traditions when addressing the relationship between unpleasant and pleasant emotions and the perception of pain[11] as well as the psychosocial interpretations of pain.[12] George Engel maintained that, while physical pain may result from underlying pathophysiology, the interpretation of pain is a psychological phenomenon.[13] He also noted that certain diagnoses, including depression, hysteria, and hypochondriasis in the American Psychiatric Association's newly created *Diagnostic and Statistical Manual of Mental Disorders*[14] were relatively common in people experiencing chronic pain.[13] The development of the Minnesota Multiphasic Personality Inventory (MMPI)[15] led to a plethora of research seeking to use psychometric tests to quantify these early theories.

Minnesota Multiphasic Personality Inventory and Chronic Pain

One of the first studies to use the MMPI in an attempt to characterize chronic pain patients found a pattern of responses that was described as the "conversion-V" or "neurotic triad." In the neurotic triad, scales for hypochondriasis (Hy), depression (D), and hysteria (Hs) are all significantly elevated, with the hypochondriasis and hysteria scales more elevated relative to depression.[16] This was interpreted to support earlier theories that individuals with emotional distress, predominantly depression, were channeling that distress into more socially acceptable physical symptoms such as physical pain.[16] Subsequent studies sought to support[17,18] or refute[19,20] this finding as an explanation for chronic pain that could not be explained on the basis of pathophysiology. The MMPI was also used in an attempt to predict treatment outcomes from spine surgery,[21,22] multidisciplinary treatment programs,[23] and the liklihood of disability.[24]

Newer versions of the MMPI (MMPI-2; MMPI-2-RF) have been validated in chronic pain patients.[25] The MMPI-2-RF has recently been studied for its efficacy in determining satisfaction and outcome with spinal cord stimulators and spinal surgery.[26]

Despite the hundreds of studies using the MMPI and its successors, there continues to be controversy regarding the applicability and appropriateness of its use in the chronic pain population.[27,28]

There are a number of other psychological inventories that have been used in an attempt to describe and characterize individuals with chronic pain and to predict treatment outcomes. Some of these measures include the Neuroticism-Extroversion-Openness Personality Inventory (NEO-PI) and its revisions,[29-31] the Millon Clinical Multiaxial Inventory[32] and subsequent revisions (MCMI-IV),[33] and the Temperament and Character Inventory (TCI).[34]

While the various iterations of the MMPI and other psychological inventories have investigated different personality characteristics as they relate to pain, relatively few studies have investigated PDs in chronic pain. Before a review of those studies, it is important for the reader to have a basic understanding of the difference between personality traits, characteristics, and disorders, as well as the potential impact immediate clinical states and psychosocial stressors may have on the expression of personality, PDs, and pain.

BASIC CONCEPTS OF PERSONALITY AND PERSONALITY DISORDERS

Personality refers to the constellation of nonpathological characteristics in an individual's patterns of thought, emotion, and behavior. Personality traits account for individual differences in behavior and intrapsychic function but are within the scope of normal human experience.

A popular model of personality posits that it is the composition of both temperament and character dimensions.[34] Temperament is relatively stable and is described as largely biological. Character is shaped during childhood and is largely shaped by social influences and maturity.[34] The concept of both temperament and character has been much studied in chronic pain.[35-37] In a seminal study, Conrad et al.[35] found that 41% of chronic pain patients met criteria for at least one PD. Because of the impact of clinical states such as depression and anxiety that are common in chronic pain, the authors separately looked at those PD chronic pain patients with and without anxiety or depression and found that 44% of those with a PD met criteria for a current mood disorder compared with 46% without a PD. Similarly, 20% of the chronic pain patients with a PD met the criteria for a current anxiety disorder compared with 25% without a PD. Another study found that factors such as depression and anxiety often affected personality traits in chronic pain patients.[27] Future research, including prospective studies, are needed in order to better understand possible causal relationships between chronic pain, emotional states, and PD diagnosis.[38]

In contrast to personality, the *Diagnostic and Statistical Manual of Mental Disorders* (DSM) defines a PD as "an enduring pattern of inner experience and behavior that deviates markedly from the expectations of the individual's culture, is pervasive and inflexible, has an onset in adolescence or early adulthood, is stable over time, and leads to distress or impairment."[39] Thus, the essential difference between a trait and disorder is the degree of distress and disruption caused.

PDs fall into three categories: Cluster A, the "odd-eccentric" cluster, includes paranoid, schizoid, and schizotypal PDs; cluster B, the dramatic, emotional cluster, includes antisocial, borderline, histrionic, and narcissistic PDs; and cluster C, the anxious-fearful cluster, includes avoidant, dependent, and obsessive-compulsive PDs.

DIATHESIS-STRESS MODEL
OF PERSONALITY DISORDERS

Personality and PDs are likely the combination of biological, developmental, and environmental factors that are influenced by state-dependent variables such as mood and anxiety. The diathesis-stress model purports that individuals have underlying genetic vulnerabilities and possibly early life experiences that interact with stressors the individual encounters later in life.[40] Depending on the nature of the stressors and the individual's ability to cope with such stressors, the vulnerability may or may not become expressed as a disease process. The diathesis-stress model was first applied to explain schizophrenia[40] and depression[41] and has also been used to explain why some individuals develop chronic back pain while others do not.[42,43] It has also been applied to the development of depression in chronic pain patients.[2] Similarly, this model has been proposed to apply to PDs in chronic pain patients.[44] Thus, combined with underlying traits and ongoing situational stressors brought on by chronic pain, an individual's underlying personality traits and characteristics may become magnified to the extent that the individual meets criteria for a PD.

EPIDEMIOLOGY OF PERSONALITY DISORDERS

Not until the DSM-III[45] was the definition of PDs formed and the reliable assessment with structured interviews of PDs developed.[46] These definitions were modified and included in subsequent DSM manuals, but the prevalence of PDs was primarily estimated from early community studies in the 1950s.[47]

A number of studies in the early 2000s sought to estimate the prevalence of PDs in the general population. Studies have generally found the prevalence rates to be between 9 and 16%.[47–49] In its most recent edition (DSM-V), the American Psychiatric Association cites data from a national epidemiologic survey suggesting approximately 15% of US adults meet criteria for at least one PD.[50] Prevalence estimates for the different clusters suggest 5.7% for disorders in cluster A, 1.5% for disorders in cluster B, 6.0% for disorders in cluster C and 9.1% for any PD, indicating frequent co-occurrence of disorders from different clusters.[48]

PREVALENCE OF PERSONALITY DISORDERS IN CHRONIC PAIN

There are relatively few studies that have investigated the prevalence of PDs in the chronic, noncancerous pain population. Of those studies that have been conducted, a wide variety of methods have been used to diagnose PDs, including patient self-report measures, clinical interviews, and structured and semistructured interviews. All studies were retrospective rather than prospective in design, thereby limiting any causal statements that can be made about the nature of the interaction between PDs and chronic pain. With the advent of the DSM-III came more rigorous diagnostic criteria and methods for diagnosis. The first published study using a semistructured interview to diagnose DSM-III PD criteria found that 37% of their chronic pain sample met criteria for at least one PD, with the most common diagnoses being histrionic PD (14%), dependent PD (12%), and borderline PD (7%).[51] Another study using a different semistructured interview found that 40% of their chronic pain sample met criteria for at least one PD, with mixed PD (22%) and dependent PD (10%) being most prevalent.[52] Reich and Thompson[53] compared prevalence rates of PDs in those with chronic pain with psychiatric patients applying for disability and with individuals undergoing competency hearings. Using semistructured interviews, they found that patients in the chronic pain group were more likely to have a PD than those in the group undergoing mental competency hearings (37% vs. 12%). Fishbain et al.,[54] using a semistructured interview to diagnosis both DSM-III Axis I and Axis II disorders, found that 59% of their chronic pain sample met criteria for a PD, with most common diagnoses being dependent PD (17%), passive-aggressive PD (15%), and histrionic PD (12%).

Weisberg et al.[55] used a combination of clinical interview, treatment notes, and both patient and family self-report measures to assess PDs in 55 chronic pain patients with pain who were evaluated and treated at a comprehensive outpatient pain management program. They found that 31% met criteria for at least one PD, and an additional 27% met criteria for PD not otherwise specified (PD-NOS), which is used when an individual meets incomplete criteria for two or more PDs. The most common diagnoses were borderline PD (13%) and dependent PD (11%). These researchers suggest that obtaining longitudinal information from both the patient and an individual with a long-standing relationship with the patient might provide a more thorough assessment of the impact of state factors such as mood, anxiety, and stress on the presentation of personality.[55] In a study using the Structured Clinical Interview for DSM-III-R Axis II Disorders[56] (SCID-II) to diagnose PD in a relatively large sample of chronic low back pain patients, the authors found that 51% met criteria for a PD, with the most common diagnoses being paranoid PD (33%), borderline PD (15%), and avoidant PD (14%).[57] In another study of 50 chronic temporomandibular joint disorder patients administered the SCID-II, 18% met criteria for paranoid PD, 15% met criteria for borderline PD, and 14% met criteria for avoidant PD.[58] In a study that used the SCID-II to assess DSM-III-R PDs in a group of patients with complex regional pain syndrome (CRPS) type I and a group with disk-related radiculopathy (DRR), of those patients who did not meet criteria for Axis I clinical disorders, 60% of the CRPS patients and 64% of the DRR patients met criteria for at least one PD.[59] The previously mentioned study by Conrad et al.[35] found that 41% of chronic pain patients met criteria for a PD diagnoses compared with 7% of the control group. The most common diagnoses were borderline PD (11%) and paranoid PD (12%). The authors found that clinical disorders, such as depression at a equally high rate, gave more credence to the importance of assessing personality in context of state factors. Fischer-Kern et al.[60] used the SCID-II to investigate the prevalence of both clinical and PD diagnoses in a university-based behavioral medicine pain clinic and found that approximately 63% of their sample of 43 patients met criteria for at least one PD, while 37.2% met criteria for two PDs and 16.3% met criteria for three or more PDs. A recent Turkish study using the SCID-II found PDs in 81% of their sample of chronic migraine sufferers. Highest rates were of obsessive-compulsive PD (50%), dependent PD (19%), avoidant PD (19%), and passive-aggressive PD (13%).[61]

In summary, the relatively few studies that have investigated PDs in various chronic pain samples have found prevalence rates from 31% to more than 80% (Table 20.1). However, as has been noted by previous researchers,

Table 20.1 PERSONALITY DISORDER IN CHRONIC PAIN

Study*	DSM version	Participants	Diagnostic measure	Axis II disorder[†]	Most prevalent Axis II disorder
Reich, Tupin, & Abramowitz (1983)	DSM-III	43 with mixed chronic pain	Unpublished semistructured interview	37%	Histrionic (14%) Dependent (12%) Borderline (7%)
Large (1986)	DSM-III	50 with mixed chronic pain	Maudsley-based semistructured interview	40%	Mixed (22%) Dependent (10%)
Fishbain et al. (1986)	DSM-III	283 with mixed chronic pain	Unpublished semistructured interview	59%	Dependent (17%) Passive-aggressive (15%) Histrionic (12%)
Reich & Thompson (1987)	DSM-III	43 with mixed chronic pain[‡] 390 forensic; 55 with disability	Unpublished semistructured interview	37%	Cluster A = 2.3% Cluster B = 21% Cluster C = 14%
Polatin et al. (1993)	DSM-III-R	200 with chronic low back pain	SCID-II	51%	Paranoid (33%) Borderline (15%) Avoidant (14%)
Gatchel et al. (1996)	DSM-III-R	50 with chronic TMD	SCID-II	Not reported	Paranoid (18%) Borderline (10%) Obsessive-compulsive (10%)
Weisberg et al. (1996)	DSM-IV	50 with mixed chronic pain	Clinical interview Chart review Family interview	31%	PD-NOS (27%) Borderline (13%) Dependent (11%)
Monti et al. (1998)	DSM-III-R	25 with CRPS 25 with DRR	SCID-II	60% (CRPS) 64% (DRR)	Obsessive-compulsive (28% CRPS; 12% DRR) Self-defeating (20% CRPS; 12% DRR) Mixed PD (20% DRR)

(continued)

Table 20.1 CONTINUED

Study*	DSM version	Participants	Diagnostic measure	Axis II disorder†	Most prevalent Axis II disorder
Conrad et al. (2007)	DSM-IV	207 with mixed chronic pain	SCID-II	41%	Paranoid (12%) Borderline (11%) Avoidant (8%) Passive-aggressive (8%)
Fischer-Kern et al. (2011)	DSM-IV	43 with mixed chronic pain	SCID-II	63%	Obsessive-compulsive (28%) Borderline (26%) Paranoid (16%)
Kayhan & Ilik (2016)	DSM=III-R	105 with chronic migraine	SCID-II	81%	OCDP (50%) Dependent PD (19%) Avoidant PD (19%) Passive-aggressive PD (13%)
Wilsey et al. (2008)	DSM-IV	113 emergency department patients with chronic pain	Personality Diagnostic Questionnaire 4th edition	18%	Not reported
Barry et al. (2016)	DSM-IV-TR	170 chronic pain patients with opioid use disorder	Diagnostic Interview for DSM-IV Personality Disorders (DIDP-IV)	52%	Antisocial (22%) Avoidant (19%) Paranoid (16%)

* Only aspects relevant to Axis II diagnosis in these studies are included in the table.

† Personality disorder rates are rounded to the nearest whole number.

‡ Pain subjects appear to be the same subjects from Reich, Tupin, & Abramowitz (1983).

CRPS = complex regional pain syndrome; DRR = disk-related radiculopathy; DSM = *Diagnostic and Statistical Manual of Mental Disorders*; SCID = Structured Clinical Interview for DSM-III-R; PD = personality disorder; PD-NOS = personality disorder not otherwise specified (used when individual has features of more than one personality disorder but fails to meet full criteria for any personality disorder); TMD = temporomandibular disorder.

owing to a variety of factors, including state-dependent variables, stressors unique to chronic pain, genetic and developmental influences, and other known and unknown factors, significant caution must be heeded when making a PD diagnosis in the chronic pain patient. In addition, knowing premorbid functioning is crucial to understanding the multifactorial nature of the observed behavior. Nontheless, the presence of a PD increases the liklihood of comorbid conditions, such as substance misuse and abuse, and makes treatment of chronic pain that much more challenging to the pain clinician.

COMORBID SUBSTANCE ABUSE AND PERSONALITY DISORDERS IN CHRONIC PAIN

There has been a relative paucity of research on the interaction between PDs and substance abuse in chronic pain. One study investigated psychological comorbidities, including PDs, in chronic pain sufferers presenting to a university emergency department and an urgent care clinic requesting opioids.[62] Pertinent results demonstrated that 18% likely had a PD diagnosis and found that PD was significantly related to opioid abuse.[62] A recent study found the incidence of PDs to be 52% in those with co-occurring chronic pain and substance use disorders.[5] The most common PD was antisocial PD (22%), followed by avoidant PD (19%) and paranoid PD (16%). Although there is little literature on this topic, both these studies suggest that PDs may be a moderating variable in the incidence of substance use disorders in chronic pain.

TREATMENT OF PERSONALITY DISORDERS IN CHRONIC PAIN

While both chronic pain and PDs can prove to be daunting to the clinician separately, the combination can pose unique challenges and opportunities in regard to treatment. While the patient's maladaptive behaviors are by definition problematic in a variety of settings, the patient's legitimate concerns are often disregarded as secondary to the manifestations of their PDs or simply being "difficult." Indeed, the pain clinician may be the first provider to have an overarching view and appreciation of both conditions.

The need to screen for PDs by the pain clinician is rooted in the understanding that the manifestations of the PD in the chronic pain patient can be exacerbated or unmasked by the patient's pain condition according to the diathesis-stress model.[44] In addition, the need for vigilance and awareness with these conditions is considerable because these patients are at higher risk for various adverse outcomes, including substance use disorders.[62] Attempting to detangle the PD from the chronic pain state with the goal of treating one or the other may be difficult at best.

Cognitive behavioral therapy for chronic pain (CBT-CP) has been well documented in the literature as one of the most effective treatments for chronic pain.[63-65] Acceptance and commitment therapy (ACT)[66] has been shown to benefit patients with PDs who had failed previous treatment resulting in significant improvements in personality pathology and quality of life.[67] ACT for chronic pain has also been effective in decreasing pain intensity, anxiety, and disability.[68] The use of CBT-CP and ACT may be a potential avenue for treatment, but research specifically aimed at the coexisting pain and PD population is lacking.

Dialectical behavior therapy (DBT), a current mainstay of treatment of borderline PD, focuses on the development of emotional skills with the ultimate goal of improving emotional regulation and control,[69] and it encourages goal-oriented behavior aimed at increasing functionality. It should be noted, as with other therapy modalities, that there is minimal evidence on the use of DBT in the pain patient with comorbid PD.

Given the common elements between CBT and DBT, it stands to reason that a hybrid model combining elements of both CBT-CP and DBT might be a highly successful approach to maximizing treatment potential in patients with comorbid chronic pain and PDs, especially borderline PD.

CONCLUSION

In this chapter, we provided a background to the importance of addressing PDs in the chronic pain population. The application of the diathesis-stress model was introduced as a way to better incorporate the relative contributions of genetic vulnerability, early life experience, and the multiple stressors to which individuals with chronic pain are exposed in order to explain the high prevalence of PDs found in the chronic pain population. We addressed the prevalence of PD in the chronic pain population and introduced the reader to the current state of treatment of PDs. Understanding the role PDs may play in the expression of behaviors observed in a substantial proportion of chronic pain sufferers should result in the tailoring of multimodal treatments for chronic pain that emphasize nonopioid medical management and cognitive behavioral and physical therapies.

REFERENCES

1. Institute of Medicine. *Relieving Pain in America: A Blueprint for Transforming Prevention, Care, Education, and Research.* Washington, DC: Author; 2011.
2. Banks SM, Kerns RD. Explaining the high rates of depression in chronic pain: A diathesis-stress framework. *Psychol Bull.* 1996;119(1):95–110.
3. McWilliams LA, Cox BJ, Enns MW. Mood and anxiety disorders associated with chronic pain: An examination in a nationally representative sample. *Pain.* 2003;106(1–2):127–133.
4. Weisberg JN. Personality and personality disorders in chronic pain. *Curr Rev Pain.* 2000;4(1):60–70.
5. Barry DT, Cutter CJ, Beitel M, Kerns RD, Liong C, Schottenfeld RS. Psychiatric disorders among patients seeking treatment for co-occurring chronic pain and opioid use disorder. *J Clin Psychiatry.* 2016;77(10):1413–1419.
6. Martel MO, Shir Y, Ware MA. Substance-related disorders: A review of prevalence and correlates among patients with chronic pain. *Prog Neuropsychopharmacol Biol Psychiatry.* 2018;87(part B):245–254.
7. Rudd RA, Seth P, David F, Scholl L. Increases in drug and opioid-involved overdose deaths—United States, 2010–2015. *MMWR Morb Mortal Wkly Rep.* 2016;65(5051):1445–1452.
8. Naylor B, Boag S, Gustin SM. New evidence for a pain personality? A critical review of the last 120 years of pain and personality. *Scand J Pain.* 2017;17:58–67.
9. Rey R. *The History of Pain.* Cambridge, MA: Harvard University Press; 1998.
10. Breuer J, Freud S. *Studies on Hysteria: (1893–1895).* London, UK: Hogarth Press/Institute of Psycho-Analysis; 1995.
11. Cabot RC. *Differential Diagnosis.* Philadelphia: W. B. Saunders; 1911.
12. Szasz TS. *Pain and Pleasure: A Study of Bodily Feelings.* London, UK: Tavistock; 1957.
13. Engel GL. Psychogenic pain and pain-prone patient. *Am J Med.* 1959;26(6):899–918.
14. American Psychiatric Association. *Diagnostic and statistical manual of mental disorders.* 1st ed. Washington, DC: Author; 1952.
15. Hathaway SR, McKinley J. *Minnesota Multiphasic Personality Inventory.* Minneapolis, MN: University of Minnesota Press; 1943.
16. Hanvik LJ. MMPI profiles in patients with low-back pain. *J Consult Psychol.* 1951;15(4):350–353.
17. Gentry WD, Shows WD, Thomas M. Chronic low back pain: A psychological profile. *Psychosomatics.* 1974;XV:174–177.
18. McCreary C, Turner J, Dawson E. Differences between functional versus organic low back pain patients. *Pain.* 1977;4:73–78.
19. Bradley LA, Prokop CK, Margolis R, Gentry WD. Multivariate analyses of the MMPI profiles of low back pain patients. *J Behav Med.* 1978;1(3):253–272.
20. Sternbach RA, Wolf SR, Murphy RW, Akeson WH. Traits of pain patients: The low-back "loser." *Psychosomatics.* 1973;14(4):226–229.
21. Waring EM, Weisz GM, Bailey SI. Predictive factors in the treatment of low back pain by surgical intervention. In: Bonica JJ, Albe-Fessard D, eds. *Advances in Pain Research and Therapy.* Vol 1. New York, NY: Raven Press; 1976.

22. Block AR, Ohnmeiss DD, Guyer RD, Rashbaum RF, Hochschuler SH. The use of presurgical psychological screening to predict the outcome of spine surgery. *Spine J.* 2001;1(4):274–282.

23. Kleinke CL, Spangler AS Jr. Predicting treatment outcome of chronic back pain patients in a multidisciplinary pain clinic: Methodological issues and treatment implications. *Pain.* 1988;33(1):41–48.

24. Gatchel RJ, Polatin PB, Mayer TG. The dominant role of psychosocial risk factors in the development of chronic low back pain disability. *Spine.* 1995;20(24):2702–2709.

25. Tarescavage AM, Scheman J, Ben-Porath YS. Reliability and validity of the Minnesota Multiphasic Personality Inventory-2-Restructured Form (MMPI-2-RF) in evaluations of chronic low back pain patients. *Psychol Assess.* 2015;27(2):433–446.

26. Block AR, Marek RJ, Ben-Porath YS, Kukal D. Associations between pre-implant psychosocial factors and spinal cord stimulation outcome: Evaluation using the MMPI-2-RF. *Assessment.* 2017;24(1):60–70.

27. Fishbain D, Cole B, Cutler R, Lewis J, Rosomoff H, Rosomoff R. Chronic pain and the measurement of personality: Do states influence traits? *Pain Medicine.* 2006;7(6):509–529.

28. Turk DC, Fernandez E. Personality assessment and the Minnesota Multiphasic Personality Inventory in chronic pain: Underdeveloped and overexposed. *Pain Forum.* 1995;4(2):104–107.

29. Costa PT, McCrae RR. *The NEO Personality Inventory Manual.* Orlando, FL: Psychological Assessment Resources; 1985.

30. Costa PT, McCrae RR. *Revised NEO Personality Inventory (NEO–PI–R) and NEO Five-Factor Inventory (NEO–FFI) Professional Manual.* Odessa, FL: Psychological Assessment Resources; 1992.

31. McCrae RR, Costa PT Jr., Martin TA. The NEO-PI-3: A more readable revised NEO Personality Inventory. *J Pers Assess.* 2005;84(3):261–270.

32. Millon T. *Millon Clinical Multiaxial Inventory.* Minneapolis, MN: National Computer Systems; 1977.

33. Millon T, Grossman S, Millon C. *Millon Clinical Multiaxial Inventory-IV: MCMI-IV.* Bloomington: NCS Pearson; 2015.

34. Cloninger C, Svrakic, DM., Przybeck, TR. A psychobiological model of temperament and character. *Arch Gen Psychiatry.* 1993;50:975–990.

35. Conrad R, Schilling G, Bausch C, et al. Temperament and character personality profiles and personality disorders in chronic pain patients. *Pain.* 2007;133(1–3):197–209.

36. Garcia-Fontanals A, Garcia-Blanco S, Portell M, et al. Cloninger's psychobiological model of personality and psychological distress in fibromyalgia. *Int J Rheum Dis.* 2016;19(9):852–863.

37. Gencay-Can A, Can SS. Temperament and character profile of patients with fibromyalgia. *Rheumatol Int.* 2012;32(12):3957–3961.

38. Weisberg JN, Boatwright BA. Mood, anxiety and personality traits and states in chronic pain. *Pain.* 2007;133(1–3):1–2.

39. American Psychiatric Association. *Diagnostic and Statistical Manual of Mental Disorders.* 5th ed. Washington, DC: Author; 2013.

40. Meehl PE. Schizotaxia, schizotypy, schizophrenia. *Am Psychologist.* 1962;17:827–838.

41. Monroe SM, Simons AD. Diathesis-stress theories in the context of life stress research: Implications for the depressive disorders. *Psychol Bull.* 1991;110(3):406–425.
42. Flor H, Turk DC. Etiological theories and treatments for chronic back pain. I. Somatic models and interventions. *Pain.* 1984;19(2):105–121.
43. Turk DC, Flor H. Etiological theories and treatment for chronic back pain. II. Psychological models and interventions. *Pain.* 1984;19:209–233.
44. Weisberg JN, Keefe FJ. Personality disorders in the chronic pain population: Basic concepts, empirical findings, and clinical implications. *Pain Forum.* 1997;6(1):1–9.
45. American Psychiatric Association. *Diagnostic and Statistical Manual of Mental Disorders.* 3rd ed. Washington, DC: Author; 1980.
46. Lenzenweger MF. The longitudinal study of personality disorders: History, design considerations, and initial findings. *J Pers Disord.* 2006;20(6):645–670.
47. Lenzenweger MF. Epidemiology of personality disorders. *Psychiatr Clin North Am.* 2008;31(3):395–403, vi.
48. Lenzenweger MF, Lane MC, Loranger AW, Kessler RC. DSM-IV personality disorders in the National Comorbidity Survey Replication. *Biol Psychiatry.* 2007;62(6):553–564.
49. Torgersen S, Kringlen E, Cramer V. The prevalence of personality disorders in a community sample. *Arch Gen Psychiatry.* 2001;58(6):590–596.
50. Grant BF, Hasin DS, Stinson FS, et al. Prevalence, correlates, and disability of personality disorders in the United States: Results from the national epidemiologic survey on alcohol and related conditions. *J Clin Psychiatry.* 2004;65(7):948–958.
51. Reich J, Tupin JP, Abramowitz SI. Psychiatric diagnosis of chronic pain patients. *Am J Psychiatry.* 1983;140(11):1495–1498.
52. Large RG. DSM-III diagnoses in chronic pain: Confusion or clarity? *J Nerv Ment Dis.* 1986;174(5):295–303.
53. Reich J, Thompson WD. DSM-III personality disorder clusters in three populations. *Br J Psychiatry.* 1987;150:471–475.
54. Fishbain DA, Goldberg M, Meagher BR, Steele R, Rosomoff H. Male and female chronic pain patients categorized by DSM-III psychiatric diagnostic criteria. *Pain.* 1986;26(2):181–197.
55. Weisberg JN, Gallagher RM, Gorin A. Personality disorder in chronic pain: A longitudinal approach to validation of diagnosis. Paper presented at: 15th Annual Scientific Meeting of the American Pain Society; November 1996; Washington, DC.
56. Spitzer RL, Williams JB, Gibbon M, First MB. *Structured Clinical Interview for DSM-III-R.* New York, NY: New York State Psychiatric Institute; 1988.
57. Polatin PB, Kinney RK, Gatchel RJ, Lillo E, Mayer TG. Psychiatric illness and chronic low-back pain: The mind and the spine—which goes first? *Spine.* 1993;18(1):66–71.
58. Gatchel RJ, Garofalo JP, Ellis E, Holt C. Major psychological disorders in acute and chronic TMD: An initial examination. *J Am Dent Assoc.* 1996;127(9):1365–1370, 1372, 1374.
59. Monti DA, Herring CL, Schwartzman RJ, Marchese M. Personality assessment of patients with complex regional pain syndrome type I. *Clin J Pain.* 1998;14(4):295–302.
60. Fischer-Kern M, Kapusta ND, Doering S, Hörz S, Mikutta C, Aigner M. The relationship between personality organization and psychiatric classification in chronic pain patients. *Psychopathology.* 2011;44(1):21–26.

61. Kayhan F, Ilik F. Prevalence of personality disorders in patients with chronic migraine. *Compr Psychiatry*. 2016;68:60–64.
62. Wilsey BL, Fishman SM, Tsodikov A, Ogden C, Symreng I, Ernst A. Psychological comorbidities predicting prescription opioid abuse among patients in chronic pain presenting to the emergency department. *Pain Med*. 2008;9(8):1107–1117.
63. Majeed MH, Sudak DM. Cognitive behavioral therapy for chronic pain: One therapeutic approach for the opioid epidemic. *J Psychiatr Pract*. 2017;23(6):409–414.
64. Ehde DM, Dillworth TM, Turner JA. Cognitive-behavioral therapy for individuals with chronic pain: Efficacy, innovations, and directions for research. *Am Psychol*. 2014;69(2):153–166.
65. Knoerl R, Lavoie Smith EM, Weisberg J. Chronic pain and cognitive behavioral therapy: An integrative review. *West J Nurs Res*. 2016;38(5):596–628.
66. Cederberg JT, Cernvall M, Dahl J, von Essen L, Ljungman G. Acceptance as a mediator for change in acceptance and commitment therapy for persons with chronic pain? *Int J Behav Med*. 2016;23(1):21–29.
67. Chakhssi F, Janssen W, Pol SM, van Dreumel M, Westerhof GJ. Acceptance and commitment therapy group-treatment for non-responsive patients with personality disorders: An exploratory study. *Personal Ment Health*. 2015;9(4):345–356.
68. McCracken LM. Learning to live with the pain: Acceptance of pain predicts adjustment in persons with chronic pain. *Pain*. 1998;74(1):21–27.
69. Wilks CR, Korslund KE, Harned MS, Linehan MM. Dialectical behavior therapy and domains of functioning over two years. *Behav Res Ther*. 2016;77:162–169.

21

Pain and Comorbid Psychiatric Illnesses in Elderly People

A Fitful Marriage and Its Management

MELLAR P. DAVIS AND JOHN L. SHUSTER, JR. ■

INTRODUCTION

Until recently, pain was considered a natural part of aging and was rarely investigated in elderly people. The reported prevalence of pain in elderly people is highly variable. Pain prevalence differs depending on the country surveyed, study date, type of study, population considered "elderly," pain definition and chronicity, study design, sites of pain. and number of painful sites present. Pain domains described in prevalence studies are acute, chronic, intensity, interference, episodic, "persistent," regional, multiple, or "widespread." Time periods described are current; 1, 3, 6, or 12 months' duration; or life time prevalence.[1] Current pain occurs in 28 to 73% of elderly people (defined here as age ≥65 years); chronic pain occurs in 25 to 76% of community-dwelling elderly people and in 83 to 93% of those in residential care. In most studies, pain prevalence is greater in women. More than 20% of elderly Americans use analgesic medications on a daily basis.[2] Under-recognized and undertreated pain in older patient patients is distressingly problematic, with as many as three of every four elderly patients who have chronic pain suffering without treatment and with the majority reporting inadequate relief.[3] A significant number do not volunteer pain and assume that it is part of growing old. Physicians frequently do not screen for pain in patient encounters.

PAIN AND MENTAL ILLNESS IN ELDERLY PEOPLE

The relationship between pain and depression is complex; the presence of both makes managing each difficult. Long-term opioids lead to pain and depression and reduce the pain-relieving benefits of analgesics and compliance prescriptions. There is a risk that a depressed patient will either overdose on analgesics or misuse analgesics for depression and the rewarding effects of opioids. Depression may occur at any time during the course of pain: concurrent with, before, or after the onset of pain.[4] Two-thirds of individuals with depression somatize their pain, which misleads physicians into thinking that the pain is physical. Opioids may be used by depressed patients for sleep disturbances. Clinicians should be aware that depression may facilitate the development of pain refractory to analgesics.[5] Depression accompanying pain decreases pain tolerance and lowers pain thresholds.[6] It is worth noting that depression is accompanied by loss of appetite, loss of energy, and pain as presenting symptoms, which can be mistaken for analgesic side effects.

The co-occurrence of depression and pain appears to be the result of a common neurobiological substrate.[7] In a study of individuals older than 50 years with osteoarthritis and depressive symptoms, pain severity was out of proportion to radiographic changes.[8] Among elderly people, poor self-rated health was not mediated by the comorbidities but by pain and pain interference.[9,10]

Psychiatric disorders are highly associated with chronic pain. Pain is associated with mental disorders (66.7%), of which 50% are mood disorders, 33.3% anxiety disorder, 20% somatoform disorder, and 17% substance abuse disorder. Greater pain severity is associated with a greater incidence of depression, anxiety, and insomnia.[11] Chronic pain predicts the number of psychiatric comorbidities (odds ration [OR] = 1.4–4.39).[12] Although anxiety and depression were less frequently found in older than younger individuals, those with psychiatric illnesses were more likely to have physical conditions that were painful.[13] The OR of having pain with anxiety and/or depression ranges between 1.48 and 3.86.[14] Anxiety and/or depression with pain impairs recovery from depression and predicts poorer analgesic outcomes, greater pain intensity, interference with daily activities, and greater health care expenditures than either pain or depression or anxiety alone.[15] Patients with depression and pain have a greater number of painful sites than those without depression or anxiety.[16] The paucity of objective physical and radiographic findings accompanying severe pain should be a clue that the individual is depressed.[17]

Pain-processing disorders such as fibromyalgia occur with greater frequency (OR > 2) in those with major depressive disorder.[18] Compared with nonpainful comorbidities, the suicide risk (ideation, plan, and attempts) is significantly greater with pain and depression relative to depression alone (OR = 1.4).[19]

A small survey (N = 89) focused on elderly people with chronic pain, with an average duration of pain of 5.5 years and with one-fourth of respondents reporting more than one pain site. Nearly two-thirds had a psychiatric disorder, most commonly depression (41.6%), somatoform disorders (33.7%), anxiety (18%), and drug abuse disorders. The younger the age at pain onset, the greater the pain intensity and the more likely an accompanying psychiatric illness. For every 10-mm increase in Visual Analog Scale–rated pain severity (0–100 mm), there was a 54% increased likelihood of a psychiatric disorder. Depression increased the perception that pain could not be controlled. Severity predicted greater pain interference and increased dependence on others for daily activities.[20]

WHY DO PAIN AND DEPRESSION OCCUR TOGETHER?

A common neural substrate for pain and depression includes shared neuroanatomical organization, neurotransmission, and neurotrophins within the central nervous system. Both are associated with dysregulation of the hypothalamic-pituitary-adrenal axis and neuroinflammation.[21] Because there is a shared neurobiological basis between pain and depression, single classes of medications such as tricyclic antidepressants, selective serotonin/norepinephrine reuptake inhibitors, opioids, classic and nonclassic cannabinoid agonists, and N-methyl-D-aspartate receptor antagonists may be effective in treating both.

TREATMENT OF COMORBID PAIN AND PSYCHIATRIC ILLNESS IN ELDERLY PEOPLE

Physiological changes in elderly people influence drug pharmacodynamics and pharmacokinetics. Gastric emptying is often delayed, and gastric acidity is reduced, which will influence the rate and amount of drug absorption based on drug pKa (the pH at which ionized and un-ionized drug are in equilibrium). Peristalsis and blood flow to the gut are delayed, which further influences drug absorption. Body fat increases as muscle mass diminishes, which alters the volume of distribution of hydrophilic drugs. Lower doses of hydrophilic drugs produce the same responses as higher doses in young people—hence the dosing strategy of "starting low and going slow." Reduced hepatic blood flow and liver mass reduces first-pass hepatic clearance. This means greater drug bioavailability per dose and greater systemic exposure for drugs with a high first-pass clearance. Reduced renal blood flow and glomerular filtration rate results in drug accumulation for those medications requiring renal clearance. With reduced muscle mass, there is a reduced correlation of serum creatinine to glomerular filtration rate. Adjusting drug doses to creatinine clearance is less accurate in elderly people. There are reduced opioid receptor density and changes in receptor sensitivity, which alter response compared with younger individuals.[22]

The health state of the elderly is highly variable from individual to individual, which makes choosing initial drug doses and titration to get a response less predictable. In general, however, the dose at which toxicity occurs moves closer to the dose that is therapeutic, resulting in a narrower therapeutic index. The ability to tolerate medications is vastly different in healthy than in frail elderly people.[23] Unfortunately, in analgesic trials, very few individuals are older than 65 years, despite the high prevalence of pain in that population, and elderly patients are often excluded because of comorbid illnesses or psychiatric disorders.[24] Chronological age, drug metabolism, drug clearance, and drug responses poorly correlate.[25] Consequently, undertreatment of pain and psychiatric illness in elderly patients results from the fear of severe adverse events.[26]

There is little evidence on which to base analgesics choices. There are few trials of oral opioids that exclusively study elderly patients. Two trials studied transdermal fentanyl: one with a high placebo response, and an open-label study demonstrating a high response rate.[27] There are a number of trials using buprenorphine, which included a significant number of elderly people.[28] Choices of adjuvants may be made based on accompanying psychological symptoms. Table 21.1 reviews psychotropics and lists their associated psychological benefits.

With these limitations, the American Geriatrics Society has recommended a primary role for carefully selected opioids, given the limitations of alternative drug classes (e.g., nonsteroidal anti-inflammatory drugs [NSAIDs]).[29]

Consensus recommendations are that treatment must be individualized. Buprenorphine, based on consensus, is a reasonable choice in elderly patients with neuropathic pain.[30]

From a safety point of view, both fentanyl and buprenorphine have reduced gastrointestinal side effects relative to morphine.[30] Buprenorphine is associated with reduced falls compared with other opioids[31] and with fewer drug interactions than oxycodone, methadone, and fentanyl. Fentanyl should be avoided in patients with hepatic failure because CYP3A4 is reduced in liver

Table 21.1 Psychotropics that treat both pain and psychological symptoms

Drug	Mechanism	Dose	Toxicity	Added benefits
Amitriptyline	Norepinephrine/serotonin reuptake inhibitor, sodium channel blocker, NMDA receptor antagonist	10–25 mg at bedtime, titrate to 200 mg over 4 weeks as tolerated, lower doses needed for pain than depression	Orthostatic hypotension, somnolence, fatigue, urinary retention, sexual dysfunction, increased intraocular pressures, arrhythmia. Needs CYP2D6 genotype	Antidepressant, antianxiety, sleep
Nortriptyline	Same as amitriptyline	Same as amitriptyline	Similar to amitriptyline, less anticholinergic side effects	Same as amitriptyline
Desipramine	Same as amitriptyline	Same as amitriptyline	Same as nortriptyline	Same as amitriptyline
Gabapentin	Calcium channel blocker	300 mg at bedtime day1, titrated to 300 mg tid by day 3, and increased by 300 mg every 4 days with a goal of 1800 mg/day. Maximum 3600 mg/day limited by GI absorption	Dizziness, somnolence, fatigue, GI upset, ataxia, abnormal vision and gait, nystagmus, headache, cognitive dysfunction, potential for abuse and used to potential opioid rewarding effects by addicts	Sleep, antianxiety, potential mood stabilizer, nausea, hiccoughs, intractable cough, seizures, uremic pruritus
Pregabalin	Calcium channel blocker	75 mg day1, titrate every 4 days by 75 mg up to 300 mg/day, maximum dose 600 mg/day. Not limited by GI absorption and incomplete cross tolerance to gabapentin	Similar to gabapentin plus edema and weight gain	Similar to gabapentin
Duloxetine	Serotonin, norepinephrine reuptake inhibitor	20–30 mg daily week 1, increased to 60 mg/day week 2, rarely titrate to 120 mg/day. Take in the morning.	Nausea, somnolence, tremor, sweating, blurry vision, anxiety	Depression, chemotherapy-related neuropathy (only proven adjuvant)
Venlafaxine	Same as duloxetine at doses of 150 mg/day or higher	75 mg in the morning day1, titrate weekly to a maximum of 225 mg/day	Similar to duloxetine plus hypertension at higher doses	Depression, acute pain from taxanes or oxaliplatin

(continued)

Table 21.1 CONTINUED

Drug	Mechanism	Dose	Toxicity	Added benefits
Mirtazapine	Selective serotonin, norepinephrine neurotransmitter facilitator via blockade of autoreceptors and serotonin receptors 2 and 3	15 mg at night, increase every week up to a maximum of 45 mg at bedtime	Somnolence, dry mouth, morning hangover, impaired psychomotor coordination, which may impair driving. Evidence for analgesia is weak	Sleep, depression, antianxiety, few drug interactions
Carbamazepine	Sodium channel clocker	100 mg day 1, titrate weekly by 100 mg up to 200 mg three times daily	Rash, photosensitivity, drowsiness, hyponatremia, nausea, aplastic anemia. Stimulates CYP3A$ leading to multiple drug interactions	Mood stabilizer, first-line analgesic for trigeminal neuralgia
Oxcarbazepine	Sodium channel blocker	150 mg day 1, titrate every 4 days to 600 mg twice daily	Hyponatremia, somnolence, drowsiness, ataxia, tremor. Fewer drug interactions than carbamazepine	Mood stabilizer
Lamotrigine	Sodium channel blocker	25 mg day 1, titrate by 25 mg weekly to 200 mg/day	Stevens-Johnsons syndrome, dizziness, somnolence, GI disturbance, abnormal vision, gait disturbance	Mood stabilizer
Topiramate	Sodium channel blocker	25 mg day 1, titrate every 4 days by 25 mg up to 100 mg twice daily, maximum dose 200 mg twice daily	Dizziness, somnolence, ataxia, tremor, gait disturbance, weight loss, nephrolithiasis	Antidepressant augmentation for refractory depression
Valproic acid	Increases CNS GABA neurotransmission	750 mg day 1 in divided doses, titrate up to 1500–2000 mg/day	Thrombocytopenia, hepatitis, pancreatitis, hypothyroidism, hyperammonemia, somnolence, drug interactions via CYP3A4 inhibition	Aggressive behavior, bipolar disorders, sleep, anxiety, hyperalert delirium

GABA = gamma-aminobutyric acid; GI = gastrointestinal; NMDA = N-methyl-D-aspartate.

disease, whereas glucuronidated metabolized opioids are safer in patients with moderate hepatic failure. In elderly patients with renal failure, buprenorphine is preferred because its clearance is independent of renal function. Sedatives such as benzodiazepines should be avoided in patients since the combination further increases the risk for opioid-related falls, confusion, and respiratory failure. Buprenorphine, hydromorphone, and oxycodone are less immunosuppressive than morphine and fentanyl.[32]

Levorphanol is an old opioid that was neglected or underutilized after sustained-release opioids appeared on the market. It is a safer alternative to methadone[33] and is an effective analgesic for neuropathic pain.[34] Although there are no specific trials in elderly patients, there are potential benefits in this population. It is glucuronidated and not subject to P-glycoprotein efflux and hence will have fewer drug interactions relative to fentanyl, oxycodone, methadone, and morphine. The pharmacokinetics of levorphanol is much more predictable than that of methadone.[35]

Tapentadol has several advantages compared with oxycodone. It is less constipating and has fewer drug interactions because it is conjugated rather than metabolized by the cytochrome P450 system.[36] Tramadol requires conversion to desmethyl-tramadol by CYP2D6 and has been associated with seizures in elderly people.[37] Tapentadol does not require this conversion, and the parent drug is active. Data pooled from three randomized trials specifically assessed tapentadol in those 75 years and older. The comparison was between tapentadol and oxycodone and placebo. Tapentadol had lower gastrointestinal toxicity than oxycodone and had equivalent analgesia.[38]

Acetaminophen is the first-line nonopioid drug of choice for older individuals with musculoskeletal pain. Patients weighing less than 50 kg and malnourished patients should have doses limited to 2 g/day.[39] The volume of distribution is reduced in frail elderly patients compared with healthy elderly patients; frailty is associated with decreased total clearance of acetaminophen and a prolonged half-life.[40] Interestingly, elderly people are less likely to generate the toxic metabolite NAPQI, which is responsible for liver failure.[41]

NSAIDs are more effective for persistent inflammatory musculoskeletal disorders than acetaminophen. Chronic use is to be avoided in elderly patients because of gastrointestinal and renal toxicity, and short-term use should only be pursued with great caution in older patients. NSAIDs account for 25% of hospitalizations for adverse drug events in elderly patients.[42] Gastrointestinal adverse effects are reduced by misoprostol or proton pump inhibitors. Bleeding events increase with age, particularly when combined with antithrombotic agents.[43] Renal vascular constriction and sodium retention occur, which worsens renal function and hypertension and is particularly problematic when individuals are taking angiotensin-converting enzyme inhibitors and diuretics.

Diclofenac epolamine 1.3% topical patch is an excellent alternative to systematic NSAIDs in elderly patients and is recommended by most guidelines.[44] It is approved for treatment of acute pain associated with sprains, strains, and contusions.[45] The patch delivers effective concentrations at the site of injury, with minimal (1%) systemic levels relative to oral delivery (75 mg of diclofenac).[46] Topical NSAIDs are better analgesics than oral acetaminophen and improve function and joint stiffness better than systemic opioids and intra-articular corticosteroids.[47]

Corticosteroids are sometimes used as analgesics or co-analgesics. However, elderly people have reduced clearance of certain corticosteroids, such as methylprednisolone, and experience greater immunosuppression than younger individuals and greater hypothalamic pituitary adrenal suppression.[48]

Antidepressants and anticonvulsants are used as adjuvants; these are reviewed in Table 21.1.

Transdermal 5% lidocaine patches have largely been utilized for postherpetic neuralgia. The lidocaine patch is a better analgesic than pregabalin for postherpetic neuralgia and is equally effective as pregabalin in the treatment of diabetic neuropathy.[49] It is not systematically absorbed and therefore has few adverse drug effects and drug interactions. Patches can be left on for 24 hours. A o1-hour topical application of 8% capsaicin plaster relieves localized neuropathic pain for more than 13 weeks. Pre-emptive topical analgesia should be applied before capsaicin. Topical capsaicin cream has been used for osteoarthritis, but many cannot tolerate it.[50]

Vitamin D replacement (50,000 IU) relieves knee pain in individuals who are deficient in vitamin D. Vitamin D is given weekly. Not only does pain improve, but quadriceps strength also improves.[51]

CONCLUSION

Pain in elderly people with coexisting psychological symptoms is a challenge to treat. Tolerance to opioid analgesics and adjuvants is reduced with age. The question is whether to treat the psychological symptom with a nonopioid analgesic or adjuvant, which also may treat the pain, and hope that both symptoms will respond, or to treat the pain with an opioid such as buprenorphine, which also can treat depression. There are large gaps in our understanding of pain in elderly people, and there are few evidence-based guidelines to give direction. As the population ages, the combination of pain and depression in elderly people will increase. This is an important area that needs research.

REFERENCES

1. Abdulla A, Adams N, Bone M, et al. Guidance on the management of pain in older people. *Age Ageing*. 2013;42(suppl 1):i1–57.
2. Gibson SJ. Pain and aging: The pain experience over the adult life span. *Proc 10th World Congr Pain*. 2003;24:767–790.
3. Arneric SP, Laird JMA, Chappell AS, Kennedy JD. Tailoring chronic pain treatments for the elderly: Are we prepared for the challenge? *Drug Discov Today*. 2014;19(1):8–17.
4. Barkin RL, Barkin SJ, Barkin DS. Perception, assessment, treatment, and management of pain in the elderly. *Clin Geriatr Med*. 2005;21(3):465–490, v.
5. Perahia DG, Kajdasz DK, Royer MG, Walker DJ, Raskin J. Duloxetine in the treatment of major depressive disorder: An assessment of the relationship between outcomes and episode characteristics. *Int Clin Psychopharmacol*. 2006;21(5):285–295.
6. Raskin J, Wiltse CG, Siegal A, et al. Efficacy of duloxetine on cognition, depression, and pain in elderly patients with major depressive disorder: An 8-week, double-blind, placebo-controlled trial. *Am J Psychiatry*. 2007;164(6):900–909.
7. Knaster P, Karlsson H, Estlander AM, Kalso E. Psychiatric disorders as assessed with SCID in chronic pain patients: The anxiety disorders precede the onset of pain. *Gen Hosp Psychiatry*. 2012;34(1):46–52.
8. Han HS, Lee JY, Kang SB, Chang CB. The relationship between the presence of depressive symptoms and the severity of self-reported knee pain in the middle aged and elderly. *Knee Surg Sports Traumatol Arthrosc*. 2016;24(5):1634–1642.
9. Nutzel A, Dahlhaus A, Fuchs A, et al. Self-rated health in multimorbid older general practice patients: A cross-sectional study in Germany. *BMC Fam Pract*. 2014;15:1.
10. Molarius A, Janson S. Self-rated health, chronic diseases, and symptoms among middle-aged and elderly men and women. *J Clin Epidemiol*. 2002;55(4):364–370.
11. Annagur BB, Uguz F, Apiliogullari S, Kara I, Gunduz S. Psychiatric disorders and association with quality of sleep and quality of life in patients with chronic pain: A SCID-based study. *Pain Med*. 2014;15(5):772–781.
12. Dominick CH, Blyth FM, Nicholas MK. Unpacking the burden: Understanding the relationships between chronic pain and comorbidity in the general population. *Pain*. 2012;153(2):293–304.
13. Scott KM, Von Korff M, Alonso J, et al. Age patterns in the prevalence of DSM-IV depressive/anxiety disorders with and without physical co-morbidity. *Psychol Med*. 2008;38(11):1659–1669.
14. McWilliams LA, Goodwin RD, Cox BJ. Depression and anxiety associated with three pain conditions: Results from a nationally representative sample. *Pain*. 2004;111(1–2):77–83.
15. Bair MJ, Robinson RL, Katon W, Kroenke K. Depression and pain comorbidity: A literature review. *Arch Intern Med*. 2003;163(20):2433–2445.
16. Docking RE, Beasley M, Steinerowski A, et al. The epidemiology of regional and widespread musculoskeletal pain in rural versus urban settings in those >/=55 years. *Br J Pain*. 2015;9(2):86–95.

17. Hans H, Lone A, Aksenov V, Rollo CD. Impacts of metformin and aspirin on life history features and longevity of crickets: Trade-offs versus cost-free life extension? *Age.* 2015;37(2):31.

18. Demyttenaere K, Bruffaerts R, Lee S, et al. Mental disorders among persons with chronic back or neck pain: Results from the World Mental Health Surveys. *Pain.* 2007;129(3):332–342.

19. Braden JB, Sullivan MD. Suicidal thoughts and behavior among adults with self-reported pain conditions in the national comorbidity survey replication. *J Pain.* 2008;9(12):1106–1115.

20. Ho PT, Li CF, Ng YK, Tsui SL, Ng KF. Prevalence of and factors associated with psychiatric morbidity in chronic pain patients. *J Psychosom Res.* 2011;70(6):541–547.

21. Blackburn-Munro G. Hypothalamo-pituitary-adrenal axis dysfunction as a contributory factor to chronic pain and depression. *Curr Pain Headache Rep.* 2004;8(2):116–124.

22. Calsini P, Mocchegiani E, Fabris N. The pharmacodynamics of thymomodulin in elderly humans. *Drug Exp Clin Res.* 1985;11(9):671–674.

23. McLachlan AJ, Hilmer SN, Le Couteur DG. Variability in response to medicines in older people: Phenotypic and genotypic factors. *Clin Pharmacol Therapeut.* 2009;85(4):431–433.

24. Rochon PA, Fortin PR, Dear KBG, Minaker KL, Chalmers TC. Reporting of age data in clinical-trials of arthritis: Deficiencies and solutions. *Arch Intern Med.* 1993;153(2):243–248.

25. Butler JM, Begg EJ. Free drug metabolic clearance in elderly people. *Clin Pharmacokinet.* 2008;47(5):297–321.

26. Teno J, Casey V, Rochon T, Mor V, Wright R. Resident assessment of pain management: A new tool to examine pain management in NH. *Gerontologist.* 2004;44:508.

27. Kongsgaard UE, Poulain P. Transdermal fentanyl for pain control in adults with chronic cancer pain. *Eur J Pain.* 1998;2(1):53–62.

28. Likar R, Kayser H, Sittl R. Long-term management of chronic pain with transdermal buprenorphine: A multicenter, open-label, follow-up study in patients from three short-term clinical trials. *Clin Therapeut.* 2006;28(6):943–952.

29. Ferrell B, Argoff CE, Epplin J, et al. Pharmacological management of persistent pain in older persons. *J Am Geriatr Soc.* 2009;57(8):1331–1346.

30. Pergolizzi J, Boger RH, Budd K, et al. Opioids and the management of chronic severe pain in the elderly: Consensus statement of an International Expert Panel with focus on the six clinically most often used World Health Organization Step III opioids (buprenorphine, fentanyl, hydromorphone, methadone, morphine, oxycodone). *Pain Pract.* 2008;8(4):287–313.

31. Vestergaard P, Rejnmark L, Mosekilde L. Anxiolytics, sedatives, antidepressants, neuroleptics and the risk of fracture. *Osteoporos Int.* 2006;17(6):807–816.

32. Martucci C, Panerai AE, Sacerdote P. Chronic fentanyl or buprenorphine infusion in the mouse: Similar analgesic profile but different effects on immune responses. *Pain.* 2004;110(1–2):385–392.

33. McNulty JP. Chronic pain: Levorphanol, methadone, and the N-methyl-D-aspartate receptor. *J Palliat Med.* 2009;12(9):765–766.

34. Rowbotham MC, Twilling L, Davies PS, Reisner L, Taylor K, Mohr D. Oral opioid therapy for chronic peripheral and central neuropathic pain. *N Engl J Med.* 2003;348(13):1223–1232.

35. Atkinson TJ, Fudin J, Pandula A, Mirza M. Medication pain management in the elderly: Unique and underutilized analgesic treatment options. *Clin Therapeut.* 2013;35(11):1669–1689.

36. Terlinden R, Ossig J, Fliegert F, Lange C, Gohler K. Absorption, metabolism, and excretion of 14C-labeled tapentadol HCl in healthy male subjects. *Eur J Drug Metab Pharmacokinet.* 2007;32(3):163–169.

37. Boyd IW. Tramadol and seizures. *Med J Aust.* 2005;182(11):595–596.

38. Biondi DM, Xiang J, Etropolski M, Moskovitz B. Tolerability and efficacy of tapentadol extended release in elderly patients >/=75 years of age with chronic osteoarthritis knee or low back pain. *J Opioid Manage.* 2015;11(5):393–403.

39. Claridge LC, Eksteen B, Smith A, Shah T, Holt AP. Acute liver failure after administration of paracetamol at the maximum recommended daily dose in adults. *BMJ.* 2010;341:c6764.

40. McLachlan AJ, Bath S, Naganathan V, et al. Clinical pharmacology of analgesic medicines in older people: Impact of frailty and cognitive impairment. *Br J Clin Pharmacol.* 2011;71(3):351–364.

41. Mitchell SJ, Hilmer SNAP. Drug-induced liver injury in older adults. *Ther Adv Drug Saf.* 2010;1(2):65–77.

42. Berthold HK, Steinhagen-Thiessen E. Drug therapy in the elderly. *Internist.* 2009;50(12):1415–1423.

43. Abdulla A, Adams N, Bone M, et al. Guidance on the management of pain in older people. *Age Ageing.* 2013;42:I1–I57.

44. Petersen B, Rovati S. Diclofenac epolamine (Flector (R)) patch evidence for topical activity. *Clin Drug Invest.* 2009;29(1):1–9.

45. Lionberger DR, Brennan MJ. Topical nonsteroidal anti-inflammatory drugs for the treatment of pain due to soft tissue injury: Diclofenac epolamine topical patch. *J Pain Res.* 2010;3:223–233.

46. Brunner M, Dehghanyar P, Seigfried B, Martin W, Menke G, Muller M. Favourable dermal penetration of diclofenac after administration to the skin using a novel spray gel formulation. *Br J Clin Pharmacol.* 2005;60(5):573–577.

47. Zhang W, Nuki G, Moskowitz RW, et al. OARSI recommendations for the management of hip and knee osteoarthritis Part III: Changes in evidence following systematic cumulative update of research published through January 2009. *Osteoarthritis Cartilage.* 2010;18(4):476–499.

48. Tornatore KM, Logue G, Venuto RC, Davis PJ. Pharmacokinetics of methylprednisolone in elderly and young healthy males. *J Am Geriatr Soc.* 1994;42(10):1118–1122.

49. Baron R, Tolle TR, Gockel U, Brosz M, Freynhagen R. A cross-sectional cohort survey in 2100 patients with painful diabetic neuropathy and postherpetic neuralgia: Differences in demographic data and sensory symptoms. *Pain.* 2009;146(1-2):34–40.

50. Backonja M, Wallace MS, Blonsky ER, et al. NGX-4010, a high-concentration cap-saicin patch, for the treatment of postherpetic neuralgia: A randomised, double-blind study. *Lancet Neurol.* 2008;7(12):1106–1112.
51. Heidari B, Javadian Y, Babaei M, Yousef-Ghahari B. Restorative effect of vitamin D deficiency on knee pain and quadriceps muscle strength in knee osteoarthritis. *Acta Med Iran.* 2015;53(8):466–470.

22

Does Self-Injury Hurt?

Understanding the Experience and Potential Functions of Pain in Self-Injury

AMY KRANZLER, KARA B. FEHLING, JULIA BRILLANTE, AND EDWARD A. SELBY ■

SELF-INJURY: THE PARADOXICAL ROLE OF PAIN AND PSYCHIATRIC CONSIDERATIONS

A central principle in the study of pain is the assumption that people generally strive to avoid or minimize experiences of pain and to maximize experiences of pleasure.[1] It may therefore seem paradoxical that some individuals intentionally and repeatedly inflict physical pain on their bodies. Yet research has demonstrated that growing numbers of adolescents and adults engage in nonsuicidal self-injury (NSSI), which is the deliberate and direct destruction of bodily tissue without the presence of lethal intent.[2,3] The most common form of NSSI is intentional cutting, frequently of the arms and legs, but other common behaviors include burning, banging one's head, punching oneself or another object, severe scratching, swallowing dangerous substances, and biting, with individuals deliberately engaging in these behaviors despite, or because of, the pain they elicit. NSSI typically does not include culturally sanctioned behaviors, including traditional cultural tattooing, piercing, or other physical alterations of the body[4]; however, in Western cultures, some who self-injure do sometimes use tattooing as a form of self-injury along with other self-injurious behaviors.[5]

Recent studies have found that as many as 35.6% of adolescents[6] and 43.6% of young adults[7] engage in NSSI. As a result, the importance of understanding this behavior has been increasingly recognized, leading to growing impetus to include NSSI as a distinct psychiatric diagnosis in a future version of the *Diagnostic and Statistical Manual of Mental Disorders* (DSM).[8,9] The purpose of this chapter is to review existing understandings about the experience and potential functions of pain in NSSI.

Is Nonsuicidal Self-Injury Experienced as Painful?

One of the central questions in the study of NSSI is how individuals who engage in this behavior overcome the natural instinct to avoid pain. One possibility may be that those who engage in NSSI may naturally have, or may develop, reduced pain perception and therefore actually experience these behaviors as less painful than those who do not regularly engage in NSSI.[10] According to this "pain analgesia" hypothesis,[3] pain may not pose a barrier to engaging in NSSI for these individuals because they do not experience NSSI as painful. Consistent with this hypothesis, some studies have found that those who engage in NSSI often report experiencing little or no pain while engaging in these behaviors.[11,12]

Several laboratory studies have also found that individuals who engage in NSSI have higher pain tolerance.[13,14] Hooley and colleagues[14] found that people who engage in NSSI had higher pain thresholds (demonstrating higher levels at which a stimulus is subjectively experienced as painful), higher pain tolerance (taking longer to discontinue exposure to painful stimuli), and higher pain endurance (being willing to continue for longer after initially experiencing a stimulus as painful) than those who do not engage in NSSI. Furthermore, a recent meta-analysis similarly found that across studies, individuals who engage in NSSI report greater pain threshold, greater pain tolerance, and lower pain intensity (experiencing pain as less intense) compared with controls.[15] Together, these studies suggest that individuals who engage in NSSI often demonstrate altered pain processing, if they feel pain at all.

To date, the reasons that some self-injurers may not experience as much (or any) pain while engaging in NSSI are not yet clear. One possibility may be that individuals who engage in NSSI habituate to pain over time with repeated exposure, thereby altering their pain sensitivity through recurrent exposure to pain. However, Nock and colleagues[16] found that lifetime frequency of self-injury was not associated with the experience of pain. Another possible mechanism may be through endogenous opioids or endorphins, which are the body's natural pain killers, are released following NSSI behaviors, and may reduce experiences of pain and elicit feelings of euphoria.[17] It is thought that individuals who engage in NSSI may have higher levels of endorphins, or that engaging in NSSI may increase baseline levels of endorphins, resulting in this decreased pain sensitivity.[3] Research examining this mechanism, however, has been inconsistent, and further studies are needed.[3]

However, although several studies have documented the absence of pain during self-injury for some self-injurers, other studies have shown that many self-injurers do in fact experience pain while engaging in NSSI. For example, one study found that more than half of a sample of adolescent self-injurers reported feeling at least some to severe pain while engaging in NSSI.[16] In another study, 24% of participants reported engaging in NSSI specifically with the intention of feeling pain, and even more participants (31%) reported actually feeling pain while engaging in NSSI.[12] Furthermore, this study found that experiencing pain while engaging in NSSI was associated with greater NSSI frequency over a 2-week monitoring period. This finding suggests that not only does the experience of pain appear to be an insufficient barrier to NSSI but also that, for some individuals, the pain experienced during NSSI may be actually be particularly reinforcing, increasing the likelihood that they will continue to engage in the behavior. As such, it is critical to understand the ways in which pain may serve desirable functions for at least a subset of individuals engaging in NSSI.

Does Pain Associated With Nonsuicidal Self-Injury Serve a Desired Function? A Review of Laboratory Studies

For the subset of individuals who do report experiencing pain when engaging in NSSI, pain may play a role in facilitating the emotion regulation functions of NSSI. Researchers and clinicians have long hypothesized that people engage in NSSI primarily for emotion regulation functions or to cope with stress.[18] Accordingly, although most self-injurers report a variety of motivations for self-injuring, they most commonly report that they engage in NSSI in order to reduce negative emotion.[19] Unfortunately, research in this area has been significantly limited by the fact that self-injury cannot be observed directly in lab-based settings because of ethical considerations.

One of the primary ways researchers have circumvented this ethical stymie is by employing guided imagery with self-injurious content. These experiments attempt to recreate and study the types of emotional and physical effects that actually accompany real-life self-injury by asking self-injurious participants to create personalized scripts of NSSI behaviors and then having them relive NSSI experiences by reading these scripts. Using this methodology, Haines and colleagues[20] discovered that self-injuring participants experienced high levels of physical tension (as measured by self-report and psychophysiological measures [e.g., heart rate and respiration]) and negative affect while they imagined the time leading up to self-injury, and then experienced significant reductions in physical tension and negative affect while imagining self-injury and the time after self-injury. Non–self-injuring control participants did not show this pattern for NSSI scripts, and no participants showed this pattern when imagining control scripts (e.g., accidental injuries or aggressive interpersonal situations). Later, Brain and colleagues[21] and Welch and colleagues[22] largely corroborated these results. These studies suggest that even imagining NSSI can decrease affective and physiological distress and lends support to the idea that individuals may engage in NSSI for these emotion regulation effects.

However, given the limitations of studying the effects of NSSI via responses to NSSI imagery, other research has employed various self-injury proxies (e.g., electrical shocks) in order to more accurately mimic real-world NSSI and the pain that may accompany it. Research has shown that lab-induced pain can significantly reduce response to in-lab emotional manipulations[23] and that lab-induced pain can significantly reduce the experience of preexisting negative emotions.[24] Research on self-injurers has utilized these methods to examine the potential emotional regulatory function of pain in NSSI specifically. Many of these studies have found that self-injuring participants do report reduced negative emotion and arousal in response to NSSI proxies like a cold pressor task,[25] shock,[26,27] heat stimulation,[28] and pressure stimulation.[29] Furthermore, while there is contradicting evidence,[29] one study demonstrated that pain in NSSI might also function as an emotion regulation strategy by increasing positive emotion, in addition to reducing negative emotion.[27]

Several of these studies revealed that non–self-injuring participants also experienced reductions in self-reported negative affect in response to the NSSI proxies.[28,29] Other research, however, suggests that self-injurers and non–self-injurers respond to pain differently. For example, even when both self-injuring and non–self-injuring participants report reduced negative emotion in response to NSSI proxies, self-injuring participants report greater reductions in negative emotion.[26,29] Additionally, some research suggests that non–self-injurers experience reductions in negative emotion in response to nonpainful stimulation, while self-injurers do not.[28] Furthermore, Schmahl and colleagues[30] performed a functional magnetic resonance imaging study demonstrating that self-injuring participants' brains reacted differently to pain than the brains of non–self-injuring participants, including decreased activation in the amygdala and anterior cingulate cortex (suggesting downregulation of emotions). Although there continues to be some ambiguity in overall findings from these studies, together they suggest that for individuals who engage in NSSI, pain may serve a distinctly beneficial role and, in particular, may function as a maladaptive, though effective, method of emotion regulation.

How Does Pain Help Regulate Affect?

Although laboratory studies have demonstrated the effects of pain on reducing negative affect, less is known about the mechanisms of this effect. Biological theories of NSSI suggest that the act of self-injury serves as a soothing behavior because the injury and pain may result in subsequent physiological homeostasis reactions that counteract pain, particularly the release of endorphins. As discussed previously, endorphins are endogenous opioids that stimulate pain analgesia effects in damaged tissues while also having the potential to induce feelings of euphoria.[31] The involvement of endogenous opioids has been linked to NSSI behavior[32] and may account for why a number of individuals who self-injure report that they do not feel pain during self-injury—because the release of endorphins may ameliorate pain and provide emotional relief. However, despite the link between endogenous opioids and NSSI, treatments focusing on opioid antagonist medications as a treatment for NSSI have had mixed results in reducing NSSI, suggesting that more biological and psychological factors may contribute to the behavior.

Another recent physiological theoretical approach to understanding the role of pain in NSSI comes from the pain offset relief model.[33] This model proposes that the emotional coping benefits of NSSI may not be due to the pain itself but rather to the removal of pain immediately after NSSI behavior has been completed. The pain offset relief model builds off of the well-established biological effect that occurs when pain, which is typically aversive, is removed from an individual, resulting in that individual experiencing pleasant feelings in response.[34] This is in line with a psychological mechanism know as an "opponent process," whereby when one physiological or psychological process ceases being activated, the contrasting process response then "kicks in" as the system responds to the change.[34] In regard to self-injury, an individual may experience negative emotion, engage in NSSI that results in pain during the act of self-injury, and then experience a subsequent feeling of relief on cessation of the self-injury. Over time, then, self-injurious behavior may become paired with reward-processing activation in the brain, leading people to seek out self-injury more actively.[33] The pain offset relief model appears to be promising and may work in unison with opioid responses in contributing to the biological foundations of NSSI.

Although biology likely plays a major role in the function and maintenance of NSSI, biological processes probably occur along with psychological responses to self-injury. One psychological theory that aims to address the role of pain in NSSI is the experiential avoidance model.[2] *Experiential avoidance* refers to the use of a behavior to avoid or escape from an unwanted internal experience, such as emotional distress.[35] The experiential avoidance model of self-injury suggests that when individuals who self-injure experience emotional or cognitive stressors, they respond by engaging in NSSI as a way of "escaping" the negative thoughts and emotions that they are experiencing. Self-injury is thought to help those who self-injure avoid emotional distress by changing the individual's physiological response (possibly through the release of endorphins), distraction, and self-punishment. Changing these factors and subsequently reducing emotional distress then negatively reinforce the self-injury, which means that the self-injurer becomes more ready and willing to use self-injury to avoid future emotional distress. This trend continues to the point that NSSI comes to be used to avoid even more mild emotional distress, solidifying NSSI's effects as a maladaptive coping mechanism.

A related psychological theory that addresses the use of NSSI as a way to cope with upsetting emotions is the emotional cascade model.[36-38] This model highlights the role of pain in self-injury, suggesting that the pain is specifically what is desired in the process of self-injury. The model suggests that those who self-injure experience an extremely volatile and intense emotional experience, referred to as an "emotional cascade." During an emotional cascade, the self-injuring individual responds to an upsetting emotional event by ruminating, or constantly and repetitively thinking about the causes and consequences of a problem, in a manner that serves to progressively increase emotional distress. In turn, as emotional distress begins to escalate, the individual begins to ruminate even more intensely, creating a positive feedback cycle between rumination and negative emotion that leads to the experience of an intense and aversive emotional state.[39,40] It is in the apex of this process that self-injury may occur because the pain of self-injury is thought to serve as a powerful physical sensation on which the individual can focus attention instead of ruminate, thus short-circuiting the emotional cascade and resulting in feelings of relief as the negative emotion subsides. The emotional cascade model highlights the role of pain more so than other theoretical approaches, indicating that the pain itself is what is sought after in NSSI, owing to its potent effect as a distractor. This is consistent with reports that many of those who self-injure feel pain at the time of the self-injury.[12]

Self-injury is a complex behavior that is unlikely to have one single function with regard to pain, which is itself a complex phenomenon. Ultimately, it is likely that both biological and psychological theories play a role in the onset and maintenance of self-injury, wherein people may initially try self-injury as an experimental coping method and experience rewarding biological and psychological effects, despite the pain and relative to the previous emotional distress. Over time, as self-injury is employed more regularly, both the biological and psychological processes involved are likely to change as well, as is the experience of pain during self-injury, potentially engraining self-injury as a preferred coping method for emotional distress.

Clinical Implications

Understanding the role of pain in NSSI has important treatment implications. Treatment providers, including nurses, emergency department physicians, and psychologists, often stigmatize and have negative attitudes toward those who engage in NSSI, in part because it can appear so paradoxical to desire or intentionally elicit pain.[41,42] In particular, attributing personal control and responsibility to self-injurers, without understanding the factors that predispose and reinforce these behaviors, can increase negative attitudes and discrimination.[43] As a result, a majority of self-injurers report being dissatisfied with their treatment experiences following episodes of NSSI, reducing the likelihood that they will seek treatment in the future.[44,45] It is therefore critical that mental health clinicians, as well as nurses and doctors who encounter self-injurers in medical and emergency department settings, receive training and understand the functions of these behaviors and the way individuals may struggle to cease engaging in them despite, or because of, the pain they elicit. By recognizing the way pain elicited by NSSI can serve important emotion regulation functions, treatment providers are better posed to provide more empathetic, nonjudgmental, and effective treatments.

In particular, treatments may benefit by providing self-injurers with alternative, more adaptive strategies for emotion regulation that do not involve pain or physical injury. In recognition of the emotion regulation functions served by NSSI, several treatment approaches specifically target NSSI by teaching alternative adaptive emotion regulation strategies. For example, dialectical behavior therapy (DBT),[46] a treatment initially developed for clients with borderline personality disorder, is often used to treat NSSI and includes a focus on four modules of skills: emotion regulation, distress tolerance, mindfulness, and interpersonal effectiveness. Individuals are taught to notice urges to engage in NSSI and to increasingly use alternative effective emotion regulation strategies (e.g., distraction and self-soothing skills) instead of acting on these urges. Similarly, emotion regulation group therapy (ERGT)[47] was developed as a more clinically feasible short-term group treatment specifically targeting NSSI. ERGT is a 14-week, acceptance-based behavioral group that focuses on a range of emotion regulation skills, including emotional awareness, acceptance of difficult emotions, and nonavoidant emotion regulation strategies, among others. Other approaches include mentalization-based treatment (MBT),[48] a psychodynamic treatment that strengthens individuals' ability to understand their own and others' mental states in the context of attachment, and a manualized, short-term cognitive behavioral therapy (CBT) intervention[49] that focuses on addressing suicidal and negative thinking and problem-solving deficits. Across these different clinical approaches, in order to help patients change this behavior, clinicians first need to understand the way behaviors that would appear painful and aversive can serve important functions in helping individuals cope with difficult emotional and/or interpersonal experiences. Understanding the role of pain within NSSI enables clinicians to validate its effectiveness and help patients identify reasons that, *despite* its short-term effectiveness, they may want to change this behavior.

Unfortunately, despite the many deleterious consequences of NSSI, there is a paucity of research examining treatment outcomes of interventions specifically targeting NSSI,[50] and as such, there are few empirical data offering guidelines for the treatment or prevention of NSSI.[3] This is due in large part to NSSI frequently being categorized together with suicidal behaviors under the umbrella term of "parasuicidal" behaviors, leaving it unclear how effective treatments are at specifically reducing NSSI behaviors.[51] Understanding the distinct role of pain in NSSI helps distinguish this behavior from suicidal behaviors, with the impact of NSSI being an immediate and short-lasting experience,[52] and highlights the potentially distinct treatment needs in addressing these behaviors. As such, although there are several promising treatment approaches, there is a pressing need for increased evaluation of treatments specifically targeting NSSI behaviors.

REFERENCES

1. Van Orden KA, Witte TK, Cukrowicz KC, Braithwaite SR, Selby EA, Joiner TE Jr. The interpersonal theory of suicide. *Psychol Rev*. 2010;117(2):575–600.
2. Chapman AL, Gratz KL, Brown MZ. Solving the puzzle of deliberate self-harm: The experiential avoidance model. *Behav Res Ther*. 2006;44:371–394.
3. Nock MK. Self-injury. *Ann Rev Clin Psychol*. 2010;6:339–363.
4. Wohlrab S, Stahl J, Kappeler PM. Modifying the body: Motivations for getting tattooed and pierced. *Body Image*. 2007;4(1):87–95.
5. Stirn A, Hinz A. Tattoos, body piercings, and self-injury: Is there a connection? Investigations on a core group of participants practicing body modification. *Psychother Res*. 2008;18(3):326–333.
6. Zetterqvist M, Lundh LG, Dahlström Ö, Svedin CG. Prevalence and function of non-suicidal self-injury (NSSI) in a community sample of adolescents, using suggested DSM-5 criteria for a potential NSSI disorder. *J Abnorm Child Psychol*. 2013;41(5):759–773.

7. Hasking P, Momeni R, Swannell S, Chia S. The nature and extent of non-suicidal self-injury in a non-clinical sample of young adults. *Arch Suicide Res.* 2008;12(3):208–218.

8. American Psychiatric Association. *Diagnostic and Statistical Manual of Mental Disorder.* 5th ed. Washington, DC: Author; 2013.

9. Selby EA, Kranzler A, Fehling KB, Panza E. Nonsuicidal self-injury disorder: The path to diagnostic validity and final obstacles. *Clin Psychol Rev.* 2015;38:79–91.

10. Franklin JC, Aaron RV, Arthur MS, Shorkey SP, Prinstein MJ. Nonsuicidal self-injury and diminished pain perception: The role of emotion dysregulation. *Comprehension Psychiatry.* 2012;53(6):691–700.

11. Nock MK, Prinstein MJ. Contextual features and behavioral functions of self-mutilation among adolescents. *J Abnorm Psychol.* 2005;114(1):140.

12. Selby EA, Nock MK, Kranzler A. How does self-injury feel? Examining automatic positive reinforcement in adolescent self-injurers with experience sampling. *Psychiatry Res.* 2014;215(2):417–423.

13. Russ MJ, Campbell SS, Kakuma T, Harrison K, Zanine E. EEG theta activity and pain sensitivity in self-injurious borderline patients. *Psychiatry Res.* 1999;89:201–214.

14. Hooley JM, Ho DT, Slater J, Lockshin A. Pain perception and nonsuicidal self-injury: A laboratory investigation. *Personality Disord.* 2010;1(3):170.

15. Koenig J, Thayer JF, Kaess M. A meta-analysis on pain sensitivity in self-injury. *Psychol Med.* 2016;46(8):1597–1612.

16. Nock MK, Joiner TE, Gordon KH, Lloyd-Richardson EE, Prinstein MJ. Non-suicidal self-injury among adolescents: Diagnostic correlates and relation to suicide attempts. *Psychiatry Res.* 2006;144:65–72.

17. Van Ree JM, Niesink RJ, Van Wolfswinkel L, et al. Endogenous opioids and reward. *Eur J Pharmacol.* 2000;405(1):89–101.

18. Klonsky ED. The functions of deliberate self-injury: A review of the evidence. *Clin Psychol Rev.* 2007;27(2):226–239.

19. Nock MK, Prinstein MJ, Sterba SK. Revealing the form and function of self-injurious thoughts and behaviors: A real-time ecological assessment study among adolescents and young adults. *J Abnorm Psycho.* 2009;118(4):816–827.

20. Haines J, Williams CL, Brain KL, Wilson GV. The psychophysiology of self-mutilation. *J Abnorm Psychol.* 1995;104(3):471.

21. Brain KL, Haines J, Williams CL. The psychophysiology of self-mutilation: Evidence of tension reduction. *Arch Suicide Res.* 1998;4(3):227–242.

22. Welch SS, Linehan MM, Sylvers P, Chittams J, Rizvi SL. Emotional responses to self-injury imagery among adults with borderline personality disorder. *J Consult Clin Psychol.* 2008;76(1), 45.

23. Hollin GJ, Derbyshire SW. Cold pressor pain reduces phobic fear but fear does not reduce pain. *J Pain.* 2009;10(10):1058–1064.

24. Bresin K, Gordon KH, Bender TW, Gordon LJ, Joiner TE Jr. No pain, no change: Reductions in prior negative affect following physical pain. *Motivation Emotion.* 2010;34(3):280–287.

25. Russ MJ, Roth SD, Lerman A, et al. Pain perception in self-injurious patients with borderline personality disorder. *Biol Psychiatry.* 1992;32(6):501–511.

26. Weinberg A, Klonsky ED. The effects of self-injury on acute negative arousal: A laboratory simulation. *Motivation Emotion.* 2012;36(2):242–254.
27. Franklin JC, Lee KM, Hanna EK, Prinstein MJ. Feeling worse to feel better pain-offset relief simultaneously stimulates positive affect and reduces negative affect. *Psychol Sci.* 2013;24(4):521–529.
28. Bresin K, Gordon KH. Changes in negative affect following pain (vs. nonpainful) stimulation in individuals with and without a history of nonsuicidal self-injury. *Personality Disord.* 2013;4(1):62.
29. Schoenleber M, Berenbaum H, Motl R. Shame-related functions of and motivations for self-injurious behavior. *Personality Disord.* 2014;5(2):204.
30. Schmahl C, Bohus M, Esposito F, et al. Neural correlates of antinociception in borderline personality disorder. *Arch Gen Psychiatry.* 2006;63(6):659–666.
31. Bresin K, Gordon KH. Endogenous opioids and nonsuicidal self-injury: A mechanism of affect regulation. *Neurosci Biobehav Rev.* 2013;37:374–383.
32. Stanley B, Sher L, Wilson S, Ekman R, Huang YY, Mann JJ. Non-suicidal self-injurious behavior, endogenous opioids and monoamine neurotransmitters. *J Affect Disord.* 2010;124(1):134–140.
33. Franklin JC, Puzia ME, Lee KM, et al. The nature of pain offset relief in nonsuicidal self-injury: A laboratory study. *Clin Psychol Sci.* 2013;1:110–119.
34. Franklin JC, Hessel ET, Aaron RV, Arthur MS, Heilbron N, Prinstein MJ. The functions of nonsuicidal self-injury: Support for cognitive-affective regulation and opponent processes from a novel psychophysiological paradigm. *J Abnorm Psychol.* 2010;119:850–862.
35. Hayes SC, Wilson KG, Gifford EV, Follette VM, Strosahl K. Experiential avoidance and behavioral disorders: A functional dimensional approach to diagnosis and treatment. *J Consult Clin Psychol.* 1996;64:1152–1168.
36. Selby EA, Anestis MD, Joiner TE. Understanding the relationship between emotional and behavioral dysregulation: Emotional cascades. *Behav Res Ther.* 2008;46(5):593–611.
37. Selby EA, Joiner Jr TE. Cascades of emotion: The emergence of borderline personality disorder from emotional and behavioral dysregulation. *Rev Gen Psychol.* 2009;13:219–229.
38. Selby EA, Joiner TE Jr. Emotional cascades as prospective predictors of dysregulated behaviors in borderline personality disorder. *Personality Disord.* 2013;4(2):168–174.
39. Selby EA, Fehling KB, Panza EA, Kranzler A. Rumination, mindfulness, and borderline personality disorder symptoms. *Mindfulness.* 2016;7(1):228–235.
40. Selby EA, Kranzler A, Panza E, Fehling KB. Bidirectional-compounding effects of rumination and negative emotion in predicting impulsive behavior: Implications for emotional cascades. *J Personality.* 2016;84:139–153.
41. McAllister M, Creedy D, Moyle W, Farrugia C. Nurses' attitudes towards clients who self-harm. *J Adv Nurs.* 2002;40(5):578–586.
42. Saunders KE, Hawton K, Fortune S, Farrell S. Attitudes and knowledge of clinical staff regarding people who self-harm: A systematic review. *J Affect Disord.* 2012;139(3):205–216.

43. Law GU, Rostill-Brookes H, Goodman D. Public stigma in health and non-healthcare students: Attributions, emotions and willingness to help with adolescent self-harm. *Int J Nurs Stud*. 2009;46(1):108–119.

44. Arnold L. *Women and Self-Injury: A Survey of 76 Women*. Bristol, UK: Bristol Crisis Service for Women; 1995.

45. Taylor TL, Hawton K, Fortune S, Kapur N. Attitudes towards clinical services among people who self-harm: Systematic review. *Br J Psychiatry*. 2009;194(2):104–110.

46. Linehan MM. *Cognitive-Behavioral Treatment of Personality Disorder*. New York, NYL Guilford Press; 1993.

47. Gratz KL, Gunderson JG. Preliminary data on an acceptance-based emotion regulation group intervention for deliberate self-harm among women with borderline personality disorder. *Behav Ther*. 2006;37(1):25–35.

48. Bateman A, Fonagy P. Randomized controlled trial of outpatient mentalization-based treatment versus structured clinical management for borderline personality disorder. *Am J Psychiatry*. 2009;166(12):1355–1364.

49. Slee N, Garnefski N, van der Leeden R, Arensman E, Spinhoven P. Cognitive-behavioural intervention for self-harm: Randomised controlled trial. *Br J Psychiatry*. 2008;192(3):202–211.

50. Calati R, Courtet P. Is psychotherapy effective for reducing suicide attempt and non-suicidal self-injury rates? Meta-analysis and meta-regression of literature data. *J Psychiatr Res*. 2016;79:8–20.

51. Glenn CR, Franklin JC, Nock MK. Evidence-based psychosocial treatments for self-injurious thoughts and behaviors in youth. *J Clin Child Adolesc Psychol*. 2014;44(1):1–29.

52. Shaffer D, Jacobson C. Proposal to the DSM-V childhood disorder and mood disorder work groups to include non-suicidal self-injury (NSSI) as a DSM-V disorder. American Psychiatric Association; 2009: 1–21.

PART IV

Treatment Strategies

23

Innovative Management of Chronic Pain and Psychiatric Comorbidities

J. GREGORY HOBELMANN AND MICHAEL R. CLARK ■

INTRODUCTION

Patients who suffer from physical pain and psychiatric comorbidity are affected not only physically but also emotionally, cognitively, and spiritually. This can make caring for them challenging. Practitioners who treat pain emanate from a variety of disciplines (medicine, anesthesiology, psychiatry, psychology, physiatry, surgery, nursing) and may feel underqualified to address complaints of pain in a comprehensive manner.[1] In addition, their approach to the treatment of pain is often mirrored by their training. Regardless of their background, practitioners should be aware of the high prevalence of chronic pain and psychiatric comorbidity and the profound effects that psychiatric comorbidity has on outcomes in chronic pain. Patients who do not respond to treatment in the expected manner require further evaluation and changes in treatment.

This chapter will review the innovative management of patients with both disorders, reviewing the key concepts in the evaluation and focusing on comprehensive (interdisciplinary) treatment. Although interdisciplinary treatment is not an innovative concept in the medical world, it is in this case.

Comprehensive treatment for patients with chronic pain were abundant, for a period during the 1960s through the 1980s, and were shown to have successful outcomes. For a variety of reasons, they became financially unsustainable as the national reimbursement environment evolved. Treatment for patients with chronic pain was subsequently focused primarily on the physical aspects of pain, which included procedural interventions and medical management. In addition, reimbursement for "cognitive specialties" was limited to such an extent that patients suffering from chronic pain rarely received psychological intervention for treatment of pain complaints. Finally, "innovative therapies," such as novel medications, acupuncture, massage, and meditation, have been underutilized because of insufficient reimbursement, but often have as much proven efficacy as many of the medically accepted treatments, such as epidural steroid injections.

Comprehensive pain recovery programs typically consist of providers from multiple backgrounds, including pain medicine, other medical backgrounds, psychologists, psychiatrists, physical therapists, occupational therapists, addiction counselors/specialists, vocational rehabilitation specialists, and others, working together on a common treatment plan for the patient. Comprehensive treatment begins with a thorough evaluation. This was discussed in depth in Chapter 6. After assessing for chronic pain and comorbid psychiatric issues, a treatment plan is created, taking into account the physical, emotional, cognitive, and spiritual maladies. Finally, a solid continuing care plan is developed, taking into account the cognitive and behavioral changes needed to sustain lasting improvement.

THE PAIN PATIENT

Chronic pain becomes particularly debilitating when a person's primary identity has become that of a "pain patient." The best predictor of acute pain transitioning to chronic pain is a negative emotional response to the pain. As pain persists, function can deteriorate, leading to a lower perceived quality of life. With this comes a diminished capacity to tolerate pain, which in turn continues to worsen function and quality of life even more. Over time, the pain becomes the primary focus of life, and the assumed identity has changed to that of a person suffering with chronic pain.

In that role, both primary and secondary gains are often present. *Primary gain* refers to the internal factors that maintain pain. For example, having pain reduces the emotional strain of not being able to function as the patient was once able to function. *Secondary gain* refers to external factors that are often easier to identify. For example, continued pain excuses the patient from previous responsibilities, such as work or duties at home.

Furthermore, people suffering with debilitating chronic pain tend to lose their sense of self-efficacy. The patient's locus of control may transform from internal to external. With an external locus of control, patients feel that everything is done to them rather than having a sense that outcomes in life are directly related to their thoughts and behaviors. This results in a feeling of victimization.

Caring for the patient can become the primary focus of the family, making chronic pain a true family illness. The patients' repertoire of activities narrows as they minimize social activities and no longer participate in previously enjoyable endeavors. This can lead to a feeling of isolation, and in this setting, psychiatric comorbidities may evolve or worsen. In particular, affective and anxiety disorders are frequently recognized.

The development of the role of a "pain patient" is insidious and often goes unrecognized by both the person and the people who care for him. Patients are not actively seeking this role and should not be blamed for its evolution. True progress can be made when patients realize that external forces cannot simply fix them. They realize that what they have been doing is not working and that fundamental change in thinking and behavior are needed to improve their situation. Taking ownership of their pain and playing an active role in their recovery can lead to remarkable results.

COMPREHENSIVE PAIN RECOVERY

Physical Modalities

It is only when pain persists longer than would be expected for tissue healing that it becomes chronic. Of course, all efforts should be made to resolve the physical defect causing the pain if it can be identified. Even when the pain persists, there can be areas of pathology that should continue to be addressed. This section will review an algorithmic approach to the treatment of the physical components of chronic pain. The details of each modality are discussed elsewhere.

A full interventional workup should be completed to evaluate for surgeries, injections, or other procedures that may help attenuate the pain. Several injections can be performed for diagnostic as well as therapeutic purposes. Many of these procedures can be repeated, such as facet blocks and epidural steroid injections, to help manage the pain over time. Surgical procedures, such a diskectomy and spinal fusion, are meant to be more definitive but are not always successful. Spinal cord stimulators are reserved for refractory cases of radiculopathy and complex regional pain syndrome and have demonstrated moderate effect.[2]

Procedural interventions should be performed in conjunction with the optimization of medical management, which is an ongoing process. The general classes of medication that have been shown to be beneficial in the management of chronic pain include anti-inflammatory medications, antidepressants, anticonvulsants (membrane stabilizing medication), muscle relaxants, topical agents (i.e., local anesthetics, capsaicin) and opioids. Opioids deserve special attention because controversy surrounds long-term treatment owing to concerns for long-term efficacy and safety, in particular tolerance, dependence, abuse, overdose, and opioid-induced hyperalgesia. In individuals with psychiatric comorbidity, opioid use must be considered even more carefully because opioids may exacerbate depressive and anxiety disorders.[3] Pain typically improves when opioids are discontinued in patients who have been using them for long-term treatment.[4] Hence, discontinuation of opioids is an important initial step in a comprehensive treatment program.

There have been no novel analgesics approved for clinical use over the past 3 decades, despite the widely accepted need for medications that are both effective and safe. Several potential targets have been identified for the development of new analgesic medications, including nerve growth factor (NGF), 1.7-selective voltage-gated sodium channels, N-type voltage-gated calcium channels, and angiotensin II AT_2 receptors.[5] NGF is a major mediator of inflammatory and neuropathic pain.[6] NGF inhibitors, such as tanezumab and fulranumab, are potential prospects as novel analgesics, and tanezumab has entered the stage of clinical development. Preliminary studies have shown mixed results for a variety of pain conditions, but the long-term efficacy and safety has yet to be determined.[7] Tumor necrosis factor-α (TNF-α) has been implicated to play a pivotal role at both the peripheral and central levels of pain sensitization. Anti–TNF-α therapy has not been shown to be efficacious in alleviating radicular pain, but it has inspired interest in evaluating its potential use in other neuropathic pain syndromes.[8] Despite being counterintuitive, the use of low-dose naltrexone, an opioid antagonist, has been demonstrated to reduce symptom severity in a variety of conditions, such as fibromyalgia, Crohn disease, multiple sclerosis, and complex regional pain syndrome. More evidence is needed to verify that it is superior to placebo, however.[9] With so many potential targets and such a great perceived need, it is likely that novel medications will continue to emerge.

As pain persists, activity is often reduced, resulting in becoming deconditioned. The deconditioning and worsening of pain, in turn, result in less activity. As such, resuming normal activity should be an immediate goal (conditioning). Delaying the resumption of normal activity may lead to greater disability.[10] Treatment with physical therapy aims to reduce disability and suffering by reducing pain and increasing tolerance to movement.[11] Physical therapy, aqua therapy, and exercise to improve range of motion and strength can improve function, pain, and quality of life in patients with chronic pain. Mood and levels of anxiety may also improve.[1] An in-depth discussion of particular modalities will not be undertaken here, but the importance of physical therapy and exercise must be stressed as an essential component of a comprehensive pain recovery program.

There are several "alternative treatments" that are frequently utilized in comprehensive treatment programs. These are therapies that are not typically taught in medical school because their safety and efficacy have not been well established. In addition, they often are not reimbursed by insurance companies. However, anecdotally, they can be very effective in well selected individuals. These therapies include acupuncture, massage, music, and transcutaneous electrical nerve stimulation (TENS). Recently, there has been interest in the analgesic effect of repetitive transcranial magnetic stimulation (rTMS); however, more evidence is needed to determine a more solid basis for it clinical application as an analgesic.[12]

Emotional Modalities

Chronic pain has a clear negative impact on emotions. There is ample literature to link depressive and anxiety symptoms to pain. The relationship is complex and difficult to fully characterize, however. Patients with depression or anxiety symptoms are more likely than patients without those symptoms to report pain for a given physical problem. Conversely, patients with chronic pain are more likely to report depressive or anxiety symptoms.[13] Additionally, unpleasant affective states have been found to decrease pain thresholds, and vice versa.[14] Pain, depression, and anxiety can also all negatively affect sleep and coping mechanisms. Furthermore, multiple studies have shown that patients with chronic pain are at greater risk for suicidal ideation, suicide attempts, and suicide completions.[15] Most clinical diagnoses of pain conditions have been associated with increased risk for suicide.[16]

It is prudent to begin by distinguishing between depressed or anxious mood and the clinical syndromes of major depression and anxiety disorders. Up to 30% of chronic pain patients meet criteria for an anxiety disorder such as generalized anxiety disorder, panic disorder, and post-traumatic stress disorder.[17] Anxiety disorders frequently accompany other affective disorders, such as major depression, so clinicians should remain alert to the possibility of a mood disorder when patients complain of severe anxiety. In general, the approach is to diagnose and treat initially the most prominent disorder in a patient, whether it be depression or anxiety.

Depression and pain are linked neuroanatomically. Brain structures involved in emotion are also involved in pain modulation. Pain and depression also share common neurochemical pathways because both serotonin and norepinephrine are involved in depression, anxiety, and the modulation of pain signals.[13] This close association is evidenced by the fact that in some cultures, depression is more likely to be reported as a physical symptom rather than an emotional experience.[18] Anxiety and pain are also linked to several physiological phenomena, such as muscle tension and tachycardia, and can worsen both conditions. Treating anxiety in patients with somatic complaints reduces the intensity of pain.[19]

Pain, depression, and anxiety are mutually maintaining, and treatment of both pain and comorbid psychiatric symptoms is necessary to achieve optimal outcomes. Many medications used primarily to treat psychiatric conditions also alleviate pain. These include antidepressants primarily, but in some cases, mood stabilizers (anticonvulsants) may be of benefit.

For patients with co-occurring pain and depression or anxiety, treatment with antidepressants that increase serotonin and norepinephrine in the synaptic cleft is appropriate. Tricyclic antidepressants (TCAs), such as amitriptyline, nortriptyline, and desipramine, have a well-established record for treating neuropathic pain.[20] Anticholinergic effects (dry mouth, constipation), antihistaminic effects (sedation), and adrenergic effects (orthostatic hypotension) are common with TCAs and may limit their use, especially in elderly patients. Serotonin/norepinephrine reuptake inhibitors, like TCAs, increase the availability of monoamines in the synaptic cleft. They have been shown to be effective in a variety of pain conditions and have the advantage of better side-effect profiles. They are also less lethal in overdose, which is a source of concern when treating patients with depression.

Antidepressant medication can effectively treat depression in the presence of chronic pain, but there is some evidence that depression with comorbid pain is more resistant to treatment.[21] When mood disorders accompany chronic pain, as when pain accompanies other chronic medical disorders, there may be some extra hurdles for treatment to overcome. These include aversive physical symptoms, severe deactivation, vocational dysfunction, marital conflict, social isolation, and concurrent medications. Comprehensive assessment of these issues and formulation of a treatment plan that takes them into account increase the likelihood of successful depression treatment in the chronic pain patient. Pain often subsides with improvement in depressive symptoms.[22] Patients will typically report that they may still have pain but that they can tolerate it better. This statement indicates that the affective component of pain has significantly improved.

Mood stabilizers work to reduce pain through varied mechanisms, but they all essentially decrease excitation in neurons, which is thought to provide their analgesic effects. In addition, they are effective for the treatment of bipolar affective disorder. The commonly used mood stabilizers that also have demonstrated analgesic effect include valproic acid, carbamazepine, lithium, gabapentin, and pregabalin. Valproic acid reduces the frequency and intensity of migraine headache and has been used as abortive therapy for a variety of headache conditions.[23] Carbamazepine is a first-line agent for the treatment of trigeminal neuralgia and is effective in a variety of chronic pain conditions.[24] Lithium has been used to treat cluster headaches but is not a first-line or second-line treatment.[25] Gabapentin and pregabalin, which are not particularly effective as mood stabilizers, are effective for a variety of chronic pain conditions. These conditions include painful diabetic neuropathy, postherpetic neuralgia, fibromyalgia, postamputation phantom limb pain, and central neuropathic pain.[26] Care must be taken when prescribing any of these medications to evaluate for side effects and interactions with other medications.

Chronic pain is frequently associated with insomnia and anxiety. It is, therefore, common that patients are also using benzodiazepines or other sedatives. These medications mask some symptoms of depression (e.g., initial insomnia, agitation), but they are not adequate treatments for depression. In fact, dangerous levels of depression can develop under the cover of benzodiazepines. It has been suggested that benzodiazepines can induce depression with chronic use, but the evidence for this is not strong.[27] More important is the masking of depression by benzodiazepines. Nearly all patients with chronic pain should be tapered off benzodiazepines because few conditions exist for which chronic benzodiazepines are the treatment of choice.[28] Despite the lack of evidence for their efficacy, many patients with chronic pain are still treated with opioids, and the combination of opioid and benzodiazepine therapy is associated with large increases in mortality risk.[29]

In situations of treatment-resistant depression, studies have indicated that electroconvulsive therapy (ECT) can be useful for treatment of depression and pain, across a variety of painful disorders.[30] However, no carefully controlled studies demonstrate the clear effectiveness of ECT for treatment of chronic pain. ECT should be reserved for refractory cases of co-occurring mood disorder and chronic pain.

In addition to medical and interventional modalities, psychotherapeutic approaches are essential in optimal treatment of the emotional aspects of chronic pain. The clinical art of emotional treatment for those with chronic pain consists of establishing a solid therapeutic alliance around those problems.

Psychodynamic therapy may be beneficial in the treatment of chronic pain, but there is a larger body of evidence to support the use of cognitive behavioral therapy (CBT) for both emotional disturbances and chronic pain. Since the initial applications of CBT to chronic pain, much research has established the importance of cognitive and behavioral processes in how individuals adapt to chronic pain. Over the past 3 decades, CBT has become a first-line treatment for individuals with chronic pain. There is ample evidence of its efficacy in improving pain and pain-related problems across a wide spectrum of chronic pain syndromes.[31] The benefits of CBT have been found to continue up to 6 months after the completion of active treatment sessions.[32]

Although CBT has clear efficacy in the treatment of pain and emotional disturbances, more information is needed about dose and delivery method. Traditional CBT has been performed in a face-to-face setting. However, Internet-based CBT and telemedicine are becoming more frequently utilized. This method of delivery has been shown to be as effective as in-person CBT and has the advantages of improving access to care and increasing cost-effectiveness.[33] There are novel types of therapy that show promise as well, such as interoceptive exposure (IE). IE is a therapy that exposes individuals to feared bodily sensations associated with arousal. It helps people realize that although pain sensations are uncomfortable, they are not necessarily harmful.[34]

Cognitive Modalities

Pain processing can interfere with cognitive processing, and vice versa, because pain and cognition share common substrates. Several studies have demonstrated a deficit in cognitive processing in people suffering from chronic pain.[35] Problems with concentration, decision-making, and even forgetfulness are typical in patients suffering with chronic pain. Furthermore, negative thinking can lead to pessimism, poor self-esteem, excessive guilt, and self-criticism, all of which are characteristic of depression as well. People with chronic pain tend to think about their pain, even if they are thinking about solutions for their pain.

Education is a cornerstone of treating chronic pain. Patients often carry the acute pain construct with them while living with chronic pain. This may lead to a desire to protect their body by avoiding certain movements necessary to ultimately improve their condition. Identifying misinformation and educating the patient can lead to a perception of increased control of pain, resolution of depression, and promotion of healthy activities like exercise and relaxation.[36] Education includes not only the patient but also loved ones. There is ample evidence that patients do better when families are engaged in the rehabilitation process.[37] Families should be encouraged to support and validate the patient's experience and return them to their appropriate relational role, which helps to restore that vital identity.

CBT plays an important part in improving cognitions as well. Maladaptive thoughts lead to negative feelings and worsening of pain. CBT is designed to address this maladaptive pattern by addressing these cognitive distortions about the pain experience to enable the patient to change the behaviors related to it. One of the most effective CBT methods in pain patients is to combine coping skills training focusing on fear of pain, reinjury, and movement with gradual activity and movement-based physical therapy.[38] The cognitive behavioral therapist attempts to assist patients to try new behaviors and to adopt more adaptive modes of thinking.

Spiritual Modalities

Spirituality is difficult to define because it has different meaning to individuals depending on multiple factors, including cultural background and religion. However, it can be described in general as the core of a person's identity and motivation for life. As described previously, chronic pain slowly and insidiously transforms a person's identity until the person is left with the identity of a person in pain. This can result in drastic changes in motivation for living. A person who was once motivated to have a family, build a career, and develop meaningful relationships can be reduced to being motivated solely to cope with the pain and distress. The person is left asking questions such as, "Why me?" and "Who or what would let this happen?" In this state, the person tends to lose connection to others and is left feeling isolated, whether or not there is a strong support system. The person's ability to cope and tolerate distress is much diminished.

Spiritual therapy can be defined as any modality that will help return meaning and purpose to one's life and reshape one's identity. Spiritual care may provide insight, may inspire hope, and is thought to mediate mental and physical health for patients.[39] There is a paucity of research in this area, but it makes intuitive sense that this is beneficial in patients with pain with or without comorbid psychiatric illness.

Group therapy has fallen out of favor for many psychiatric conditions other than substance use disorder, but it can be invaluable in treating patients with chronic debilitating pain. Being with others who can empathize can create social connections that combat the feeling of isolation. Seeing others who have progressed and hearing how they are coping can provide a renewed sense of hope. Having cognitive distortions challenged by a peer can be a powerful means of both gaining insight and empowering individuals to take ownership of their recovery. A renewed sense of self-efficacy can be promoted in this setting.

Meditation has been shown in several studies to inhibit or relieve pain perception.[40] It can be defined as a form of mental training that aims to improve an individual's core psychological capabilities, such as attentional and emotion regulation. In particular, mindfulness meditation has received much attention lately. There is mounting evidence of the therapeutic effects of mindfulness on pain, stress, negative emotion, and addictive processes.[41] Meditation can help focus patients on the present and provide inspiration for their immediate recovery needs.

CONCLUSION

Comprehensive pain programs are not innovative in the sense that they are not novel, but they are innovative in the sense that they are only recently re-emerging as a standard of care. There certainly have been innovations in treatment since comprehensive programs were abundant in the past, and those novel approaches should be incorporated into programs as they are developed. We know that comprehensive pain rehabilitation programs can be effective. They have been shown to be very effective in improving pain, mood, and function in patients with chronic pain.[42] Among all pain-related treatments, comprehensive rehabilitation is the only approach that has consistently been shown to be associated with return to work, reduction in hospitalization over a 10-year period, and meaningful, sustained improvement in pain and function.[37] This improvement has been shown to persist for up to 13 years.[43] A return to comprehensive pain rehabilitation can make great strides in reducing pain intensity, improving function, and increasing quality of life.

REFERENCES

1. Nicolson SE, Caplan, JP, Williams DE, Stern TA. Comorbid pain, depression, and anxiety: Multifaceted pathology allows for multifaceted treatment. *Harv Rev Psychiatry*. 2009;17(6):407–420.
2. Song JJ, Popescu A, Bell RL. Present and potential use of spinal cord stimulation to control chronic pain. *Pain Physician*. 2014;17(3):235–246.
3. Scherrer JF, Salas J, Copeland LA, et al. Increased risk of depression recurrence after initiation of prescription opioids in noncancer pain patients. *J Pain*. 2016;17(4):473–482.
4. Criostomo RA, Schmidt JE, Hooten WM, et al. Withdrawal of analgesic medication for chronic low-back pain patients: Improvement in outcomes of multidisciplinary rehabilitation regardless of surgical history. *Am J Phys Med Rehabil*. 2008;87:527–536.

5. Salat K, Kowalczyk P, Grylo B, et al. New investigational drugs for the treatment of neuropathic pain. *Expert Opin Investig Drugs.* 2014;23(8):1093–1104.

6. Mizumura K, Murase S. Role of nerve growth factor in pain. *Handb Exp Pharmacol.* 2015;227:57–77.

7. Bannwarth B, Kostine M. Targeting nerve growth factor (NGF) for pain management: What does the future hold for NGF antagonists? *Drugs.* 2014;74(6):619–626.

8. Pimentel DC, El Abd O, Benyamin RM, et al. Anti-tumor necrosis factor antagonists in the treatment of low back pain and radiculopathy: A systematic review and meta-analysis. *Pain Physician.* 2014;17(1):E27–E44.

9. Piesner KB, Vaegter HB, Handberg G. Low dose naltrexone for pain. *Ugeskr Laeger.* 2015;177(43):V03150248.

10. Nicholas MK. Pain management in musculoskeletal conditions. *Best Pract Res Clin Rheumatol.* 2008;22:451–470.

11. Egan M, Seeger D, Schops P. Physiotherapy and physical therapy in pain management. *Schmerz.* 2015;29(5):562–568.

12. Galhardoni R, Correia GS, Araujo H, et al. Repetitive transcranial magnetic stimulation in chronic pain: A review of the literature. *Arch Phys Med Rehabil.* 2015;96(suppl 4):S156–S172.

13. Bair MJ, Robinson RL, Katon W, Kroenke K. Depression and pain comorbidity: A literature review. *Arch Intern Med.* 2003;163:2433–2445.

14. Stanos S, Houle TT. Multidisciplinary and interdisciplinary management of chronic pain. *Phys Med Rehabil Clin N Am.* 2006;17:435–450.

15. Fishbain D. Approaches to treatment decisions for psychiatric comorbidity in the management of the chronic pain patient. *Med Clin North Am.* 1999;83(3):737–759.

16. Ilgen MA, Zivin K, McCammon RJ, et al. Pain and suicidal thoughts, plans and attempts in the United States. *Gen Hosp Psychiatry.* 2008;30:521–527.

17. Outcalt SD, Kroenke K, Chambler NR, et al. Chronic pain and comorbid mental health conditions: Independent associations of posttraumatic stress disorder and depression with pain, disability, and quality of life. *J Behav Med.* 2015;38(3):535–543.

18. Stahl S, Briley M. Understanding pain in depression. *Hum Psychopharmacol.* 2004;19(suppl 1):S9–S13.

19. Lenze EJ, Karp JF, Muslant BH, et al. Somatic symptoms in late-life anxiety: Treatment issues. *J Geriatr Psychiatry Neurol.* 2005;18:89–96.

20. Dosenovic S, Jelicic Kadic A, Mijanovic M, et al. Interventions for neuropathic pain: An overview of systematic reviews. *Anesth Analg.* 2017;125(2):643–652.

21. Kroenke K, Shen J, Oxman TE, Williams JW, Dietrich AJ. Impact of pain on the outcomes of depression treatment: Results from the RESPECT trial. *Pain.* 2008;134:209–215.

22. Salerno SM, Browning R, Jackson JL. The effect of antidepressant treatment on chronic back pain: A meta-analysis. *Arch Intern Med.* 2002;162(1):19–24.

23. Stillman MJ, Zajac D, Rybicki LA. Treatment of primary headache disorders with intravenous valproate: Initial patient experience. *Headache.* 2004;44:65–69.

24. Wiffen PJ, Rees J. Lamotrigine for acute and chronic pain. *Cochrane Database Syst Rev.* 2007;2:CD006044.

25. Ekbom K. Lithium for cluster headache: Review of the literature and preliminary results of long-term treatment. *Headache*. 1981;21:132–139.

26. Moore, RA, Wiffen PJ, Derry S et al. Gabapentin for chronic neuropathic pain and fibromyalgia in adults. *Cochrane Database Syst Rev*. 2014;(4):CD007938.

27. Dellemijn PL, Fields HL. Do benzodiazepines have a role in chronic pain management? *Pain*. 1994;57(2):137–152.

28. Salzman C. The APA task force report on benzodiazepine dependence, toxicity, and abuse. *Am J Psychiatry*. 1991;148(2):151–152.

29. Dimidjian S, Hollon SC, Dobson KS, et al. Randomized trial of behavioral activation, cognitive therapy, and antidepressant medication in the acute treatment of adults with major depression. *J Consult Clin Psychol*. 2006;74(4):658–670.

30. Wasan AD, Artin K, Clark MR. A case-matching study of the analgesic properties of electroconvulsive therapy. *Pain Med*. 2004;5(1):50–58.

31. Ehde DM, Dilworth TM, Turner JA. Cognitive-behavioral therapy for individuals with chronic pain: Efficacy, innovations, and directions for research. *Am Psychol*. 2014;69(2):153–166.

32. Kneorl R, Lavoie Smith EM, Weisberg J. Chronic pain and cognitive behavioral therapy: An integrative review. *West J Nurs Res*. 2016;38(5):596–628.

33. Cuijpers P, van Straten A, Andersson G. Internet-administered cognitive behavioral therapy for health problems: A systematic review. *J Behav Med*. 2008;31:169–177.

34. Asmundson GJG. The emotional and physical pains of trauma: Contemporary and innovative approaches for treating co-occurring PTSD and chronic pain. *Depression Anxiety*. 2014;31:717–720.

35. Moriarty O, Finn DP. Cognition and pain. *Curr Opin Support Palliat Care*. 2014;8(2):130–136.

36. Matthews M, Davin S. Chronic pain rehabilitation. *Neurosurg Clin N Am*. 2014;25:799–802.

37. Raichle KA, Romano JM, Jensen MP. Partner responses to patient pain and well behaviors and their relationship to patient pain behavior, functioning, and depression. *Pain*. 2011;152(1):82–86.

38. Brox JI, Reikeras O, Nygaard O, et al. Lumbar instrumented fusion compared with cognitive intervention and exercises in patients with chronic back pain after previous surgery for disc herniation: A prospective randomized controlled study. *Pain*. 2006;122:145–155.

39. Garschagen A, Steegers MA, van Bergen AH, et al. Is there a need for including spiritual care in interdisciplinary rehabilitation of chronic pain patients? Investigating an innovative strategy. *Pain Pract*. 2015;15(7):671–687.

40. Nakata H, Sakamoto K, Kakigi R. Meditation reduces pain-related neural activity in the anterior cingulate cortex, insula, secondary somatosensory cortex, and thalamus. *Front Psychol*. 2014;5:1489.

41. Garland EL, Black DS. Mindfulness for chronic pain and prescription opioid misuse: Novel mechanisms and unresolved issues. *Subst Use and Misuse*. 2014;49(5):608–611.

42. Gatchel RJ, Okifuji A. Evidence-based scientific data documenting the treatment and cost-effectiveness of comprehensive pain programs in chronic nonmalignant pain. *J Pain*. 2006;7(11):779–793.

43. Patrick LE, Altamaier EM, Found EM. Long-term outcomes in multidisciplinary treatment of chronic low back pain: Results of a 13-year follow-up. *Spine*. 2004;29(8):850–855.

24

Acknowledging the Clinical Effects of Words in Pain Medicine and Psychiatry

LISE BOUCHARD AND MARIO INCAYAWAR ∎

A young Ecuadorian woman suffering from depression, anxiety, and chronic back pain said: "My husband is an American young man who repeatedly insults me, it is going on for some time. It is an unbearable injury to me. I absolutely prefer suffering physical aggression because it could heal and disappear with time. The wounds caused by his verbal offenses will stay for my entire life. . . ." The American young man, in astonishment, only responded, "They are just words! I never touched her!"

This vignette depicting a young woman and her husband who visited our Cross-Cultural Clinic for Pain and Psychiatry shows how the importance given to words may vary from one culture to another. Yet, words are powerful, and they permeate every aspect of human life. Language is not only a communication tool, it is also a social instrument of power[1] used to attain or maintain domination, to persuade, to bring consolation, or to induce a certain change of behavior. We observe in fascination how carefully crafted words in poetry, the storytelling of a novel, the rhetoric of a theater play, the cutting words of satires, or the devastating curse for the *Santería* believer can generate intense emotions of sadness, joy, anger, and demoralization, combined with tears, palpitations, shaky hands, and facial flushing. Everybody knows that words of love have intense effects, both emotional and somatic, on enamored young couples. Similarly, the use of words is omnipresent in the doctor–patient relationship. Doctors' words have powerful effects on their patients, and the quality of their communication, verbal and nonverbal, plays an important role in positive and negative clinical outcomes.[2]

This chapter focuses on the overlooked effects of language on biological systems and the brain. Neurolinguistics, neurology, and neuroscience have for some time examined the impact of neurological damage on patients' linguistic capacities and performance. However, rarely has the scientific community explored in the other direction: the biological impact of words on the brain. The influence of a particular cultural view among researchers may account for this omission. It is interesting to note that in the English language, there is a children's rhyme: "Stick and stones may break my bone, but words will never hurt me," which aims to trivialize the impact of name-calling. In contrast, as we have just seen, in other countries such as Ecuador, verbal offense and abuse are considered worse than physical abuse.

CLINICAL RELEVANCE OF MEANINGFUL COMMUNICATION

Linguistic anthropologist John Gumperz[3] suggested, with his model of interactional sociolinguistics, that speaking the same language is not enough to attain a good understanding between two interlocutors. Beyond dialectal regional differences, dissimilarities in sociocultural knowledge, such as not sharing common traditions, habits, patterns, and beliefs, can cause interference and lead to miscommunication. Conversely, interlocutors who share common sociocultural knowledge make more reliable and accurate conversational inferences, hence experiencing less misunderstanding and enhanced quality of the exchange.

Meaningful words and communication between individuals have tangible biological and behavioral consequences that can be either healthy or deleterious. In the clinical setting, the consequences resulting from a successful and meaningful communication in which the parties involved share a common understanding are good doctor–patient communication, patient satisfaction, and even clinically beneficial placebo effect. In contrast, the consequences of miscommunication where the speaker unintentionally triggers a reaction in the listener, who, in turn, makes an inaccurate interpretation of the message are patients' distrust, lack of engagement, and noncompliance with treatment plans, as well as the activation of a nocebo effect.

Moreover, language plays a significant role in the establishment of a social hierarchy. As Bourdieu states, the skillful use of words allows certain individuals to gain influence and power. The rhetorical ability of a politician will help him gain leadership roles, a good verbal negotiation will help close a fruitful deal to a businessman, and the carefully chosen words of a diplomat could define peace or war during a conflict between nations. By the same token, a doctor who not only treats disease but also talks and listens carefully to his or her patients will practice quality care, will be appreciated by the patients, and will gain a well-deserved reputation. It is worth noting that social success in the form of social prestige and status appears to have biological consequences even in animals. On that point, a recent experiment done with macaques[4] remarkably shows that social status not only affects the gene expression at the baseline but also directly alters the immune system and response to infections. Social hierarchy provokes a pro-inflammatory and depressed immune response in low-status individuals, while it generates a robust antiviral immune response in high-status individuals. Researchers comment that because macaques are our close evolutionary relatives, these results likely show mechanisms that may underlie social status effects in humans.

In sum, despite the fact that language is generally relegated to the background and is seldom the object of dedicated studies in the medical arena,[5] it has nevertheless an actual impact on human health. An example of this is a recent study showing that for elderly patients, having a female doctor could significate lower mortality and hospital readmission rates.[6] The authors explain that female physician practice is characterized by more use of patient-centered communication and psychosocial counseling. They thus commit more time to patients and have more verbal exchanges with them. This suggests that differences in practice between female and male physician patterns, clearly involving the use of language, may have important clinical implications for patient outcomes.

INSIGHTS FROM BIOMEDICAL RESEARCH

Language is omnipresent in cognitive, emotional, and psychological processes. Several studies appear to reveal the biological and behavioral effects of writing, verbal communication, and reading.

Writing

Intriguing research has shown that writing memories or a journal helps individuals go through hardship, cope with psychological trauma, and alleviate physical symptoms and pain. Indeed, the writing exercise allows the individual to organize his or her thoughts and envision potential solutions. Smyth et al. have demonstrated the amazing effects of words on chronic physical conditions. Their unique study of patients suffering from asthma and rheumatoid arthritis[7] has revealed that writing about stressful life experiences resulted in symptom reduction. Furthermore, according to Spiegel,[8] who examined the link between emotional expression and disease outcome, finding meaning in a stressful situation may thwart the hypothalamic-pituitary-adrenal axis dysregulation ensuing from cumulative stress. Once again, given that the process of finding meaning is related to semantics, which is a domain of linguistics, Spiegel's research shows the important effect of words on biology.

Moreover, it has been shown that writing style changes can help to predict behavioral therapy outcomes. An example is the interesting recent research carried out by Doogan and Warren,[9] which showed that language can be a predictor of the reincarceration outcome of therapeutic community graduates. In that study, therapeutic community residents were asked to make written communications to co-residents. Amazingly, the residents who changed their expression patterns throughout the therapy sessions presented a lower rate of reincarceration than individuals who showed little or no change. Thus, these results revealed that changes in semantic networks have a noticeable relationship with reincarceration risk.

Verbal Communication

Beyond the emotional responses that words can provoke, which we all have experienced, research has unveiled important biological impacts of verbal exchanges. Parents all over the world use verbal comforting to calm a child who is in pain. When they fall, children tend to respond very well to this kind of intervention and usually quickly stop crying. Astonishingly, in a recent study of the hormonal profile of children exposed to a stressful social situation, Seltzer, Ziegler, and Pollak[10] found that verbal interaction can have biological effects as much as touch can. They observed that young girls who received only vocal comfort from their mothers released the same amount of oxytocin as girls who received vocal comfort plus the presence of their mothers. This shows once again the power of speech.

Furthermore, the words we choose when talking seem to have an impact not only on our interlocutors but also on ourselves. In that vein, Monin et al.[11] observed that caregiving spouses who used more positive emotion-processing words showed lower heart rate reactivity when talking about their partners' suffering. This is a remarkable example of the impact of linguistic markers of emotion regulation on cardiovascular reactivity.

Placebo and Nocebo Effects

The language also plays a critical role in the placebo and nocebo phenomena. It usually takes the form of verbal suggestions that influence the outcome positively (placebo) or negatively (nocebo). The placebo effect is commonly obtained when a simple sugar pill is presented with words of persuasion, making it a valuable medicine in the eyes of the patient. Astoundingly, though, the influence of words can be so compelling that a recent study carried out with patients suffering from chronic low back pain revealed that the beneficial effect endured even when the patients knew for a fact that they were taking a placebo.[12]

Likewise, negative words can have a tangible biological impact. They can even interfere with clinical treatment. On this point, in their review of the nocebo effect of expectations on clinical outcomes, Benedetti et al.[13] mentioned that negative verbal suggestions provoke a state of anxiety that leads to the release of cholecystokinin, which enhances pain transmission and therefore induces hyperalgesia.

Reading

Everyone has experienced the influence that the words we read can have on our mood. We become happy as we read a letter containing good news and sad when, on the contrary, it carries gloomy information. Books can also inspire readers to act in positive or negative ways. More direct effects on the brain of words we read have been recently published. Using functional magnetic resonance imaging (fMRI), Berns et al. showed that there is short-term increased brain connectivity in the left angular/supramarginal gyri and right posterior temporal gyri after reading a novel. Interestingly, they also observed changes in the bilateral somatosensory cortex that persisted several days; however, its significance remains unknown.[14]

Another study using positive and negative emotional words as input examined the activity in the regions of the brain involved in the interaction between self-related and emotional processing. Researchers observed that self-referential condition activated the right dorsomedial prefrontal cortex, with positive words causing a stronger effect. There were also reductions in the insula, temporal, and occipital regions associated with both positive and negative words, and in the inferior parietal regions associated with negative words.[15]

Pain Words, Emotional Pain, and Physical Pain

Neuroscientists and brain imaging researchers have found a direct effect of verbal pain descriptors on pain-related regions in the brain. For instance, Kelly et al.

found that reminding oneself of painful events activates the anterior cingulate cortex and inferior frontal gyrus,[16] and the study of Osaka et al. showed that words expressing affective pain activate the anterior cingulate cortex as physical pain does.[17] For their part, in an interesting twist, Richter et al.[18] observed that regions of the brain associated with the pain matrix were activated by pain-related words, especially when participants were focusing their attention on those words. It is also fascinating to learn that swearing appears to decrease perceived pain and increase tolerance to cold-pressor pain; thus, this form of speech has been presented as having hypoalgesic effects.[19]

Furthermore, the link between depression and physical pain has been established for a time. A large number of patients with depression, up to 80%, present with mainly physical symptoms, including pain.[20] In fact, physicians frequently prescribe tricyclic antidepressants to alleviate pain syndromes such as fibromyalgia.[21] Interestingly, a study revealed that these drugs work better than relaxation, which is a words-based strategy, for patients with chronic tension headaches. However, when the relaxation and antidepressants are combined, they have a synergistic effect.[22] The pain neuronal matrix is thus involved in the processing of both emotional and physical pain. Supporting further this point, the results of an fMRI study revealed that social rejection, which it is worth noting, often takes place through speech, activates two brain regions that are key in the response to physical pain: the anterior cingulate cortex and the right ventral prefrontal cortex.[23] The first area operates as an alarm system that sends signals to higher brain regions that urge the individual to take action to stop the pain. The second area acts to decrease the emotional suffering caused by the pain. In the study, the anterior cingulate cortex became more active as the participant experienced a more intense sensation of being excluded. In contrast, the right ventral prefrontal cortex was more active as the participant felt more included. Intriguingly, the administration of acetaminophen seems capable of alleviating the behavioral and neural responses associated with the pain of social rejection.[24] Once more, this gives evidence of the biological impact of words on the brain.

Bullying, Racist Attacks, and Biological and Epigenetic Changes

The nocebo effect of threatening or demoralizing words can be devastating, as can also be verbal abuse occurring within the family or the community at large, such as insults and verbal racist attacks. They can provoke noticeable physical reactions in the individual, as illustrated in the following case:

> An indigenous teenager from a Quichua community told us how he was suffering from anxiety when he was going to high school in the neighboring

town of Otavalo, in northern Ecuador. As he was approaching the town, always dreading the usual daily insults and racist attacks, he felt his heart beating rapidly and his hands becoming sweaty.

An important component of bullying is the use of language to intimidate and/or denigrate a person. In fact, when done through the Internet, bullying can even be entirely verbal. In recent years, there have been several reports in the news of teenagers who committed suicide after being victims of harassment by their peers at school and through email and social media. However, verbal abuse also has an insidious impact. Basic research takes us one step further in understanding the influence of language on our biology at the cellular, molecular, and genetic levels. A study carried out by Graham et al. showed that the use of meaning-making words during a conflictive marital discussion is associated with smaller increases in serum interleukin-6 and tumor necrosis factor-α pro-inflammatory cytokines over 24 hours.[25] Furthermore, Perroud et al.'s seminal study revealed that childhood maltreatment may cause epigenetic modifications such as increased methylation of glucocorticoid receptor gene (NR3C1) and downregulation of brain-derived neurotrophic factor (BDNF) gene expression that is linked to adult psychopathology.[26] Early maltreatment, including physical and emotional abuse and neglect, has also been associated with shorter telomere length, higher mitochondrial DNA copy numbers (altered mitochondrial biogenesis), and subsequent cellular aging and psychopathology.[27] In this line of inquiry, another study on the effect of racial discrimination on African American men, which frequently occurs through speech, revealed that it is associated with reduced telomere length, suggesting accelerated biological aging and vulnerability to mental illness. The striking effects are even stronger when racial discrimination and internalization of racial bias, a process also occurring through language, are both present.[28]

CONTRIBUTIONS FROM PSYCHIATRIC RESEARCH

Words and Psychopathology

Language is ubiquitous and widely used in psychiatric therapy, especially psychotherapy.[29] It also appears to play an important role in psychopathology. For instance, parental verbal aggression in childhood appears to be more strongly associated with depression and anger-hostility than is parental physical abuse. A fascinating study conducted by Teicher et al. found that verbal abuse of children, perpetrated by parents or peers, is a devastating type of maltreatment associated with higher rates of psychopathology in adulthood and serious alterations of the brain structure, namely the corpus callosum. In fact, individuals who had suffered such mistreatment, especially during middle school years, had underdeveloped connections between the two brain hemispheres.[30] It seems that the impact was stronger at that age because it constitutes a sensitive period for neural connections development and insulation with myelin.[31]

In another study examining abnormal moral reasoning with complete and partial callosotomy patients, participants were asked to judge the action of a person in a fictive scenario. The results showed that all patients based their judgments on the outcomes and disregarded the beliefs of the agent. In other words, they did not take into account the intention (good or bad) of the individual realizing the action. So, if the outcomes were good, they considered the person had done a nice thing even when they were aware that, in fact, the person wanted to do harm. The researchers concluded that their findings suggest that normal judgments of morality require full interhemispheric integration of information, or in other terms full connections between the right temporoparietal junction and right frontal processes.[32] On the basis of these two studies, Fields[33] proposes that verbal abuse of children, which causes underdeveloped connections of the corpus callosum, could lead to adults having abnormal moral reasoning, with the harmful societal consequences that this could bring.

Biological Effects of Talkative Psychotherapy

As its name indicates, language is at the core of talkative psychotherapy. Studies on the shared underlying biological effects of psychotherapy compared with pharmacological treatments are compelling and help us realize once again the impressive biological impact of words.

Among them, a review of 101 trials compared the efficacy of pharmacological, psychological, and self-help interventions in the treatment of social anxiety disorders in adults. The authors concluded that pharmacological and individual cognitive behavioral therapy were both equally effective, but psychological therapy had a lower risk for side effects and should thus be preferred.[34] Moreover, another study carried out by Knoerl et al.[35] has shown that in 43% of the trials examined, psychotherapy was effective at reducing pain intensity.

Remarkably, the efficacy was comparable between face-to-face and online formats of treatment. These results highlight further the important influence of language on biological systems and the brain. Furthermore, in a study on gene expression, it was found that patients suffering from post-traumatic stress disorder who showed improvement after cognitive behavioral therapy had an increased expression of FKBP5 protein and an increased hippocampal volume.[36] Finally, a captivating study on psychotherapy in borderline personality disorder revealed that, amazingly, talkative therapy was able to reverse the methylation status of the BDNF gene, showing once again the capability of language to induce epigenetic changes and restore function and mental health.[37]

FINAL REMARKS

Through these studies, we have seen that language is a powerful double-edged sword. It can be a meaning carrier associated with deleterious psychological and biological effects that can ultimately make the victim vulnerable to physical or mental disorders. Conversely, it appears that words might also have the power of reversing psychopathology and biological damages and relieving physical pain through psychotherapy and other forms of verbal exchanges. Beyond the obvious psychological and social benefits of a humane conversational exchange, words appear to have a non-negligible biological effect. The beneficial and deleterious effects seemingly occur at the cellular and molecular levels. This is the main reason why words and a positive doctor–patient communication should matter in a high-quality medical encounter.

Hence, the main contribution of medical linguistics to pain medicine and psychiatry could be to help comply with the bioethical principle, "First, do no harm," by avoiding not only bad prescription of medicines or medical interventions but also inappropriate words. Poor or failed communications with patients could potentially induce iatrogenic effects. The biological impact of words is a serious matter that cannot be overlooked anymore. As Holmes et al. stated, "we need to know . . . how one human talking to another brings changes in brain activity and cure or ease mental disorders."[38] Medical linguistics could contribute to a better understanding of the sociocultural and linguistic factors at play during the verbal exchange. It could develop conversational strategies to help physicians and psychotherapists improve communication skills that lead to the restoration of function and wellbeing in their patients.

Medical schools should attach all due importance to developing their students' communication skills. They should instill in them the sound knowledge that communication is as serious and impactful as other clinical skills they learn.

REFERENCES

1. Bourdieu P, Thompson JB. *Language and Symbolic Power.* Cambridge, MA: Harvard University Press; 1991.

2. Benedetti F. Placebo and the new physiology of the doctor-patient relationship. *Physiol Reviews*. 2013;93(3):1207–1246.

3. Gumperz JJ. Sociocultural knowledge in conversational inference. In: Saville-Troike M, ed. *Georgetown University Roundtable on Languages and Linguistics*. Washington, DC: Georgetown University Press; 1977:191–212.

4. Snyder-Mackler N. Social status alters immune regulation and response to infection in macaques. *Science*. 2016;354(6315):1041–1045.

5. Thomas P, Fraser W. Linguistics, human communication and psychiatry. *Br J Psychiatry*. 1994;165:585–592.

6. Tsugawa Y, Jena A, Figueroa J, Orav E, Blumenthal D, Jha A. Comparison of hospital mortality and readmission rates for medicare patients treated by male vs female physicians. *JAMA Intern Med*. 2017;177(2):206–213.

7. Smyth JM, Stone AA, Hurewitz A, Kaell A. Effects of writing about stressful experiences on symptom reduction in patients with asthma or rheumatoid arthritis: A randomized trial. *JAMA*. 1999;281(14):1304–1309.

8. Spiegel D. Healing words: Emotional expression and disease outcome. *JAMA*. 1999;281(14):1328–1329.

9. Doogan NJ, Warren K. Semantic networks, schema change, and reincarceration outcomes of therapeutic community graduates. *J Subst Abuse Treat*. 2016;70:7–13.

10. Seltzer LJ, Ziegler TE, Pollak SD. Social vocalizations can release oxytocin in humans. *Proc Biol Sci*. 2010;277(1694):2661–2666.

11. Monin JK, Shultz R, Lemay EP Jr, Cook TB. Linguistic markers of emotion regulation and cardiovascular reactivity among older caregiving spouses. *Psychol Aging*. 2012;27(4):903–911.

12. Carvalho C, Caetano, JM, Cunh LA, Rebouta P, Kaptchuk TJ, Kirsch I. Open-label placebo treatment in chronic low back pain. *Pain*. 2016;157(12):2766–2772.

13. Benedetti F, Lanotte M, Lopiano L, Colloca L. When words are painful: Unraveling the mechanisms of the nocebo effect. *Neuroscience*. 2007;147(2):260–271.

14. Berns GS, Blaine K, Prietula MJ, Pye BE. Short- and long-term effects of a novel on connectivity in the brain. *Brain Connect*. 2013;3(6):590–600.

15. Fossati P, Hevenor SJ, Graham SJ, et al. In search of the emotional self: An fMRI study using positive and negative emotional words. *Am J Psychiatry*. 2003;160(11):1938–1945.

16. Kelly S, Lloyd D, Nurmikko T, Roberts N. Retrieving autobiographical memories of painful events activates the anterior cingulate cortex and inferior frontal gyrus. *J Pain*. 2007;8(4):307–314.

17. Osaka N, Osaka M, Morishita M, Kondo H, Fukuyama H. A word expressing affective pain activates the anterior cingulate cortex in the human brain: An fMRI study. *Behav Brain Res*. 2004;153(1):123–127.

18. Richter M, Eck J, Straube T, Miltner WH, Weiss T. Do words hurt? Brain activation during the processing of pain-related words. *Pain*. 2010;148(2):198–205.

19. Stephens R, Atkins J, Kingston A. Swearing as a response to pain. *Neuroreport*. 2009;20(12):1056–1060.

20. Kirmayer LJ RJ, Dworkind M, Yaffe MJ. Somatization and the recognition of depression and anxiety in primary care. *Am J Psychiatry*. 1993;150(5):734–741.

21. Carter GT SM. Antidepressants in pain management. *Curr Opin Investig Drugs.* 2002;3(3):454–458.
22. Holroyd KA, O'Donnell FJ, Stensland M, Lipchik GL, Cordingley GE, Carlson BW. Management of chronic tension-type headache with tricyclic antidepressant medication, stress management therapy, and their combination: A randomized controlled trial. *JAMA.* 2001;285(17):2208–2215.
23. Eisenberger NI, Lieberman MD, Williams KD. Does rejection hurt? An fMRI study of social exclusion. *Science.* 2003;302(5643):290–292.
24. Dewall CN, Macdonald G, Webster GD, et al. Acetaminophen reduces social pain: Behavioral and neural evidence. *Psychol Sci.* 2010;21(7):931–937.
25. Graham JE, Glaser R, Loving TJ, Malarkey WB, Stowell JR, Kiecolt-Glaser JK. Cognitive word use during marital conflict and increases in proinflammatory cytokines. *Health Psychol.* 2009;28(5):621–630.
26. Perroud N, Paoloni-Giacobino A, Prada P, et al. Increased methylation of glucocorticoid receptor gene (NR3C1) in adults with a history of childhood maltreatment: a link with the severity and type of trauma. *Transl Psychiatry.* 2011;1:e59.
27. Tyrka AR, Price LH, Kao HT, Porton B, Marsella SA, Carpenter LL. Childhood maltreatment and telomere shortening: preliminary support for an effect of early stress on cellular aging. *Biol Psychiatry.* 2010;67(6):531–534.
28. Chae DH, Nuru-Jeter AM, Adler NE, et al. Discrimination, racial bias, and telomere length in African-American men. *Am J Prev Med* 2014;46(2):103–111.
29. van Staden W. Language, mind, and world. *Philos Psychiatr Psychol.* 2005;12(1):77–78.
30. Teicher MH, Samson JA, Sheu YS, Polcari A, McGreenery CE. Hurtful words: Association of exposure to peer verbal abuse with elevated psychiatric symptom scores and corpus callosum abnormalities. *Am J Psychiatry.* 2010;167:1464–1471.
31. Fields R. Sticks and stones: Hurtful words damage the brain. *New Brain.* 2010. https://www.psychologytoday.com/blog/the-new-brain/201010/sticks-and-stones-hurtful-words-damage-the-brain. Accessed April 15, 2020.
32. Miller MB, Sinnott-Armstrong W, Young L, et al. Abnormal moral reasoning in complete and partial callosotomy patients. *Neuropsychologia.* 2010;48(7):2215–2220.
33. Fields R. Of two minds on morality. *Blog* 2010. http://www.huffingtonpost.com/dr-douglas-fields/of-two-minds-on-morality_b_738916.html. Accessed April 15, 2020.
34. Mayo-Wilson E, Dias S, Mavranezouli I, et al. Psychological and pharmacological interventions for social anxiety disorder in adults: A systematic review and network meta-analysis. *Lancet Psychiatry.* 2014;1(5):368–376.
35. Knoerl R, Lavoie Smith EM, Weisberg J. Chronic pain and cognitive behavioral therapy: An integrative review. *West J Nurs Res.* 2016;38(5):596–628.
36. Levy-Gigi E, Szabo C, Kelemen O, Keri S. Association among clinical response, hippocampal volume, and FKBP5 gene expression in individuals with posttraumatic stress disorder receiving cognitive behavioral therapy. *Biol Psychiatry.* 2013;74(11):793–800.

37. Perroud N, Salzmann A, Prada P, et al. Response to psychotherapy in borderline personality disorder and methylation status of the BDNF gene. *Transl Psychiatry.* 2013;3:e207.

38. Holmes EA, Craske MG, Graybiel AM. Psychological treatments: A call for mental-health science. *Nature.* 2014;511(7509):287–289.

25

Detecting and Managing the Untreated Pain in Dementia

ANNE CORBETT ■

INTRODUCTION

Dementia is a devastating neurodegenerative condition characterized by progressive cognitive decline that leads to the loss of function and independence, changes in behavior, loss of communication, and eventually death. There are more than 30 million people worldwide with dementia, and this number is set to rise as populations become increasingly dominated by an ageing profile, with prevalence expected to reach 100 million by 2050.[1] Prevalence of dementia in people 60 years and older in global regions varies from 4.6% in Central Europe to 8.7% in North Africa, with all other regions falling between 5.6% and 7.6%. Fifty-eight percent of people with dementia live in low- and middle-income countries.[2] Dementia is distressing for the individual affected, particularly since there are currently few treatments and no cure. The condition also exerts considerable burden on informal carers who support their relatives and friends to live at home. The overall cost of dementia is enormous, reaching more than $818 billion worldwide each year. Long-term residential care is a major driver of cost in dementia care, with about one-third of people living in nursing homes or care homes.[2]

Dementia represents a complex clinical challenge for treatment and care. In addition to cognitive and functional decline, patients are often frail and present with a number of comorbidities that complicate decision-making and lead to unique mosaics of symptoms and treatment needs. This challenge is combined with the increasing loss of insight and self-care ability in the patient and is exacerbated further by the gradual loss of language and communication ability that is inherent in the condition.[3] There is therefore a high risk for unmet need in people with dementia, which affects quality of life and well-being[4] and can be a trigger for the emergence of behavioral and psychological symptoms of dementia (BPSD), such as agitation, aggression, and psychosis.[5] BPSD are a particular challenge for treatment and may lead to institutionalization or prescription of potentially harmful antipsychotic medications. It is important to differentiate dementia and associated BPSD from delirium, which is common in older adults in acute hospital settings, particularly in the context of postoperative care and infection. Delirium is a short-lived confusional state, whereas dementia is a progressive neurodegenerative condition. However, BPSD can represent an overlap between these states, and it is critical that accurate assessment is completed to identify and treat delirium where it arises. A major element of unmet need, and a known trigger for BPSD, is pain.[6]

Pain is common in people with dementia and if left untreated can have severe and long-term impacts on the individual. Although these issues are well-documented, there is a lack of clear guidance on how pain should be both assessed and managed in the context of dementia. This chapter aims to provide a summary of the current evidence pertaining to pain management in dementia and to provide recommendations for clinicians working with this patient group.

EPIDEMIOLOGY OF PAIN IN DEMENTIA

Prevalence of Pain

Approximately 50% of people with dementia experience regular pain.[7] As this prevalence increases with severity of cognitive and functional impairment, this figure is higher in care home settings, reaching about 80% of residents with dementia.[8] These figures are based on a considerable evidence base of clinical trials and epidemiological studies that have used pain assessment and proxy measures to estimate pain prevalence. It should be noted that because off challenges in the assessment of pain, all estimates should be treated with some caution.

Nature and Type of Pain

The nature of pain in dementia varies according to the causality, but people with dementia commonly experience persistent pain (lasting more than 3 months). The most common cause is musculoskeletal pain as a result of arthritic conditions, particularly osteoarthritis, which affects more than 60% of people with dementia.[9] Pain can also arise from a wide range of conditions and complications in these patients, including infections, of which genitourinary tract infection and respiratory conditions are particularly common; gastrointestinal complains, such as peptic ulcers and intestinal obstructions; and falls.[10] In the later stages of dementia, pressure ulcers are a particular source of pain as a result of patients spending long periods in bed.[11] Neuropathic pain is also common, arising from underlying long-term conditions such as diabetes and cardiovascular disease.

Impact of Pain

Pain is an unpleasant experience that causes distress and discomfort, particularly if left untreated for long periods. In addition to these subjective impacts, untreated pain also has tangible repercussions on the clinical and psychological health of people with dementia. These include reduced mobility, muscle weakness and falls, and depression, apathy, and anxiety. Pain is also associated with reduced quality of life.[12] Importantly, pain is also a major underpinning cause of BPSD, often leading to agitation, aggression, apathy, and depression.[13] BPSD are challenging to treat and are often treated with antipsychotic medications despite the significant side effects associated with these drugs. Detection and prompt treatment of pain is therefore a critical factor in avoiding unnecessary prescriptions of this nature.

BIOLOGY OF PAIN IN DEMENTIA

Despite the prevalence of pain in people with dementia, the associated biology is not yet fully understood. This is an important area of research since the underlying biology of pain, and how it is affected by dementia conditions such as Alzheimer disease, may play a critical role in how a patient perceives and responds to pain and how it is subsequently reported, assessed, and treated. There is a widespread assumption that the neuropathology of dementia leads to a reduction in pain perception. In part, this is supported by work in animal models and in small cohorts of people with dementia who appear to show higher pain tolerance or a reduced response to painful stimuli compared with cognitively healthy controls.[14,15] However, the literature hints at considerable complexity depending on specific pathways affected and the type of pain stimulus used.[16] It is also not clear if or how different types of pain may be altered, and whether this varies between different dementia subtypes. However, the current evidence suggests alterations in the neuropathological and emotional perception of pain and how these are processed. Preliminary work also suggests that people with Alzheimer disease pathology may show differential responses to individual analgesics such as opioids and anti-inflammatory medications. Furthermore, there is emerging evidence suggesting that peripheral inflammation in conditions such as osteoarthritis may have a direct impact on neuroinflammation in Alzheimer disease, and thus a potential role in the progression of the disease.[17] These early indications highlight the importance of ongoing research into this area and emphasize the need for a judicious, prompt approach to pain management in this patient group to ensure that treatment is appropriate and effective.

GUIDANCE FOR PAIN MANAGEMENT

A number of guidance resources are available for pain management in older adults, ranging from comprehensive guidance published by the American and British Geriatric Societies[18,19] to brief pain treatment pathways for specific pain types such as neuropathic pain.[20] However, a review of guidelines conducted in 2015 reported that only four of 15 available guidelines were tailored for people with dementia. Within these, considerable gaps were identified. Guidelines focused either only on pain assessment or on pharmacological treatment, or were highly specialist in format, thus hindering their implementation into usual care. Importantly, no guidance was available for use in nursing homes or care homes, despite the high prevalence of pain in these settings. There is a clear need for evidence-based guidance on pain management for key dementia groups in community, hospital, and residential care settings. Despite this lack of usable guidance, there is robust evidence regarding appropriate pain assessment and treatment approaches, which can be applied in clinical practice.

ASSESSMENT OF PAIN IN PEOPLE WITH DEMENTIA

Accurate assessment of pain in people with dementia is essential to ensure timely and appropriate treatment, in addition to enabling monitoring of the impact of treatment approaches. However, pain assessment in dementia is not straightforward. Pain is a subjective experience, which is perceived differently between individuals. The most meaningful approach to pain assessment is therefore through self-report.[21] While self-report is largely intact and accurate in people with mild dementia,[22] it becomes increasingly hindered as the dementia progresses. In part this is due to the loss of communication and language ability that occurs in the later stages of dementia. The accuracy of self-report is further limited by impairment to short-term memory that prevents patients from reporting their experience of pain in the recent past.[23] The issue is exacerbated further by the loss of insight people experience into their own condition. As a result, numerous observational tools have been developed to measure pain where self-report is not feasible (Box 25.1).[6] Of the 35 tools that

---

Box 25.1

EXAMPLES OF TOOLS TO ASSESS PAIN IN PEOPLE WITH DEMENTIA

Tools for Self-Report of Pain (Where There Is Capacity)
- **Recommended:** Present Pain Intensity (PPI) scale, report of pain experienced now versus last week
- Visual Analog Scale, numerical and facial rating scales

Caregiver or Informant-Based Rating Scales
- **Recommended:** Abbey Pain Scale
- Pain Assessment for the Dementing Elderly (PADE) and global staff rating
- Pain Assessment Instrument in Noncommunicative Elderly persons (PAINE)

Observational Rating Scales
- **Recommended:** Mobilization-Observation-Behavior-Intensity-Dementia (MOBID-2) Pain Scale
- Discomfort Scale for Dementia of Alzheimer's Type (DS-DAT)
- Checklist of Nonverbal Pain Indicators (CNPI)
- Pain Assessment in Advanced Dementia (PAINAD)
- Elderly Caring Assessment 2 (EPCA-2)
- DOLOPLUS-2
- Non-Communicative Patient's Pain Assessment Instrument (NOPPAIN)
- Pain Assessment Checklist for Seniors With Limited Ability to Communicate (PACSLAC)
- Dutch-Translated Pain Assessment Checklist for Seniors With Limited Ability to Communicate (PACSLAC-D)

---

exist, the quality of evidence supporting their use is highly variable. The most commonly used, and best validated, tools are described next.

Self-Reported Pain Assessment

Where patients have the capacity and insight, self-report is the most meaningful approach to detecting pain in dementia. A number of tools exist, all of which use analog scales to enable patients to score their pain on a set scale. These may take the form of verbal, numerical, or facial ratings using images depicting increasing levels of pain.[21] The best validates of these is the Present Pain Intensity scale, an eight-point scale that shows good reliability and validity in dementia.[24] As would be expected, the usefulness and accuracy of this approach falls as dementia severity increases.[25]

Caregiver-Rated Pain Assessment

Informants can play a helpful role in identifying and monitoring pain in a person with dementia, particularly if they know the person well and are in regular contact, preferably daily, with them. This approach relies on the caregiver accurately remembering and reporting changes in behavior that signify the presence of pain, including facial expressions, body movements, verbalizations, and changes in activities or mood. Taken together, these changes are described as pain-related behaviors and are often unique to the individual. The most commonly used and well-validated assessment tool of this type is the Abbey Pain Scale,[26] a six-item scale that captures caregiver-reported changes or events relating to the main pain-related behaviors described previously, in addition to a subjective rating of the intensity of the pain. This tool is particularly well-validated for use in people with severe dementia and is often the tool of choice when assessing pain in residents with extremely limited capacity. Its simplicity means that the Abbey scale can also be administered by trained care staff in residential settings. Additional caregiver-rated pain assessment tools include the 24-item Pain Assessment for the Dementing Elderly and the 22-item Pain Assessment in Non-Communicative Elderly Scale. A new approach to caregiver-rated pain assessment is to consider the impact of pain on the patient's daily activities and well-being through a Pain Interference Scale (PIS). This approach is commonly used with cognitively healthy adults,[27] and a new dementia-specific PIS has been developed and is undergoing validation.

Observational Assessment

Observational assessment of pain uses the same approach as caregiver-rated assessment but usually involves a more complex or lengthy protocol, making them suitable for use by a specialist or in a research setting. This assessment method also detects pain through recording of pain-related behaviors and often includes the use of guided movement or monitoring during activities to identify sources and locations of pain. These observational assessment scales include the Discomfort Scale for Dementia of Alzheimer Type (DS-DAT), the Checklist of Nonverbal Pain Indicators (CNPI), the Pain Assessment in Advanced Dementia, and the DOLOPLUS-2, which have reasonable reliability data. However, these tools are complex and lengthy to use, involving long periods of intense observation, which hinders their use in clinical practice.[28] More recently, a new tool has been developed that seeks to address this issue. The Mobilization-Observation-Behavior-Intensity-Dementia Pain Scale (MOBID-2) sets out a simple protocol for brief observations of a patient at rest and during guided movements, during which pain-related responses are recorded. This instrument has shown excellent validity and appears to be more feasible for use in clinical practice than other scales, as well as providing a sensitive scale for research use.[29]

Biomarkers for Pain

There is currently no way to accurately detect pain through biomarker analysis in the clinic. However, research is ongoing into this area. There is particular interest in the use of cerebrospinal fluid as a source of markers of inflammatory pain.[30] Neuropeptides have been suggested as a means of identifying nociceptive pain.[31] However, this field of research is still relatively young, and extensive validation is needed before a biomarker test will reach the clinic. Similarly, neuroimaging is currently in use as a research tool to investigate the neurological pathways of pain, but there is no indication that imaging will be introduced as a feasible diagnostic approach for identifying pain, particularly because of the cost of this technology.

Recommendations for Pain Assessment

Physicians are recommended to follow key guiding principles when assessing pain in a person with dementia. These are summarized in Box 25.2. There are

Box 25.2

Guiding Principles for Assessing Pain in People With Dementia

- Get to know the person—person-centeredness is pivotal to accurate pain assessment
- Conduct a thorough medical review—identification of likely underlying causes of pain and pain risk will help to inform the overall pain assessment. This is particularly valuable in cases in which neuropathic pain is likely, for example, in someone with existing diabetes or a previous myocardial infarction.
- Look for change—changes in activities, mood, and overall well-being are very helpful indicators of the presence of pain.
- Assess the person's capacity for accurate self-report—if self-report is feasible, this is by far the most meaningful approach to assessment.
- Work with a carer—identify someone (a carer or family member) who knows the person well and has regular (daily) contract with the person because the carer will be able to report on any likely pain, its causes, and possible routes for treatment.
- Assess pain using one or more tools with good validity in people with dementia.
- Consult with other health professionals, including psychologists, psychiatrists, neurologists, nurses, and social workers.

a large number of pain assessment tools available, none of which have gold-standard quality evidence supporting their use.[32] Often, the best approach is for physicians to select a tool they are most comfortable with and to become very familiar with its use and interpretation. Best practice would be to use two tools in combination. These would be used for both assessment and ongoing monitoring of pain. Based on the evidence, the most accurate and meaningful tools are the following:

1. Self-report using the Present Pain Intensity scale when self-report is possible
2. Preliminary identification of pain using the Abbey Pain Scale, in partnership with a caregiver
3. In-depth exploration of the intensity, source, and location of pain using an observational tool such as the MOBID-2

TREATMENT OF PAIN IN PEOPLE WITH DEMENTIA

Timely, effective, and appropriate treatment of pain is critical to improve quality of life for people with dementia. There is a good evidence base supporting the use of different treatment approaches, often best applied by a multidisciplinary team, although these are rarely translated into practice. The fluctuating, complex nature of pain leads to the need for a tailored approach to pain treatment. The most meaningful approach is to utilize a stepped framework of escalating treatments that responds to the needs and treatment response of the individual patient. Polypharmacy is a significant risk in dementia patients because of their frequent comorbidities and frailty. As a result, nondrug approaches should always be considered as a first-line treatment in cases of mild or moderate pain, followed by an escalating ladder of analgesic medications. All treatment regimens must commence with a comprehensive needs assessment and should be informed by a medical review to ensure that any underlying medical conditions are also receiving appropriate treatment.

Nonpharmacological Treatment of Pain

Nondrug approaches to address pain are often helpful in cases in which pain is mild to moderate. Nondrug treatments should always be considered for people with dementia since they often lack the ability or capacity to take simple steps to address their own pain compared with cognitively healthy adults. There are two main approaches to nondrug treatments. The first involves direct treatment of the pain through physical therapies. The best evidence exists for heat/cold therapy, and there are also small trials that indicate the benefit of massage and transcutaneous electrical nerve stimulation treatment.[33-35] The second approach targets the psychological aspects of pain by utilizing psychosocial or environmental techniques to reduce the pain experience. This may include the use of music therapy, which has some promising initial supporting evidence,[36] or the use of structured social interaction. Adaptation to environmental issues, such as noise, light, or furniture arrangements, can also play a helpful role.

There is a need for larger, more robust trials of these approaches, but they should be considered, particularly for patients who have a history of responding well to nondrug and "comfort" approaches. The principles of person-centered care are central to these treatment options to ensure that they are appropriate and acceptable for the individual. Consultation with family or caregivers is often helpful in these cases to identify possible nondrug approaches that the person favored in the past to ameliorate pain, such as taking a hot bath for joint pain, dimming bright lights to ease a persistent headache, or taking a gentle walk to mobilize limbs.

Pharmacological Treatment of Pain

In cases of persistent or severe pain, and where first-line nondrug approaches are not suitable or effective, a stepped approach to pharmacological treatment should be taken. Prescribing audits indicate that analgesics are commonly used in people with dementia, particularly as-needed prescriptions of acetaminophen and transdermal preparations of opioids such as fentanyl.[37–40] Prevalence of analgesic use varies widely across different countries, with reports ranging from 76% in Australia to 46% in Sweden and 29% in Poland. These variations are likely largely due to reporting technique but also reflect differing guidelines and practice in these nations.[6,37,38] Comparisons with cognitively healthy adults suggest that underprescribing is not an issue per se, but they raise concerns regarding the inappropriate use of analgesics in this group. The use of opioids, which carry a considerable risk for harm in naïve, frail populations, is a particular concern. Before any analgesic prescription, a full medical review and needs assessment should be conducted in order to identify comorbidity and risk profiles that may be relevant to specific analgesics. In particular, a precision approach to analgesic prescription is key in these patients, particularly considering the potential for polypharmacy and risk with frail individuals.

The evidence supporting the use of analgesia in dementia is considerable and highlights key treatment principles for prescribers to follow. It is clear from several randomized controlled trials and additional clinical studies that stepped analgesic use is beneficial to pain and discomfort in people with established pain. The literature also supports the use of analgesics as a treatment component to address BPSD, particularly agitation. Acetaminophen is widely considered to be the most appropriate first-line analgesic because of its efficacy and safety and is often used in combination with nondrug approaches.[39] However, options for escalation in cases in which acetaminophen is not sufficient are limited and not well-supported in the literature. Nonsteroidal anti-inflammatory drugs (NSAIDs) are rarely used, despite the prevalence of inflammatory pain, because of perceived safety concerns. This warrants urgent research since the evidence supporting this assumption is limited.[40] Nonetheless, NSAIDs should be use with caution and should only be considered if risk to gastrointestinal complications is low.

Care must be taken to consider the frailty and comorbidities present in the patient, particularly when considering the use of opioid medications. There is emerging evidence that indicates elevated opioid sensitivity and increased risk for severe adverse events, including mortality, in people with dementia compared with healthy older adults.[41] For this reason, any opioid prescription should commence at a low dose, over a short period, and should be accompanied by a rigorous monitoring schedule.

Despite their frequent use in general populations, support for the use of alternative pharmacotherapy to address pain is extremely limited because of the lack of clinical studies, particularly randomized clinical trials. There is a need to investigate treatments such as anticonvulsants, antidepressants, and other novel analgesics to establish their potential value in the dementia population. This is particularly pressing given the emerging evidence that points toward a differential treatment response in dementia compared with healthy older adults.[42]

The key to good pharmacological management of pain in this group is therefore to take a judicious and cautious approach. A critical aspect of this will be to provide clear, evidence-based training for carers, particularly in residential settings, to ensure they are equipped to play an active role in pain management.[43] Prescribers should not assume that a licensed analgesic for older adults will have the same clinical effect in a person with dementia, and should impose monitoring and dosage restrictions accordingly.

Recommendations for Pain Treatment

Guiding principles for physicians in treating pain in a person with dementia are summarized in Box 25.3.

CONCLUSION

Pain is common in people with dementia and is closely related to clinically significant issues and comorbidity. Accurate assessment and prompt, appropriate treatment are essential to manage pain and avoid a host of potential impacts, including falls, behavioral symptoms, and worsening of quality of life.

Both assessment and treatment of pain should be conducted within the guiding principles of person-centered care and with careful consideration of the specific implications that the dementia condition may have on the person's pain experience and likely treatment response. Physicians must strike a careful balance between effective treatment and the risk for polypharmacy and treatment sensitivity. For this reason, monitoring is particularly critical in the dementia patient group to ensure that pharmacological treatments are effective, appropriate, and not applied for longer than necessary.

Box 25.3

Guiding Principles for Treating Pain in People With Dementia

- Use best practice for pain assessment—as described in Box 25.2.
- Conduct a thorough medical review and needs assessment—underlying comorbidities may influence the choice of treatment that is most appropriate.
- Take a person-centered approach—consult the person, carers, and family to establish preferences for treatment and what has been effective in the past.
- Consider the use of first-line nondrug approaches—where pain is mild or moderate, these treatments may be of use, particularly in cases in which there is a concern about polypharmacy or a history of response to nondrug approaches.
- Use a stepped approach to pharmacological treatment, commencing with acetaminophen (up to 1mg), unless pain is severe or causing significant distress.
- Carefully consider the implications of escalated pharmacological analgesic treatment, particularly if opioids will be used.
- Start with a low dose—if the use of opioids or other strong analgesics is warranted, this approach will help to mitigate risk for increased sensitivity.
- Monitor carefully—implement a strict monitoring regime and prepare to withdraw or reduce dose if safety concerns arise or if pain recedes.

Carers play a vital role in the well-being and overall health care of people with dementia. It is essential that they are fully involved and informed in the pain management process. This may include supporting pain assessment through their observations and knowledge of the person, supporting decision-making in treatment choices, administration of nondrug therapies, and providing ongoing monitoring of symptoms. Physicians should therefore work closely with caregivers to maximize the effectiveness of pain management plans.

REFERENCES

1. Wimo A, Jonsson L, Bond J, Prince M, Winblad B. The worldwide economic impact of dementia 2010. *Alzheimers Dement.* 2013;9(1):1–11, e13.

2. Prince M, Bryce R, Albanese E, Wimo A, Ribeiro W, Ferri CP. The global prevalence of dementia: A systematic review and metaanalysis. *Alzheimer Dement.* 2013;9(1):63–75, e62.

3. Ballard C, Corbett A, Jones EL. Dementia: Challenges and promising developments. *Lancet Neurol.* 2011;10(1):7–9.

4. Banerjee S, Samsi K, Petrie CD, et al. What do we know about quality of life in dementia? A review of the emerging evidence on the predictive and explanatory value of disease specific measures of health related quality of life in people with dementia. *Int J Geriatr Psychiatry.* 2009;24(1):15–24.

5. Ballard C, Corbett A. Management of neuropsychiatric symptoms in people with dementia. *CNS Drugs.* 2010;24(9):729–739.

6. Corbett A, Husebo B, Malcangio M, et al. Assessment and treatment of pain in people with dementia. *Nat Rev Neurol.* 2012;8(5):264–274.

7. Shega JW, Hougham GW, Stocking CB, Cox-Hayley D, Sachs GA. Pain in community-dwelling persons with dementia: Frequency, intensity, and congruence between patient and caregiver report. *J Pain Symptom Manage.* 2004;28(6):585–592.

8. Achterberg WP, Pieper MJ, van Dalen-Kok AH, et al. Pain management in patients with dementia. *Clin Intervent aging.* 2013;8:1471–1482.

9. Hunt LJ, Covinsky KE, Yaffe K, et al. Pain in community-dwelling older adults with dementia: Results from the National Health and Aging Trends Study. *J Am Geriatr Soc.* 2015;63(8):1503–1511.

10. Black BS, Finucane T, Baker A, et al. Health problems and correlates of pain in nursing home residents with advanced dementia. *Alzheimer Dis Assoc Disord.* 2006;20(4):283–290.

11. Horn SD, Bender SA, Bergstrom N, et al. Description of the national pressure ulcer long-term care study. *J Am Geriatr Soc.* 2002;50(11):1816–1825.

12. Corbett A, Husebo BS, Achterberg WP, Aarsland D, Erdal A, Flo E. The importance of pain management in older people with dementia. *Br Med Bull.* 2014;111(1):139–148.

13. Ballard C, Smith J, Husebo B, Aarsland D, Corbett A. The role of pain treatment in managing the behavioural and psychological symptoms of dementia (BPSD). *Int J Palliat Nurs.* 2011;17(9):420, 422, 424.

14. Gibson SJ, Voukelatos X, Ames D, Flicker L, Helme RD. An examination of pain perception and cerebral event-related potentials following carbon dioxide laser stimulation in patients with Alzheimer's disease and age-matched control volunteers. *Pain Res Manage.* 2001;6(3):126–132.

15. Benedetti F, Vighetti S, Ricco C, et al. Pain threshold and tolerance in Alzheimer's disease. *Pain.* 1999;80(1–2):377–382.

16. Corbett A, Husebo B, Malcangio M, et al. Assessment and treatment of pain in people with dementia. *Nat Rev Neurol.* 2012;8(5):264–274.

17. Kyrkanides S, Tallents RH, Miller JN, et al. Osteoarthritis accelerates and exacerbates Alzheimer's disease pathology in mice. *J Neuroinflamm.* 2011;8:112.

18. AGS Panel on Persistent Pain in Older Persons. The management of persistent pain in older persons. 2002;50(S6):205–224. Accessed September 23, 2015. https://doi.org/10.1046/j.1532-5415.50.6s.1.x

19. Abdulla A, Adams N, Bone M, et al. Guidance on the management of pain in older people. *Age Ageing*. 2013;42(suppl 1):i1–57.

20. Gloucestershire Hospitals NHS Foundation Trust. Neuropathic pain treatment pathway. 2013. Accessed September 23, 2015. https://www.gloshospitals.nhs.uk/gps/treatment-guidelines/pain-formulary/

21. Closs SJ, Barr B, Briggs M, Cash K, Seers K. A comparison of five pain assessment scales for nursing home residents with varying degrees of cognitive impairment. *J Pain Sympt Manage*. 2004;27(3):196–205.

22. Snow AL, Chandler JF, Kunik ME, et al. Self-reported pain in persons with dementia predicts subsequent decreased psychosocial functioning. *Am J Geriatr Psychiatry*. 2009;17(10):873–880.

23. Morrison RS, Siu AL. A comparison of pain and its treatment in advanced dementia and cognitively intact patients with hip fracture. *J Pain Sympt Manage*. 2000;19(4):240–248.

24. Zwakhalen SM, Hamers JP, Abu-Saad HH, Berger MP. Pain in elderly people with severe dementia: A systematic review of behavioural pain assessment tools. *BMC Geriatr*. 2006;6:3.

25. Cohen-Mansfield J. Relatives' assessment of pain in cognitively impaired nursing home residents. *J Pain Sympt Manage*. 2002;24(6):562–571.

26. Abbey J, Piller N, De Bellis A, et al. The Abbey Pain Scale: A 1-minute numerical indicator for people with end-stage dementia. *Int J Palliat Nurs*. 2004;10(1):6–13.

27. Tyler EJ, Jensen MP, Engel JM, Schwartz L. The reliability and validity of pain interference measures in persons with cerebral palsy. *Arch Phys Med Rehabil*. 2002;83(2):236–239.

28. Herr K, Bjoro K, Decker S. Tools for assessment of pain in nonverbal older adults with dementia: A state-of-the-science review. *J Pain Sympt Manage*. 2006;31(2):170–192.

29. Husebo BS, Ostelo R, Strand LI. The MOBID-2 pain scale: Reliability and responsiveness to pain in patients with dementia. *Eur J Pain*. 2014;18(10):1419–1430.

30. Mattsson N, Blennow K, Zetterberg H. CSF biomarkers: Pinpointing Alzheimer pathogenesis. *Ann N Y Acad Sci*. 2009;1180:28–35.

31. Calcutt NA, Stiller C, Gustafsson H, Malmberg AB. Elevated substance-P-like immunoreactivity levels in spinal dialysates during the formalin test in normal and diabetic rats. *Brain Res*. 2000;856(1–2):20–27.

32. Lichtner V, Dowding D, Allcock N, et al. The assessment and management of pain in patients with dementia in hospital settings: A multi-case exploratory study from a decision making perspective. *BMC Health Serv Res*. 2016;16:427.

33. Curkovic B, Vitulic V, Babic-Naglic D, Durrigl T. The influence of heat and cold on the pain threshold in rheumatoid arthritis. *Zeitschrift fur Rheumatologie*. 1993;52(5):289–291.

34. Cameron M, Lonergan E, Lee H. Transcutaneous electrical nerve stimulation (TENS) for dementia. *Cochrane Database Syst Rev*. 2003(3):CD004032.

35. Hodgson NA, Andersen S. The clinical efficacy of reflexology in nursing home residents with dementia. *J Altern Complement Med*. 2008;14(3):269–275.

36. Park H. Effect of music on pain for home-dwelling persons with dementia. *Pain Manage Nurs*. 2010;11(3):141–147.

37. Tan EC, Visvanathan R, Hilmer SN, et al. Analgesic use and pain in residents with and without dementia in aged care facilities: A cross-sectional study. *Australas J Ageing*. 2016;35(3):180–187.

38. Thakur ER, Amspoker AB, Sansgiry S, et al. Pain among community-dwelling older adults with dementia: Factors associated with undertreatment. *Pain Med*. 2017;18(8):1476–1484. https://doi.org/10.1093/pm/pnw225

39. American Geriatrics Society. Pharmacological management of persistent pain in older persons. 2009. *J Am Geriatr Soc*. 2009 Aug;57(8):1331–1346. doi: 10.1111/j.1532-5415.2009.02376.x. Epub 2009 Jul 2.

40. Aisen PS. Evaluation of selective COX-2 inhibitors for the treatment of Alzheimer's disease. *J Pain Sympt Manage*. 2002;23(4 suppl):S35–S40.

41. Barg J, Belcheva M, Rowinski J, et al. Opioid receptor density changes in Alzheimer amygdala and putamen. *Brain Res*. 1993;632(1–2):209–215.

42. Stubbs B, Thompson T, Solmi M, et al. Is pain sensitivity altered in people with Alzheimer's disease? A systematic review and meta-analysis of experimental pain research. *Exp Gerontol*. 2016;82:30–38.

43. Corbett A, Nunez K, Smeaton E, et al. The landscape of pain management in people with dementia living in care homes: A qualitative mixed methods study. *Int J Geriatr Psychiatry*. 2016;31(12):1354–1370.

26

Effective Management of Pain in Autism Spectrum Disorder and Intellectual Disability

DJEA SARAVANE ■

INTRODUCTION

Research has shown that people with intellectual disability (ID) or autism spectrum disorder (ASD) have markedly higher rates of chronic medical conditions than do people in the general population.[1] Relatively little empirical knowledge is available to guide our understanding and treatment of pain among people with ASD. Compounding this paucity of knowledge are notions that persons with ASD are insensitive or indifferent to pain.

Pain behavior can be ambiguous, leading to confusion and highly subjective assessments that present a tremendous challenge for clinicians, researchers, patients, and their families. Even when pain-specific behaviors are evident, they have been regarded as altered, blunted, or confused with other sources of generalized stress or arousal, or misinterpreted as indicative of general emotional stress or autonomic dysregulation (rage behaviors). This notion has been reinforced by standardized texts[2] reporting that autism is associated with "a high threshold for pain." Our understanding of pain in ASD is very limited and to a great extent based on anecdotal reports and clinical studies derived from heterogeneous populations. Yet, these individuals are often undertreated for pain or not treated for it at all because health care professionals either don't know how to assess their pain or don't recognize that certain nonverbal behaviors can be the expression of pain.

While ASD alters typical forms of communication, everyday interests, and behaviors, there are no data to support the commonly held belief that persons with an ASD experience pain any less frequently or severely than others.

Unfortunately, few studies have addressed the issue of pain assessment and treatment in people with ID or ASD. Using retrospective chart reviews, Bosch et al. considered 25 patients who engaged in self-injurious behavior and found that seven (28%) had previously undiagnosed medical conditions that could cause pain or discomfort. After these conditions were treated, self-injurious behavior decreased in six of the seven (86%).[3] The investigation of several related phenomena may lead to an understanding of possible relationships between neurodevelopment and the pain system. Together, such disparate findings are difficult to reconcile but might suggest that altered pain sensitivity in ASD may be related to differences in mode of pain expression or levels of function, coupled with an altered endogenous biological capacity to mount a nociceptive response.

EXPLORING THE EXPERIENCE OF PAIN IN AUTISM SPECTRUM DISORDER AND INTELLECTUAL DISABILITY

To date, few studies have been conducted on sensitivity to pain stimulation and pain expression in this population.

Hyporeactivity

Individuals with ASD have been described as having reduced sensitivity to pain,[4] indifference to pain,[5] and a high pain threshold.[2] Thus, these reports of altered pain sensation were based on anecdotal observations and clinical impressions.[6]

However, some experimental studies also found this hyporeactivity. Tordjman et al.[7] reported a decrease in behavioral reactivity in children with ASD compared with a control group while performing a venipuncture. Similarly, Pernon and Rattaz[8] found that children with ASD have a decrease in facial reactivity during painful stimulation compared with children without ASD.

Hyperreactivity

Tordjman et al.,[7] in their study, noted reactive behaviors immediately after venipuncture despite a decrease in motor reactivity at the time of the painful procedure. Nader et al.[5] observed greater facial reactivity in 3- to 7-year-old children with ASD during the venipuncture compared with children without ASD.

However, the use of bundling to aid in the safety of the procedure in that study limited the interpretation of this finding.[5]

Sensitivity Threshold

There has been very little research on the topic of sensitivity threshold. Clinicians and families report a high sensitivity for pain. Objective observational measures should be systematically used in studying sensitivity thresholds in ASD patients.[9]

Self-Aggression

In the clinical setting, problem behavior of a self-aggressive nature is not uncommon. Some researchers consider that self-aggression is more related to the stress associated with the examination than to pain. The link between self-harm and pain has not been clearly established. The exacerbation of self-injurious behaviors (such as head banging, hitting or biting oneself, or throwing oneself against hard objects) in people with severe cognitive impairment can be an indication of pain. Thus, the role of discomfort or pain in self-injurious behavior deserves a careful evaluation.[10]

Sleep Disorders

Sleep disorders are frequent comorbidities of ASD, and their prevalence ranges from 50 to 80% of people with autism. Tudor et al. show that the experience of pain in these people is a predictor of sleep disorders, including disruptions, the occurrence of parasomnia, and nocturnal awakenings.[11]

Gastrointestinal Tract

Gastrointestinal problems are significantly overrepresented in ASD and can often be related to problem behaviors, sensory responsivity, sleep disorders, rigid-compulsive behaviors, aggression, anxiety, and irritability.[12] In individuals with ASD, atypical presentation of common gastrointestinal problems can include the emergence or intensification of seemingly autistic behaviors such as self-harm, irritability, aggression, strange posture or movements, and pain.[13]

UNDERSTANDING THE NATURE OF PAIN
IN AUTISM SPECTRUM DISORDER AND
INTELLECTUAL DISABILITY

Several studies have reported insensitivity to pain in the autistic population compared with control groups, but the contribution of other factors that may partially explain the results is lacking. Using a sociocommunicative perspective, Craig[14] has offered an alternative explanation for the pain insensitivity in people with ASD. The altered perception of others derives from inadequate communication skills and social relatedness.

Direct links between the altered neurological substrate that underlies ASD and nociceptive systems remain elusive. Many hypotheses have been put forward to explain the difference between feeling and expressing pain in people with autism:

- **Neurochemical hypotheses with dysfunction of the opioid or serotonin system, but no conclusive data exists.** Opioid hyperfunction may account for reported pain insensitivity and may be linked to a variety of factors, including a genetic-related opioid system dysfunction that could lead to overproduction, deficient degradation, abnormal feedback, or messenger mechanisms. Research findings addressing opioid system function in ASD have been mixed. The serotoninergic hypothesis has been little studied, although selective serotonin inhibitors are used to reduce certain symptoms such as anxiety and stereotyped behaviors in ASD.
- **Sensory abnormalities in autistic people.** These anomalies concern all sensory modalities and are understood in terms of sensory hyporeactivity or hyperreactivity, decrease in the threshold of stimulus discrimination, or difficulty in modulating sensory information.
- **Abnormal social relationships, adaptive communication, and difficulties in regulating the expression of negative emotions** may explain the atypical pain expression.[15] In addition, Buie et al.[16] provide integrated modeling that takes into account the different hypotheses involving intrapersonal factors (sensory alterations, self-harm, language disorders) and environmental factors (the observer's ability to understand the message) in the perception and expression of pain.

These specific aspects of pain perception and expression should be taken into account when considering the particularities of autistic functioning such as difficulties in modulating sensory influx, somatosensory alterations, communication alterations, and abnormal social relationships. These elements have implications for the management of pain in autistic people, and more broadly for the management of problem behaviors. The most challenging task is to assess and interpret the painful symptomatology and to consider other medical conditions as causes.

PAIN ASSESSMENT

Until clinical research is conducted using a rigorous methodology, the atypical expression of pain raises the question of how to assess and manage pain in people with ASD, particularly when there are major communication disorders. The pain can be underestimated and therefore undertreated. Together, given altered facial emotional expression, social responsiveness, and appropriate use of language, it is likely that typical ASD expressions of pain are altered. In the face of acute pain, a person with ASD might not cry, use appropriate verbal communication, or seek comfort from a caregiver, leading to a perception that the person with ASD is not experiencing pain. It is important to know the patient's social network, such as family members, caregivers, nurses, and others, in order to interpret the manifestation (pleasure/displeasure, comfort/discomfort) of pain. It is recommended to use all possible means of communication (e.g., pictogram, digital tablets, computer, sign language).

Pain assessment is commonly achieved through self-report, observational, and/or proxy methods. Impaired communication skills may make self-report difficult for people with ASD.[14,17,18] Unfortunately, observational pain assessment can also be difficult because of idiosyncratic behaviors associated with ASD and/or cognitive impairment (atypical vocalizations, facial expressions) that may result in inaccurate estimates of pain by those unfamiliar with the individual's typical behavioral responses.[19] Consequently, different observers/caregivers may interpret pain behaviors differently.[20]

It is worth noting that certain behaviors may suggest an organic pathology or pain[21] such as previously acquired skills abilities, a sudden change in behavior, anger and opposition, irritability, sleep disorders, tapping the throat, eating disorders, teeth grinding, making faces, frowning, tics, self-mutilation, constant ingestion, vocalization, and moaning.

Given the complexity of these atypical manifestations of pain, Barthelemy Durand Hospital has set up care protocols tailored to individuals with ASDs. The protocols take into account the environment, sensorial approach, patience, and advance planning of the routine care. Systematic assessment of pain with methods tailored to each case is used for specific and personalized management.[21,22]

The semiological signs of pain expression in ASD identified are aggressiveness, self-harm, screaming without particular cause, sleep disorders, unexplained violent explosion, and repetitive stereotyped movements in the painful area. These signs should be considered to indicate a painful condition and require a systematic investigation into the etiology of pain.[21,23,24]

Pain Comorbidity

Comorbidities are frequent in this population, the most significant are the following:

- **Gastrointestinal symptoms**
  Gastrointestinal symptoms are significantly over-represented in ASD and are often related to behavior problems, sensory over-responsivity, dysregulated sleep, aggression, anxiety, and irritability.[13] Several studies have shown a high prevalence of gastrointestinal symptoms in children with ASD compared with children without ASD, with an odds ratio of 4.5.[25] In recent years, there has been increasing recognition of gastrointestinal comorbidities—both functional bowel problems and pathological findings—among people with ASD, including diarrhea, constipation, gastroesophageal reflux, gastritis, duodenitis, and colitis. In ASD, atypical presentation of common gastrointestinal problems can include the emergence or intensification of self-harm, irritability, aggression, strange posturing or movements, and pain. When abdominal pain or discomfort is the first event and the appropriate medical treatment is effective, the disruptive behavior may diminish.
- **Epilepsy**
  The prevalence of epilepsy is increased in ASD and is even higher in those with co-occurring ID, ranging from 5 to 46% in various studies.[26] The clinician should be careful when individuals with ASD present a family history of seizures, multiple febrile seizures, a first-time afebrile seizure, sleep disturbances, ID with or without focal neurological abnormalities, or a history of regression. Pain has been described related to epileptic seizures, most often partial and atypical.
- **Dental disease**
  Dental conditions should be considered as a source of discomfort or pain, particularly in children presenting with irritability or agitation. Cavities, dental infection, and dental erosion are common sources of pain.

- **Menstrual pain or premenstrual syndrome**

  Some medical problems that emerge in adolescence may be difficult to identify in youths with ASD, particularly those who have communication difficulties. Migraine headaches may emerge during early to mid-adolescence. Careful attention should be paid to clinical manifestations of headache, including squeezing of the head or increased sensitivity to sound and light.

  Menstrual pain is another common cause of distress in adolescent girls with ASD and is often undertreated. Premenstrual dysphoric disorders should be considered when mood fluctuation occurs just before menstruation. Clinicians should be attentive to the possibility of epilepsy during adolescence and even extending into adulthood.

Other Sources of Pain

Many other conditions can cause pain or irritability, such as pressure sores, otitis, sinusitis, or fractures and dislocations. During the clinical examination, it is imperative to detect and manage them to avoid disruptive behaviors.

PAIN ASSESSMENT TOOLS

The identification and assessment of pain is the responsibility of everyone, including those close to the person with ASD or ID, including family members, caregivers, and professionals. If pain is detected, the assessment will be challenging and require knowledge and careful observation.

The assessment must be carried out using appropriate tools. It is important to keep in mind how changes in nonverbal and social behavior and inability to develop social relationships affect the standard use of these pain assessment tools. Poor eye contact or lack of social expression could negatively influence measurements. Tools developed to identify pain in people with intellectual disabilities[27,28] may provide ways to assess pain in people with severe cognitive impairment. Thus, we can consult the GED DI (pain/intellectual disability assessment grid), the EDAAP (assessment of pain in adolescents and adults with multiple disabilities), or the ESD (a pain assessment tool for individuals with communication disorders, the EDAAP adapted for ASD).

Barthelemy Durand Hospital developed a tool to help identify potentially acute pain. This tool: ESDDA: simplified pain assessment tool for people with communication difficulties in ASD,[23] is provided in Table 26.1

Table 26.1 USER GUIDE TO THE ESDDAA PAIN SCALE

Établissement public de santé
Barthélemy Durand

ESDDA

Simplified Pain Evaluation Scale for Dyscommunicative Autism Spectrum Disorders (Echelle Simplifiée d'Evaluation de la Douleur chez les personnes Dyscommunicantes avec troubles du spectre de l'Autisme)

Instructions: Answer YES or NO for each question. More than 2 YES answers in TOTAL indicates potential pain.

INDIVIDUAL BEING EVALUATED

First Name:
Last Name:
Date of Birth:

Date of Evaluation	..../..../....		..../..../....		..../..../....		..../..../....		..../..../....		..../..../....		..../..../....	
Time	....:...		....:...		....:...		....:...		....:...		....:...		....:...	
	YES	NO	YES	NO	YES	NO	YES	NO	YES	NO	YES	NO	YES	NO
1. Behaviour *Has there been a noticeable change?*														
2. Gestures and facial expressions *Has there been a noticeable change?*														
3. Audible expressions (cries, groans, etc.) *Has there been a noticeable change?*														
4. Sleep patterns *Has there been a noticeable change?*														
5. Opposition to care														
6. Identification of a painful area upon examination														
TOTAL NUMBER OF "YES" ANSWERS	/6		/6		/6		/6		/6		/6		/6	
Completed by														

Regional Centre for Pain and Somatic Care in Mental Health and Autism - Document written by Dr Isabelle Mytych and Dr Julie Renaud-Mierzejewski - Drafted on 31 January 2017

This scale defines six items: behavior, gestures and facial expression, audible expressions (cries, groans), sleep patterns, opposition to care, and identification of a painful area on examination. More than two positive answers in total indicate a potential pain. This tool can be used by health care as well as non–health care staff, including family members, caregivers, educators, social workers, and others.

Approaches focused on sensitive and specific methods for measuring nonverbal manifestations of pain and behavioral reactivity to procedural pain have been investigated, but the clinical usefulness of these methods is yet to be proved.[29]

PAIN MANAGEMENT IN AUTISM SPECTRUM DISORDER AND INTELLECTUAL DISABILITY

The management of pain must include the identification, when possible, of the painful pathology, its evaluation, and the preparation of treatment plans aimed at reducing problem behaviors. But, even with a careful history and specific approaches investigating irritability, identifying specific sources of pain may remain difficult. A pain-related diagnosis may not always be possible; however, even after a careful empiric evaluation, an empiric medication trial and careful ongoing assessment may be the only available management options.

Therapeutic options may be based on pharmacological and non-pharmacological options.[28]

Pharmacological Treatment

Analgesic treatments are prescribed according to the modalities of use in general population. However, special precautionary measures must be taken into account:

- Oral or transdermal routes of drug administration are preferred. Intramuscular injections should be avoided, especially in the event of prolonged treatment (muscle mass may be reduced, atypical stress).
- Because of bowel movement problems and the frequency of constipation, prolonged use of opioids should be avoided and take preventive measures.
- Topical anesthetic creams may be recommended for care-induced pain (e.g., for blood sampling), or an equimolar mixture of nitrogen protoxide and oxygen may be used for clinical pain assessment examinations.

Problem behavior in ASD may be the primary or sole symptom of an underlying illness causing pain, which can be acute or chronic. When pain or discomfort is a main complaint, the implementation of inappropriate treatment, such as psychotropic medication, or of aberrant behavioral interventions, including hypostimulation or isolation rooms, is ineffective and may worsen the clinical condition.

Nonpharmacological Options

Very few studies have been conducted on the effectiveness of nonpharmacological approaches to pain management in ASD patients. Physical approaches such as massage, touch, and hot and cold physiotherapy techniques can be very helpful. Other therapeutic strategies, such as music, certain osteopathic techniques, and adaptive physical activity, can be offered.

Some video entertainment tools can also be useful (digital tablets, movies, video games).

CONCLUSION

Medical comorbidities and pain can be difficult to recognize in patients suffering from ASD or ID. The failure to identify medical illness and pain is due in part to communication impairments and sometimes aberrant symptomatology. Widespread underdiagnoses and access barriers to appropriate health care for ASD are the result of commonly held beliefs that aberrant behaviors and symptoms are "just a part of autism."

Understanding the atypicality of autistic functioning in relation to the specific characteristics of pain perception and expression in people with ASD or ID must break with the long-standing assumption that these people are insensitive to pain. Behavioral changes should be a sign that there is an underlying experience of pain. The assessment of the pain and its treatment should be a priority. This assessment must be personalized, taking into account the problem behavior and its frequency, intensity, and duration, as well as its context and associated events. Pain in people with ASD, who are vulnerable, must be taken into account and treated as in any other individual. Leaving pain untreated clearly results in health inequalities and constitutes a gross injustice to people with ASD.

REFERENCES

1. Carr EG, Owen-Deschryver JS. Physical illness, pain and problem behavior in minimally verbal people with developmental disabilities. *J Autism Dev Disord.* 2007;37(3):413–423.
2. American Psychiatric Association. *Diagnostic and statistical manual of mental disorders.* 4th ed. Washington, DC: Author; 2000.
3. Bosch J, Van Dyke DC, Smith SM, Poulton S. Role of medical conditions in the exacerbation of self-injurious behavior: An exploratory study. *Ment Retard.* 1997;35(2):124–130.
4. Baranek GT. Tactile defensiveness in children with developmental disabilities: Responsiveness and habituation. *J Autism Dev Disord.* 1994;24:457–471.
5. Nader R, Oberlander TF, Chambers CT, Craig KD. Expression of pain in children with autism. *Clin J Pain.* 2004;20:88–97.
6. Wing L. *The Autistic Spectrum: A Guide for Parents and Professionals.* London, UK: Constable and Robinson, 2002.
7. Tordjman S, Anderson GM, Bottbol M, et al. Pain reactivity and plasma beta-endorphin in children and adolescents with autistic disorders. *PloS One.* 2009;4(8)e5289.
8. Pernon E, Rattaz C. Les modes d'expression de la douleur chez l'enfant autiste: Ètude comparée. *Devenir.* 2003;15(3):263–277.
9. Sahoun L, Saravane D. Autisme et douleur: Ètat des connaissances et conséquence pratique. *Douleurs.* 2015;16(1):21–25.
10. Dubois A, Rattaz C, Pry R, Baghdadli A. Autism and pain: A literature review. *Pain Res Manage.* 2010;15:245–253.
11. Tudor ME, Walsh CE, Mulder EC, Lerner MD: Pain as predictor of sleep problems in youth with autism spectrum disorders. *Autism.* 2014;19(3);292–300.
12. Chaidez V, Hansen RL, Hertz-Picciotto L. Gastrointestinal problems in children with autism, developmental delays or typical development. *J Autism Dev Disord.* 2014;44(5);1117–1127.
13. Chandler S, Carcani- Rathwell I, Charman T, et al. Parent reported gastrointestinal symptoms in children with autism spectrum disorders. *J Autism Dev Disord.* 2013;43(12):2737–2747.
14. Craig KD. The social communication model of pain. *Pain.* 2015;156(7):1198–1199.
15. Buie T, Campbell DB, Fuch GJ, et al. Evaluation, diagnosis and treatment of gastrointestinal disorders in individuals with ASDs: A consensus report. *Pediatrics.* 2010;125(suppl 1):S1–S18.
16. Buie T, Fuchs GJ, Furuta GT, et al. Recommendations for evaluation and treatment of common gastrointestinal problems in children with ASDs. *Pediatrics.* 2010;125(suppl 1):S19–S29.
17. Gilbert-Mac Leod CA, Craig KD, Rocha EM, Mathias MD. Everyday pain responses in children with and without developmental delays. *J Pediatr Psychol.* 2000;25(5):301–308.

18. Breau LM, Burkitt C. Assessing pain in children with intellectual disabilities. *Pain Res Manage.* 2009;14(2):116–120.

19. Bottos S, Chambers CT. The epidemiology of pain in developmental disabilities In: Symons F, Oberlander T, eds. *Pain in Children and Adults With Developmental Disabilities.* Baltimore, MD: Paul H. Brookes; 2006:67–87.

20. Coll MP, Gregoire M, Latimer M, Eugene F, Jackson PL. Perception of pain in others: Implications for caregivers. *Pain Manage.* 2011;1(3):257–265.

21. Haute Autorité de Santé. Qualité de Vie: Handicap, les Problèmes Somatiques et les Phénomènes Douloureux. Saint-Denis La Plaine, France: HAS; 2017.

22. Centre régional douleur et soins somatiques en santé mentale, autisme, polyhandicap et handicap génétique rare. EPS. http://www.eps-etampes.fr/offre-de-soins/centre-regional-douleur-et-soins-somatiques-en-sante-mentale-autisme-polyhandicap-et-handicap-genetique-rare/. Accessed November 1, 2018.

23. Saravane D, Mytych I. Douleur et autisme. *Douleur et Analgesie.* 2018;31:137–148.

24. Mytych I, Da Silva S, Mercier C, Bodin J, Ducreux E. Contention pour soins somatiques dans les troubles du spectre autistique. *Ethique et Santé.* 2019;16:15–19.

25. McElhanon BO, McCracken C, Karpen S, Sharp WC. Gastrointestinal symptoms in autism spectrum disorders: A meta-analysis. *Pediatrics.* 2014;133(5):872–883.

26. Spence SJ, Schneider MT. The role of epilepsy and epileptiform EEGs in autism spectrum disorders. *Pediatr Res.* 2009;65(5):599–606.

27. Breau LM, McGrath PJ, Camfield CS, Finley GA. Psychometric properties of the non-communicating children's pain check list revised. *Pain.* 2002;99(1–2):349–357.

28. Marchand S, Saravane D, Gaumond I, eds. *Mental Health and Pain: Somatic and Psychiatric Components of Pain in Mental Health.* Paris: Springer-Verlag France; 2013.

29. Oberlander TF, O'Donnell ME, Montgomery CJ. Pain in children with significant neurological impairment. *J Dev Behav Pediatr.* 1999;20(4):235–243.

PART V

Pain Medicine, Psychiatry, and Society

27

Cultural Spectrum of Chronic Pain and Somatization Syndromes

Indian Experiences

GEETHA DESAI, SANTOSH K. CHATURVEDI, AND DINESH BHUGRA ■

INTRODUCTION

Chronic pain is a common symptom in medical, as well as psychiatric, practice in India. Like in any other part of the world, chronic pain is a symptom of psychiatric disorders like depression, anxiety, somatoform disorders, and dissociative disorders in India. Fatigue, tiredness, and sensory symptoms are other common somatization presentations. As can be expected from the nature and site of the bodily symptoms, these first present to general practitioners, physicians, surgeons, neurologists, or other specialists. First consultation with a psychiatrist is an exception rather than a rule. The chronic pain and somatic symptoms may be the tip of an iceberg of underlying psychiatric disorders. Given the existence of several health care systems in India, many chronic pain patients seek relief from alternative systems, such as AYUSH, which includes Ayurveda, Yoga, Unani, Siddha, and Homeopathy. These systems take a different approach to understanding bodily symptoms. Body–mind dualism is not endorsed by these systems, which provide culturally sanctioned explanations for patients' symptoms. For example, in terms of causation, pain patients often use explanatory theories related to diet (hot food and cold food), breathing, temperature (especially body temperature), and physical activity/inactivity. Within such systems, there are well-known popular treatments that claim to have minimal side effects. In addition to AYUSH, there are traditional and faith healing systems—organized and not organized, that are also very popular, along with complementary and alternative medicine (CAM).

CHRONIC PAIN SYNDROMES IN INDIA

Chronic pain is often the most common symptom that makes a person seek help. Chronic pain has been recognized as pain that persists past normal healing time and that lasts or recurs for more than 3 to 6 months.[1] Pain states present with various affective, cognitive, and behavioral changes in the person. Pain is classified based on the cause, duration, and organ systems that are involved.

Chronic pain is a highly prevalent condition that is associated with significant functional disability. Chronic pain syndrome is of complex history and unclear etiology and often responds poorly to treatment. It also causes significant morbidity, suffering, and disability and overutilization of health services. Prevalence of chronic pain in the general population in India varies between 10 and 40%, and a study from India reported a point prevalence of 13%.[2,3] This variation exists because studies have used different definitions, different interview methods, and different population settings.[2]

The contribution of chronic pain toward the global burden of disease has been underestimated.[3] The term "burden of disease" indicates the gap between actual and ideal health status. It is measure in disability adjusted life years (DALY). The World Health Organization predicts that by 2030, the four leading contributors of global burden of disease will be unipolar depression, coronary heart disease, cerebrovascular disease, and road traffic accidents.[4] Chronic pain is an important comorbidity associated with all of these conditions. Chronic pain is not merely a comorbidity of other identifiable disease or injury but is now acknowledged as a clinical condition underpinned by an agreed set of definitions and taxonomy.[5,6]

There have been recent advances in understanding pain mechanisms that could bring in the possibility of new treatments, but management of chronic pain is nonetheless generally unsatisfactory; two-thirds of sufferers report dissatisfaction with current treatment, and most chronic pain persists for many years.[7] Many risk factors have been identified for development of chronic pain. Risk factors include sociodemographic, clinical, psychological, and biological factors. Apart from women reporting high rates of chronic pain, women consistently report lower pain thresholds, lower pain tolerance, and greater unpleasantness (or intensity) of pain with differential analgesic sensitivity.[8]

However, the greatest gender differences are seen in the prevalence of chronic pain syndromes.[9]

Comorbid Chronic Pain and Psychiatric Disorders

Anxiety, depression, and catastrophizing beliefs about pain are common in patients with chronic pain and may contribute to poor prognosis in people with various pain conditions.[10-13] The temporal relationship between chronic pain and mental health remains unclear and is likely to be bidirectional. There is evidence that the top-down (central and cognitive) influences on pain perception may be greater than the peripheral input.

Around the world, chronic pain is associated with a number of psychiatric conditions and has been found to be the main presenting symptom in 45 to 60% of patients.[14] Chronic pain was found to be a frequent symptom in anxiety neurosis (60%), neurotic depression (45%), and hysteria (24.3%). Less than 3% of patients with psychosis reported chronic pain.[14] Pain is a common symptom of the following psychiatric illnesses[15]:

- Depressive disorders
- Anxiety disorders
- Dissociative disorders
- Hypochondriasis
- Somatization disorder
- Other somatoform disorders.
- Drug dependence
- Alcoholism
- Personality disorders

Chronic pain is the main or chief complaint in up to 15 to 20% of psychiatry outpatients in psychiatric centers and institutions.[14,15] However, in general hospital psychiatry units, almost one-third of patients report chronic pain. In medical outpatient clinics, chronic pain is the main complaint in almost two-thirds of the patients.[15,16] Many chronic pain patients seek relief from CAM, AYUSH systems, or naturopathy. Thus, the figures of magnitude mentioned previously are not a true reflection of the prevalence of chronic pain in India. One could also say the same about bodily symptoms. Fatigue, tiredness, tingling and numbness, and other sensory somatic symptoms are a common presentation in medical, psychiatric, and CAM systems.

There are few research studies on the prevalence of chronic pain in India. A recent epidemiological telephone survey consisting of 5004 respondents from eight cities across India reported an overall point prevalence of chronic pain of 13%. The mean intensity of pain on a numerical scale was 6.93, with chronic moderate and chronic severe pain reported by 37 and 63% of respondents, respectively. Pain in the knees (32%), legs (28%), and joints (22%) was most prevalent. Respondents with chronic pain were no longer able to exercise, sleep, maintain relationships with friends and family, or maintain an independent lifestyle. About 32% of patients lost 4 hours or more of work in the past 3 months.[17]

In a study on the development of a National Institute of Mental Health and Neurosciences (NIMHANS) screening tool for psychological problems, subjects were assessed on the question related to frequent experience of body ache and headache in the past 1 week in an individual setting. Study results indicated that 27% (16% female, 11% male) experienced pain in the normal general population group, whereas in clinical categories, 14.5% of those with anxiety disorder (9.5% female, 5% male), 13.9% of those with depression (8.9% female, 5% male), 17.9% of those with obsessive-compulsive disorder (OCD) (8.5% female, 9.4% male), and 13.9% of substance users reported pain in past 7 days.[18]

Prevalence and characteristics of chronic pain were evaluated and compared in patients with a psychiatric diagnosis with and without chronic pain in a psychiatric setting. Chronic pain was reported by 14.37% of psychiatric patients. Of these, 43% had dysthymic disorder, 20% had anxiety states, and 20% had somatoform disorders. Compared with the control group, chronic pain patients were more often middle-aged, female, married, and from an urban habitat. There was a marked difference in the diagnostic breakdown between pain and control groups, with a predominance of dysthymic and anxiety disorders in pain patients. Major depression was found in equal proportions in pain and nonpain patients.[19]

Patients with chronic pain have a significantly higher incidence of depression. It has been suggested that chronic pain may be a depressive equivalent. Higher rates of depressive symptoms are found in chronic pain patients than in general and medical populations. Pain is more often seen in patients with dysthymia than in those with unipolar or bipolar depression as well as more often in those who are from urban backgrounds, female, and married. Depression is an important predictor of disability in chronic pain patients as well as a predictor of motivation for treatment.[15]

The common question of whether depression is a cause or consequence of chronic pain does not have easy answer. Depression is risk factor for development of chronic pain. Depression is not just a comorbid condition of chronic pain. Depressed chronic pain patients report greater pain intensity and less life control, use poor coping strategies, experience greater interference from pain, and exhibit more pain behaviors causing significant distress to others. Depression should not be considered as an understandable consequence of chronic pain; it should be evaluated and treated effectively.[15]

The relationship between pain and depression is complicated and unclear. Depression aggravates pain, and pain aggravates depression. Pain is many times considered as an equivalent of depressive disorder for a number of reasons:

1. Pain is a common symptom of depression.
2. Depression occurs frequently in pain patients.
3. Chronic pain and depression have similar features and symptoms.
4. Chronic pain and depression are associated with similar family histories.
5. Chronic pain and depression both respond to treatment with antidepressants.

The following may be possible reasons for increased report of chronic pain in depressed patients:

1. **Decreased pain threshold**, resulting in report of even slight pain as more severe and unpleasant. Depressed chronic pain patients reported greater pain intensity, greater interference due to pain, and more pain behaviors compared with nondepressed patients.
2. **Poor coping with pain**
3. **Biological abnormalities** that occur through the serotonergic pathways of the central nervous system. Both pain and depression responds to selective serotonin reuptake inhibitors.
4. **Genetic or familial role.** Family studies have reported increased risk for depression in first-degree relatives of patients with chronic pain compared with the general population. Similarly, relatives of idiopathic pain patients showed increased prevalence of depressive symptoms. Increased frequency of pain problems is seen in families of chronic pain suffers. In one study, 40 to 60% of chronic pain patients reported having a parent with chronic pain.[20]

Anxiety is a common and expected component of acute pain, whereas anxiety disorders are common in chronic pain patients. Panic disorder and generalized anxiety disorder are commonly reported disorders among chronic pain patients. Decreased pain threshold and increased preoccupation with somatic symptoms and pain may be a reason for increased anxiety symptoms and disorders in patients with chronic pain.

Substance use disorders are quite common among patients with chronic pain. However, the association is complex because substance use may precede the onset of chronic pain or happen because of long-standing distressing pain. Increased sensitivity to pain and pain-relieving effects of the substance may reinforce the use of the substance. Chronic pain patients who are treated with opioids are at higher risk for developing substance misuse disorders. In a study of chronic pain in subjects with alcohol dependence syndrome, 18% had chronic pain, with 49% reporting it to be severe in intensity.[21] Higher rates of attempted as well as completed suicide are associated with chronic pain.[22]

Clinical Presentations

Patients can present with a single site of pain, which is usually headache, pain in the joints, or leg pain, or can present with pain at multiple sites. In a recent study, 301 patients who presented with bodily symptoms reported headache as the main pain site, which might be because of the neuropsychiatry setting.[16] Likewise, patients with chest pain are likely to visit cardiology clinics. One of the unique presentations was "half body ache," which is not anatomically a plausible presentation.[16]

The common pain presentations are shown here:

Pain Presentation	Percentage Frequency
Headache	61
Pain in extremities	20
Whole body ache	11
Neck pain	7
Backache	7
Abdominal pain, discomfort, indigestion	4
Chest pain, chest discomfort	3
Half body pain, pain in left half/right half of the body, pain in testis, teeth, gums, ears	3

A structured assessment of pain presentations using the Scale for Assessment of Somatic Symptoms (SASS) among these 301 patients showed the following distribution:

Pain-Related Somatic Symptoms	Percentage Frequency
Headache	70
Pain in extremities	30
Backache	22
Whole body ache	19
Abdominal pain	6

The frequency of these pain symptoms was daily (83%), and the intensity of symptoms was severe in 85% of the patients. The symptoms interfered with sleep and appetite in 95% of the patients, and 91% experienced occupation dysfunction.[16]

Three common unusual presentations of chronic pain in India are discussed next: whole body ache, multiples aches and pains, and idiopathic chronic pain.

WHOLE BODY ACHE

Whole body ache or pain is a common presentation in medical clinics. These patients make up about 20% of all chronic pain patients and are a challenge to manage. Of 100 patients presenting with whole body chronic pain, nearly 33% fulfilled the American College of Rheumatology (ACR) criteria for fibromyalgia. In fact, most had one or more tender points, and 33% of patients had more than 10 tender points. The tender points were more common in patients who were diagnosed with somatoform disorder, occurred more often the left side than the right side, and were reported more frequently by females than males.[23] These findings need to be replicated, and the explanation for this phenomenon is still elusive.

MULTIPLE ACHES AND PAINS

Multiple aches and pains are another common presentation of chronic pain in India. Most patients report two or three pain sites, but some have numerous pain sites. This is a unique challenge for physicians because they consider these patients as having functional pain or medically unexplained symptoms. Assessment and management of all pain sites pose many difficulties. Asking for many investigations to understand all pain sites is not only expensive but also raises ethical dilemmas.[24] Each site of pain can have many causes; if, on examination, no pathology is found, should the physician extensively investigate each site, thereby increasing the financial burden as well risks associated with invasive investigations?

IDIOPATHIC CHRONIC PAIN

Many physicians and neurologists believe that all chronic pain that does not have positive findings on investigation is likely to be functional or psychological. However, studies have shown that not all pain patients who do not have positive findings on investigation have evidence of a psychiatric disorder. Such pain patients are classified as having idiopathic chronic pain, and they make up about 7 to 10% of chronic pain patients in India. Such patients need symptomatic medical and behavioral management, as well as regular follow-up, because there is a likelihood that an underlying medical or psychiatric disorder will be uncovered in due course of time.[25]

SOMATIZATION SYNDROMES IN INDIA

The features of somatization disorder include multiple, recurrent, and variable physical symptoms for which there is no adequate pathophysiological explanation; there is a persistent refusal to accept reassurance of several physicians that there is no physical explanation for these symptoms. Somatization or somatizing behavior has been construed as a form of communication even if this is a very concrete form of communication and devoid of any symbolic psychological abstraction. This may be a means of communicating subjective perceptions of somatic sensations that accompany states of affective distress. In that sense, somatization is understood as a manifestation of an underlying psychological distress. Somatization is also understood as a cultural idiom of communicating and expressing distress. People from non-Western cultures may be lacking in the capacity to label emotional states, or expression of emotions may be inhibited in these cultures, and stigma is associated with psychiatric illness.

Current Classification Status of Somatoform Disorders

Somatoform disorders are a group of disorders that are coded as various categories in the *International Statistical Classification of Diseases and Related Health Problems*, 10th revision (ICD-10),[26] as somatization disorder, hypochondriacal disorder, somatoform autonomic dysfunction, persistent somatoform pain disorder, undifferentiated somatoform disorder, and other somatoform disorders.

The *Diagnostic and Statistical Manual of Mental Disorders*, 5th edition (DSM-5),[27] has replaced the DSM-IV disorders of somatization disorder, hypochondriasis, pain disorder, and undifferentiated somatoform disorder with the somatic symptom disorder. The somatic symptom disorder does not require the symptoms to be medically unexplained, and there is no specific requirement of symptom counts from among the four symptom groups for somatization disorder. However, somatic symptoms must be significantly distressing or disruptive to everyday life and must be accompanied by excessive thoughts, feelings, or behaviors. This change in emphasis in DSM-V removes the mind–body separation implied in DSM-IV[28] and encourages clinicians to make a comprehensive assessment and use clinical judgment. The proposed bodily distress disorder of ICD-11 will consider some of these concerns.

Epidemiology of Somatization in India

Large-community epidemiological data on the prevalence of somatoform disorder in India are lacking. Earlier studies have included it under hysteria and neurosis. The studies conducted were in medical settings, where the prevalence of common mental disorders was reported to be about 30 to 50%. The presentations of bodily symptoms varied highly, with unique symptoms like pain in the left cornea. In the study of patients with bodily symptoms, subjects were diagnosed to have anxiety, depression, and stress-related disorders.[16] The most common bodily symptoms presented were the following:

Chief Presenting Complaints	Percentage Frequency
Nerves beating, pulling sensation, numbness, reeling sensation, pulsating sensation in the head	6
Buzzing head, heaviness of head, jhum-jhum sensation in the head	6
Burning sensation in the head and other parts of the body	5
Tiredness, weakness, fatigue	5
Indigestion, abdominal discomfort	4
Chest discomfort	3
Giddiness, dizziness, heat and cold sensations, nausea	3
Bowel "inevacuation" (a sense of incomplete evacuation of bowels), constipation, palpitations, breathing difficulty, "worms crawling" sensation, left cornea pain, redness of eyes, belching, obstruction sensation in the throat, palate not felt, foul smell from mouth	Occasional

Somatic symptoms as noted by systematic assessment using SASS were as follows:

Sensory Somatic Symptoms	Percentage Frequency
Palpitations	13
Tingling, numbness	10
Sensation of gas bloating	8
Burning sensation	8
Heat and cold sensations	6

Nonspecific Somatic Symptoms	
Weakness of body	38
Giddiness, dizziness, fainting	9
Weakness of mind	5
Trembling, tremors	4
Tiredness, lethargy	4

Somatization Syndromes

The most common somatization syndromes that have been described in India are as follows:

Somatization Syndromes in India
Dhat syndrome
Female dhat syndrome
Leukorrhea
Sinking heart
Jhum-jhum syndrome
Somatic neurosis

Dhat syndrome is characterized by feelings of weakness of body and mind and attributed to loss of semen through night falls and masturbation; it leads to significant distress to the individual.[29]

Female dhat syndrome is noted in gynecological, medical, and psychiatric clinics. Women frequently attribute their physical symptoms to their passing of vaginal discharge. When the women were asked about their explanations for the cause of this white discharge per vagina, or leukorrhea, different factors were mentioned, like dietary factors, excess of heat (or cold) in the body, emotional factors and stress, physical activity of any nature, and tubectomy.[30,31]

Leukorrhea as a symptom is associated with a complex of cultural meanings as well as multiple etiologies. Prevalent etiological notions of leukorrhea include a dissolving of bones, loss of dhatu (vital fluid), and overheat.[32] Leukorrhea may represent a culturally shaped "bodily idiom of distress," in which concerns about loss of genital secretions reflect wider issues of social stress. Problems may arise when a symptom with deep cultural meaning is interpreted in a purely biomedical framework. A woman who has been experiencing bodily symptoms including excessive genital secretions might request a hysterectomy.[33]

Sinking heart is an illness in which physical sensations in the heart or in the chest are experienced, and these symptoms are thought to be caused by excessive heat, exhaustion, worry, or social failure. The Punjabi model of sinking heart offers an emic explanation of somatic symptoms. It is based on culturally specific ideas about the person, the self, and the heart and on the assumption that physical, emotional, and social symptoms of pathology accompany each other. The Punjabi model of sinking heart does not exactly correspond to medical models of heart distress. The sinking heart model bears closest resemblance to a Western model of stress. The similarity between these two models is in the form rather than in the content.[34]

Jhum-jhum syndrome is observed in medical practice in Nepal, north India, and the hilly regions of Garhwal. It presents with sensory symptoms, mainly tingling and numbness, without evidence of neurological deficits. There are no obvious social or psychological stresses. It is a form of expressing distress, dissatisfaction, and displeasure in the community and considered as an acceptable form of illness and adaptive role.[35]

Somatic neurosis was described in women presenting with multiple somatic complaints, mainly aches and pains, fatigue, and tiredness. It was seen commonly in Muslim women and later was studied and noted in Hindu women as well. There were no obvious psychosocial stresses; rather these women had an impoverished, restrictive social environment, where complaining of somatic symptoms was acceptable, without any stigma. This was subsequently confirmed in the community studies.[36]

Unusual Presentations

Postorgasmic somatic symptoms of whole body ache, feverish feeling, and tiredness were reported by an individual following sexual intercourse. He was diagnosed to have somatoform disorder.[37]

Asneezia, or the inability to sneeze, has been reported as a highly distressing symptom for which persons seek consultation. A middle-aged man who presented with headache, pain in the scar on his head, and asneezia had sought multiple consultations from physicians and was referred to psychiatry for evaluation. On assessment, abnormal illness behavior was documented.[38]

Physiokundalini entails bodily symptoms reported in relation to the "rising of kundalini" in some people who practice this type of yoga. Individuals with unexplained bodily symptoms often attribute the condition to certain foods, external forces, and spiritual experiences. In one case, a woman who had tingling and pain in her lower limbs discussed the spiritual component to which the symptoms were attributed.[39]

Treatment-seeking behaviors were also noted. The majority of patients with pain and bodily symptoms seek help from physicians and other health professionals before reaching mental health services. The most common sources of treatment are as follow:

Mode of Help Sought (Not in Decreasing Frequency)
Family doctors
Self-medication
Ayurveda
Faith healers
Religion
Homemade remedies
Homeopathy
Physiotherapy
Exercise
Herbal medicine
Reiki
Massage therapy
Acupuncture
Unani
Yoga, acupressure, naturopathy, aromatherapy

Psychiatric Assessment of Chronic Pain in India

Assessment of chronic pain and somatic symptoms is challenging because patients often meet mental health professionals after many months or years of illness. Since symptoms are subjective experiences that cause suffering to the individual, measuring and quantifying them can be a challenge for health professionals. Apart from the symptoms assessment, it is important to understand patients' explanatory models, experiences with health professionals, psychosocial risk factors, and cultural underpinnings of their symptoms.

The SASS is widely used in India to measure the somatic symptoms and their severity in clinical settings. The scale has four subscales, namely, pain-related symptoms, sensory somatic symptoms, nonspecific somatic symptoms, and biological function–related symptoms. The severity of somatic symptoms is rated form 1 to 3—1 = mild, 2 = moderate, and 3 = severe. The somatic symptoms are said to be present if the symptoms have occurred during the previous 2 weeks. It has been used in assessing somatization in different groups and cancer patients. When used for measurement of somatic symptoms in a disease like cancer, besides the severity scores, there is a provision to differentiate whether the physical symptoms are purely organic, purely psychological, both organic and psychological, or neither physical nor psychogenic (idiopathic).[40]

The SASS is also a useful scale to measure the severity and nature of pain as well as somatic or bodily symptoms.[41] Clinically, however, a visual or numerical analog scale (0 to 10, or 0 to 100) is used. Other alternatives include asking patients who have low literacy to assess severity of their pain in terms of how many paisa of a rupee (for percentage of distress). The pain behaviors of the individual often determine the ratings of pain intensity; sadly, this is an observation confirmed by our studies.[42] Pain is a subjective sensation, and hence rating of severity by objective signs of pain behaviors could lead to overestimation or underestimation of pain, which can be rectified only by training workshops on pain assessment for health professionals.

Management of Chronic Pain and Somatic Symptoms in India

Chronic pain and somatic/bodily symptoms need multidisciplinary and multipronged management. The goals of management are to maintain appropriate illness behavior, avoid doctor shopping and needless investigations, and plan rehabilitation. The final outcome of management is to live with chronic pain and bodily symptoms with as much activity as possible and as good a quality of life as possible. In the Indian setting where multiple explanatory models exist and where multiple treatment modalities are available, it is important to be aware of the same goals and incorporate a pluralistic approach into the clinical practice.

PHARMACOLOGICAL TREATMENT

Treatment of patients with chronic pain and somatic symptoms is often challenging. Symptoms often fail to respond to various treatments, and when they do, the initial response is often followed by fluctuations and exacerbations. The aims of treatment are not just symptom removal or reduction but more also reduction of psychological distress and improvement of the patient's functionality and quality of life.

Chronic pain and somatization can occur alone or with concomitant emotional or physical symptoms or comorbid psychiatric illness. A holistic treatment approach with both pharmacological and nonpharmacological components is therefore essential.

Treatment of chronic pain targets various pathophysiological central and peripheral pathways. Taking into consideration that pain symptoms are a large component of unexplained somatic/medical symptom complexes, pharmacological therapies that help pain syndromes are found to be useful in patients with medically unexplained symptoms (MUS).

A review of the pharmacological treatments in somatoform disorders and MUS concluded that the quality of research evidence available currently was low (most studies were short-term, with a relatively small number of participants and a high risk for bias).[43]

Adverse effects of pharmacological agents can further add to the distress and disability experienced by this group of patients, and the clinician must balance the risk-to-benefit ratio when prescribing. It is with this in mind that appropriate pharmacotherapy for chronic pain and MUS should take place. Psychotropic medications, especially antidepressants, have an important role in managing pain and somatization in India.

NONPHARMACOLOGICAL MANAGEMENT

Individuals suffering from chronic pain and somatic symptom disorders add a significant burden to clinical and health care providers owing to their excessive health care use. Such individuals keep changing their doctors because they have a firm belief that there is a biological cause behind their somatic symptoms and experience frustration if diagnostic evaluations fail to establish any medical cause. Standard medical care has been relatively unsuccessful in treating somatic symptoms. Psychological or psychiatric referral is often not appreciated and is considered stigmatizing because of poor psychological insight among such patients. Hence, management of somatic symptom disorder poses challenges for clinicians, and there is general agreement that such individuals are difficult to treat. Because standard medical care has been relatively unsuccessful in treating somatic symptoms, alternative behavioral and psychological interventions have been developed. These interventions can broadly be divided into two categories:

1. Those developed on the principles of behavioral and cognitive behavioral approaches delivered by trained therapists and physicians; these include cognitive behavioral therapy, reattribution therapy, and mindfulness and acceptance-based approaches
2. Those developed for the general practitioner; these include psychiatric consultation intervention and symptoms clinic intervention (SCI). SCI is comprises four key elements: recognition, explanation, action and learning. *Recognition* focuses on eliciting and actively listening to the patients' description of their illness and its consequences on daily living. The next focus is on negotiating *explanations* for symptoms in terms of biological and psychological mechanisms and adaptations and proposing *action* in terms of symptom control and management techniques. The doctor and patient reflect and *learn* what makes sense and what is helpful.[44]

COMPLEMENTARY AND ALTERNATIVE MEDICINE

Although many pharmacological and nonpharmacological management strategies have been used for chronic pain and somatization, most have shown marginal rates of effectiveness as well as poor acceptance by many patients. Also, pharmacological approaches may not help in better coping with stress. Consequently, a high proportion of these pain patients use CAM therapies, especially those who do not want medications.[45] Satisfaction with CAM therapies tends to be high, with studies showing that 63% of CAM users perceived their therapy to be extremely effective. CAM practitioners are said to take a holistic approach to treatments, treating not just the health concern but also the psychological issues that may interact with the medical problem.

In developing countries, the wide use of CAM is often attributable to its accessibility and affordability and the fact that it is firmly embedded within wider belief systems. An open-label trial of yoga-based therapeutic intervention was conducted for patients with somatoform pain disorder in India. Significant improvements were reported in pain and sleep in patients who underwent yoga-based intervention.[46] One must also be aware of the ethical dilemmas in the management of chronic pain and somatic symptoms.[24] More details on chronic pain and somatization syndromes in psychiatric patients are provided in a recently published book on chronic pain and MUS.[47]

CONCLUSION

Chronic pain is common presenting symptom of underlying psychiatric syndromes and can also be a comorbid condition. However, it is not considered as a symptom of depression or anxiety by nonpsychiatrist physicians. Unexplained chronic pain is often diagnosed as somatoform pain disorder. Another diagnostic category used when physical and psychological factors are not elicited is idiopathic pain. Classification of pain in psychiatry syndromes is challenging because pain could be comorbid with other psychiatric disorders. In many chronic pain conditions, the cause is not evident. Hence, assessment of pain as a standalone symptom might be useful. Assessment of pain is essential, including the site, location, intensity, and aggravating and relieving factors. Specific scales like SASS, which has a subscale on pain, might be useful in clinical assessments. Management of pain in psychiatric settings is essential because it is an overlooked common symptom. Further, understanding the complex relationship between pain and psychiatric syndromes will help clinicians in their appropriate management. The goal of management of the spectrum of chronic pain and somatization syndromes in India is same as elsewhere in the world—to live with pain with dignity and as good a quality of life as possible— however, management differs from person to person.

REFERENCES

1. Harvey AM. Classification of chronic pain: Descriptions of chronic pain syndromes and definitions of pain terms. *Clin J Pain*. 1995;11(2):163.
2. Verhaak PF, Kerssens JJ, Dekker J, Sorbi MJ, Bensing JM. Prevalence of chronic benign pain disorder among adults: A review of the literature. *Pain*. 199830;77(3):231–239.
3. Croft P, Blyth FM, van der Windt D. The global occurrence of chronic pain: An introduction. In: *Chronic Pain Epidemiology: From Aetiology to Public Health*. Oxford, UK: Oxford University Press; 2010:9–18.
4. World Health Organization. *The global burden of disease: 2004 update*. Geneva: WHO; 2008.
5. Turk DC, Rudy TE. Toward an empirically derived taxonomy of chronic pain patients: Integration of psychological assessment data. *J Consult Clin Psychol*. 1988;56(2):233.
6. Tracey I, Bushnell MC. How neuroimaging studies have challenged us to rethink: Is chronic pain a disease? *J Pain*. 2009;10(11):1113–1120.
7. Elliott AM, Smith BH, Hannaford PC, Smith WC, Chambers WA. The course of chronic pain in the community: Results of a 4-year follow-up study. *Pain*. 2002;99(1):299–307.
8. Greenspan JD, Craft RM, LeResche L, et al. Studying sex and gender differences in pain and analgesia: A consensus report. *Pain*. 2007;132:S26–S45.

9. Dionne C, Dunn K, Croft P. Does back pain prevalence really decrease with increasing age? A systematic review. *Age Ageing.* 2007;35:229–234.

10. Boersma K, Linton SJ. Psychological processes underlying the development of a chronic pain problem: A prospective study of the relationship between profiles of psychological variables in the fear-avoidance model and disability. *Clin J Pain.* 2006;22(2):160–166.

11. van der Windt D, Croft P, Penninx B. Neck and upper limb pain: More pain is associated with psychological distress and consultation rate in primary care. *J Rheumatol.* 2002;29(3):564–569.

12. van der Windt DA, Kuijpers T, Jellema P, van der Heijden GJ, Bouter LM. Do psychological factors predict outcome in both low-back pain and shoulder pain? *Ann Rheum Dis.* 2007;66(3):313–319.

13. Nijrolder I, van der Windt D, van der Horst H. Prediction of outcome in patients presenting with fatigue in primary care. *Br J Gen Pract.* 2009;59(561):e101–9.

14. Chaturvedi SK. Prevalence of chronic pain in psychiatric patients. *Pain.* 1987;29(2):231–237.

15. Bair MJ, Robinson RL, Katon W, Kroenke K. Depression and pain comorbidity: A literature review. *Arch Intern Med.* 2003;163(20):2433–2445.

16. Desai G. Patterns of illness behaviour among subjects with chronic non-organic pain. Unpublished doctoral dissertation; Guide SK Chaturvedi, NIMHANS. Bangalore, India: 2015.

17. Dureja GP, Jain PN, Shetty N, et al. Prevalence of chronic pain, impact on daily life, and treatment practices in India. *Pain Pract.* 2014;14(2):E51–E62.

18. Sharma MK, Chaturvedi SK. Pain in mental health setting and community: An exploration. *Indian J Psychol Med.* 2014;36(1):98.

19. Chaturvedi SK, Michael A. Chronic pain in a psychiatric clinic. *J Psychosom Res.* 1986;30(3):347–354.

20. Chaturvedi SK. Family morbidity in chronic pain patients. *Pain.* 1987;30(2):159–168.

21. Rohilla J, Desai G, Chand PK. Prevalence of chronic pain in patients with alcohol dependence syndrome in tertiary care center in India. *ASEAN Journal of Psychiatry* 2016;17(2):199–208.

22. Calati R, Bakhiyi CL, Artero S, Ilgen M, Courtet P. The impact of physical pain on suicidal thoughts and behaviors: Meta-analyses. *J Psychiatr Res.* 2015;71:16–32.

23. Somshekar BS, Chaturvedi SK, Desai G, Faruq U. Fibromyalgia tender points in chronic pain patients. *Indian J Psychiatry.* 2002;44:68.

24. Desai G, Chaturvedi SK. Ethical dilemmas of medically unexplained symptoms. *Indian J Med Ethics.* 2016;1(2):129.

25. Chaturvedi SK. Chronic idiopathic pain disorder. *J Psychosom Res.* 1986;30(2):199–203.

26. World Health Organization. *The ICD-10 Classification of Mental and Behavioural Disorders: Clinical Descriptions and Diagnostic Guidelines.* Geneva: Author; 1992.

27. American Psychiatric Association, American Psychiatric Association. *Diagnostic and Statistical Manual of Mental Disorders.* 4th ed. Washington, DC: Author; 1994:143–147.

28. American Psychiatric Association, American Psychiatric Association. *Diagnostic and Statistical Manual of Mental Disorders.* 5th ed. Washington, DC: Author; 2013.

29. Chadda RK. Dhat syndrome: Is it a distinct clinical entity?. *Acta Psychiatr Scand.* 1995;91(2):136–139.
30. Chaturvedi SK. Psychaesthenic syndrome related to leukorrhoea in Indian women. *J Psychosom Obstet Gynecol.* 1988;8(1):67–72.
31. Chaturvedi SK, Chandra PS, Isaac MK, Sudarshan CY. Somatization misattributed to non-pathological vaginal discharge. *J Psychosom Res.* 1993;37(6):575–579.
32. Nichter M. Idioms of distress: Alternatives in the expression of psychosocial distress. A case study from South India. *Cult Med Psychiatry.* 1981;5(4):379–408.
33. Trollope-Kumar K. Cultural and biomedical meanings of the complaint of leukorrhea in South Asian women. *Trop Med Int Health.* 2001;6(4):260–266.
34. Krause IB. Sinking heart: A Punjabi communication of distress. *Soc Sci Med* 1989;29(4):563–575.
35. Kohrt BA. "Somatization" and "comorbidity": A study of jhum jhum and depression in rural Nepal. *Ethos.* 2005;33(1):125–147.
36. Janakiramaiah N. Somatic neurosis in middle-aged Hindu women. *Int J Soc Psychiatry.* 1982;29(2):113–116.
37. Desai G, Chaturvedi SK, Sharma M. Medically unexplained symptoms explained!!!! A case of post orgasmic illness syndrome. *Indian J Med Case Rep.* 2013;2(1):18–20.
38. Chaturvedi SK, Desai G, Sharma MK. Asneezia: A medically unexplained symptom and abnormal illness behavior. Review of literature and a case report. *Arab J Psychiatry.* 2012;23(2):175–177.
39. Paradkar A, Chaturvedi SK. Physio-kundalini syndrome with neurocognitive deficits. *Int J Cult Ment Health.* 2010;3(1):25–33.
40. Chaturvedi SK, Hopwood P, Maguire P. Non-organic somatic symptoms in cancer. *Eur J Cancer.* 1993;29(7):1006–1008.
41. Desai G, Chaturvedi SK, Dahale A, Marimuthu P. On somatic symptoms measurement: The scale for assessment of somatic symptoms revisited. *Indian J Psychol Med.* 2015;37(1):17–19.
42. Desai G, Chaturvedi SK, Krishnaswamy L. Does pain behavior influence assessment of pain severity? *Indian J Palliat Care.* 2014;20(2):134–136.
43. Kleinstauber M, Witthoft M, Steffanowski A, et al. Pharmacological interventions for somatoform disorders in adults. *Cochrane Database Syst Rev.* 2014;(11):CD010628.
44. Burton C, Weller D, Marsden W, Worth A, Sharpe M. A primary care Symptoms Clinic for patients with medically unexplained symptoms: Pilot randomized trial. *BMJ Open.* 2012;2(1):e000513.
45. Wren AA, Wright MA, Carson JW, Keefe FJ. Yoga for persistent pain: New findings and directions for an ancient practice. *Pain.* 2011;152(3):477.
46. Sutar R, Desai G, Varambally S, Gangadhar BN. Yoga-based intervention in patients with somatoform disorders: An open label trial. *Int Rev Psychiatry.* 2016;28(3):309–315.
47. Desai G, Chaturvedi SK, eds. Medically unexplained somatic symptoms and chronic pain: Assessment and management. In: *A Primer for Healthcare Professionals.* 1st ed. Hyderabad, India: Paras Medical Publishers; 2017.

28

Jaki, a Puzzling Inca Syndrome of Comorbid Pain and Mental Illness

MARIO INCAYAWAR ■

THE NATURE OF *JAKI*

Jaki is a widespread condition among the Quichua-Inca people of the Andes in South America. It is a health condition familiar to an estimated 28 million Quichua-speaking people.[1] This culture-bound syndrome, however, is almost unknown by the local biomedically trained physicians, who are Spanish-speaking Latinos known by the Quichua people as *mishu*.* The result of this neglect is an outrageous exclusion of Indigenous Peoples from the mental health services available in the Andean countries.[2] We will approach *Jaki* from two opposed perspectives: the etic view embraced by local *mishu* doctors, mental health professionals, and policymakers, and the emic view that will reveal the theories of illness as articulated by Indigenous Peoples. Unraveling the nature

---

* *Mishu* is the Quichua term that refers to the dominant Spanish-speaking group in Latin America. They are individuals who have partial Indigenous descent but seek to identify themselves as whites and as being of European descent only, and who reject their Indigenous roots. They are also known in Spanish as *Mestizos* or *Latinos*.

of *Jaki* in a cross-cultural clinical encounter is challenging and often puts the even well-intentioned practitioner in a quandary.

The *Mishu* Perspective

The illness experience of Quichua patients and the way they express it are quite unique and bound to their culture and worldview. The clinical encounter with a Quichua patient suffering from *Jaki* could be perplexing or annoying to the *mishu* doctor. This is particularly true for a practitioner who does not speak Quichua and does not share basic values and views about illness and disease and how *Jaki* should be treated. The doctor will experience the same feelings as when dealing with a mysterious condition or when trying to understand a patient who speaks a foreign language and nobody could assist with a translation.

The symptoms presented by the Quichua patient suffering from *Jaki* are the ones we commonly encounter in general medical practice in any society. But the way they present to the physician will vary. Usually, those patients will mostly display a wide array of somatic symptoms such as headaches, fatigue, nausea, vomiting, minor fever, and migratory pain, among others. Moreover, they will rarely disclose psychological symptoms to their *mishu* doctors. With this clinical picture in hand, the physician will try to engage in symptom pattern recognition and often will fail. The practitioner will frequently have the impression that *Jaki* patients seems to have all kinds of symptoms. The doctor never gets a clear profile of symptoms or a pattern that would allow a proper diagnosis. For this reason, researchers suggest that the identification of this culture-bound syndrome should not be based on symptom configuration but rather on the local causes attributed to it.[3]

At least two factors account for the clinical conundrum experienced by the *mishu* doctor: (1) lack of knowledge regarding the nature of *Jaki*, and (2) physicians' ethnic/racial bias or poor cultural competency.

LACK OF KNOWLEDGE ABOUT *JAKI*

Despite the fact that *Jaki* is a highly prevalent condition in the Andes where millions of Quichua people live, the physicians are almost unaware of its existence. Usually, the doctors will consider in their clinical judgments the most familiar somatic symptoms presented to them. Because of linguistic and sociocultural barriers or simply the ease of disregarding a challenging case, they make a detour from a correct diagnosis. Based on a misdiagnosis such as "lack of vitamins," malnutrition, pain, and parasitic disease, among others, the treatment offered for *Jaki* will be vitamins, aspirin or combination of analgesics, and occasionally medicines against parasites. As a result of misdiagnosis and poor treatment, some patients will return complaining of the same symptoms, which could lead the doctor to dismissing the patient. Eventually, these poorly informed and culturally incompetent doctors could declare that nothing is wrong and "all is in your head." On occasions, when patients explicitly claim to have *Jaki*, physicians will argue that it is not a real illness but rather is an ailment resulting from superstition, and therefore is a complaint lacking any clinical importance. This misunderstanding reinforces the deeply held belief among the Quichua people that the *mishu* doctor knows little about *Jaki*, or is not qualified to treat it. Understandably, some patients will not return, realizing that the doctor does not give credit to their complaints and that the treatment offered does not work. Consequently, the misdiagnosis, poor-quality treatment, and plain medical errors frequently do not translate into relief for the patient. Probably because of this substandard and culturally insensitive care and a centuries-long history of neglect and conflict, most Quichua patients are fearful of seeking care from biomedically trained doctors. The doctors' lack of knowledge about *Jaki* clearly contributes to their disgraceful image and reputation within the Quichua society in the Andes.

PHYSICIANS' ETHNIC OR RACIAL BIAS

Appallingly, the World Health Organization reported that Indigenous Peoples are racially discriminated against and are treated as second-class citizens and as inferiors. Physicians in the Andes are almost exclusively unilingual Spanish speakers, and they rarely interact with the Quichua people outside the clinical field. This is one source of the serious language barrier and miscommunication between doctors and Inca patients. It is worth noting that the ruthless relationship between the first inhabitants of the Andes and the dominant *mishu* group is centuries long and is barely improving. In the biased postcolonial view, the Indigenous Peoples of the Americas, including the Quichua people of the Andes, are viewed as savages and as dangerous, dirty, unhealthy, illiterate, violent, stoic, and backward people and thus as a barrier to progress. It is not surprising to find that in many countries in the Americas, not only the military but also health policymakers will whisper that the "best Indian is a dead Indian." It is the history of brutal colonialism and oppression over the past five centuries in the Americas that have allowed the development of this imagery. These deeply entrenched and generalized prejudices in the mainstream *mishu* society enable expressions of racism, bigotry, ostracism, bias, and discrimination against the Americas' first inhabitants within all spheres of everyday life, including the medical setting. Predictably, Casagrande, an American anthropologist visiting Ecuador, stated, "Racism in Ecuador is institutionalized to a degree that would shock many oppressed peoples elsewhere."[4, p. 261]

The most dramatic manifestation of racial profiling and ostracism occurred two decades ago when an entire population was blamed for the outbreak of cholera epidemics that threatened the public health of an entire nation. For nearly a decade, in the 1990s, a particularly deadly epidemic of cholera surged in Ecuador and other neighboring countries. Thousands died, and entire communities were in a panic. Public health officials and health services in the country were overwhelmed. Shamefully, health professionals, health officials, and the lay *mishu* population accused the Quichua people of this public health crisis. Soon, on the streets, in public places, and in hospitals, *mishu* (Latinos) were blaming the Quichua people's bad costumes, hygiene, habits, values, and culture as the sole cause of the cholera epidemic. They literally blamed the victims of this deadly disease for the epidemic and deflected the responsibility of the outbreaks from the public health institutions and health officials to the Quichua victims. This phenomenon of blaming an entire group for an epidemic affected not only Ecuador but also other countries in the region, including Venezuela.[5] Many *mishu* doctors and health policymakers concluded: "If they are not able to help themselves, why should we help them?" Throughout history in Ecuador, diseases that ravaged the Quichua people, such as malnutrition, goiter, tuberculosis, and others, were attributed to their bad cultural traits and behavior rather than to consequences of the outrageous poverty, slavery, systematic blatant racism, and marginalization to which they were subjected for centuries.

The racist ideology in the Andes is equivalent to that which existed in North America in the 19th century. It was believed that the "savages," including Native Americans and African Americans, were incapable of feeling pain; only civilized whites, particularly of European origin, were highly sensitive to pain. They even made up a disease called "dysesthesia aethiopsis" or "obtuse sensibility of body" as being present among African Americans. This disease was thought to render them insensitive to pain when subjected to punishment.[6,7]

Appallingly, just months ago, I witnessed plain racial prejudice in a locally well-regarded social security hospital of Quito, Ecuador. The head of the Department of Psychiatry, during a moment of socializing, jokingly said: "I do not pay too much attention to dirt and germs in this overcrowded hospital, because I took longomycine," and laughed. "Longo" is a pejorative slur in Spanish used to insult an indigenous person, and "mycine" is a medical suffix usually added at the end of antibiotics' names, such as neomycin and erythromycin. She conveyed the idea that having lived in a dirty, nonhygienic way, as she assumes Indigenous Peoples live, she was not afraid of germs and was highly immune to infections in her hospital.

The medical encounters in the Andes between the *mishu* practitioners and the Quichua patients are troubling. One way to solve health professionals' ethnic and racial bias in the region should be through awareness and education. Doctors in South America receive no training on implicit racial bias or cultural sensitivity. Medical schools in the Andes do not require medical students to learn the Quichua language. Another way to attempt to solve the problem could be helping young Indigenous Peoples to pursue a career in medicine and the health professions. Unfortunately, this option has proved to be almost unapproachable. Thirty years ago, I was the first Quichua person to graduate from a medical school in the Andes. Today, there are only five Quichua physicians for a population of 5.5 million Quichua people in Ecuador.[8]

If we want to move to a more equitable society with better quality medical care, then the *mishu* doctors must contend with the ingrained racial bias, bigotry, and prejudice. When Quichua patients make the decision to visit a doctor, they are afraid to encounter a hostile and racist doctor. Any sign of cultural insensitivity, bias, or racial hostility will render Quichua patients suspicious and fearful. A somber intuition will develop that they will not be helped or treated respectfully but rather will be humiliated, attacked, or even killed by *mishu* health professionals.[2]

The Quichua Perspective

One of the first steps that physicians should take in a medical encounter with patients from cultural backgrounds other than their own is to learn the basics of their patients' health belief system. This will help them improve communication, both by improving their understanding of their patients' illness and symptoms description and by improving their ability to negotiate and explain appropriate treatment options to the patients. The goal of the physician in this context is not to become an anthropological expert but to become aware of cultural differences and gain some grasp of patients' theory of illness.

Jaki is a complex illness category composed of four subtypes. Contrary to Western biomedical nosology, the subtypes of *Jaki* are differentiated mainly by their causes rather than their symptoms. Moreover, according to the Quichua people, each of the subtypes of *Jaki* requires a specific treatment strategy. *Jaki* is divided into four illnesses: *mancharishca-wairashca* (victim of evil spirits; for brevity, these two illnesses are merged into one), *shungu nanay* (heart pain), and *rurashka* (sorcery).[3]

MANCHARISHCA-WAIRASHCA (VICTIM OF EVIL SPIRITS)
In this theory of illness, a person who experiences intense fright and fear can develop *mancharishca-wairashca*. This fright results in the temporary separation of the person's spirit from the body. This wandering spirit is vulnerable and

could be taken by evil spirits from nature (*cucucuna*). In the case of *wairashca*, evil winds or particles of misfortune can enter the person's body, causing illness.

In *mancharishca*, the patient's spirit leaves the body as a result of experiencing an intense fright. It is thought that at that moment, *cucucuna*, present everywhere in nature, can sequester the person's spirit and hold it captive. The separation of the spirit from the body is thought to cause the symptoms. The treatment is aimed at negotiating with the evil spirits and liberating the patient's captive spirit and reintroducing it into the body. In the case of *wairashca*, evil winds (*waira*) or particles of misfortune (*chiki*) suddenly enter the frightened person's body. A variety of signs and symptoms will follow the exposure to those evil winds or particles of misfortune.

There are many potential sources of fright. Fright can be triggered by humans, animals, plants, and inanimate objects. Some of the most severe causes of fright are inanimate objects such as waterfalls, water springs, and ditches. After a person suffers from *mancharishca*, the illness can last from 1 week to several months. *Wairashca*, on the other hand, is usually an acute illness, lasting about a week, when treated. Without treatment, however, *wairashca* is believed to become chronic, last months or years, and become resistant to treatment. The symptoms of *mancharishca-wairashca* include a wide range of psychological and somatic symptoms such as sadness, irritability, insomnia, diarrhea, back pain, fever, thirst, and tremors, among others.

SHUNGU NANAY (HEART PAIN)

Shungu nanay is an illness that originates from experiences of hardship and sorcery. A series of negative life events can lead to *shungu nanay*. Common examples of negative life events include land disputes, the death of a relative, loss of a valued animal, family plights or conflicts with *mishu* (Latinos), poverty, illness, lost harvests, marital conflicts, social exclusion, and lack of social support, among others. At first, a person may experience *pinsamintu*, a complex emotional state composed of sadness, anxiety, and anger. *Pinsamintu* can then transform into *shungu nanay*. It can take up to 1 year for the symptoms of *shungu nanay* to become noticeable, and the illness usually lasts from 1 month to several years. Many symptoms are experienced by patients suffering from *shungu nanay*. However, for the Quichua people, there are two specific symptoms that are indicative of *shungu nanay*: pain in the *shungu* (liver, lung, and heart areas) and convulsions. The traditional Quichua healers' treatment aims first to ensure that evil winds (*waira*) are not present and that the person's spirit is safe. Second, the treatment seeks to improve the emotional state of the patient. Therapies include *ñacchachi*, in which the head of the patient is rubbed systematically from the forehead to the occipital region. An infusion composed of 12 medicinal herbs used specifically for the treatment of *shungu nanay* is part of the local treatment armamentarium. Interestingly, according to the Quichua people, *shungu nanay* is the only *Jaki* subcategory for which physicians' pharmaceutical treatment is sought.

Rurashka (Sorcery)

Rurashka is an illness that could develop after a person suffers a sorcery attack. *Rurashka* occurs when a specialized healer puts a curse on a patient by request of an envious enemy. Individuals at risk for *rurashka* are those who are well-off and enjoy privileges, such as having successful harvests, a big house, connections with influential *mishu* people, or many friends, for they may spur envy in the people around them. Having a cheating spouse, conflicts with neighbors, or lawsuits can also increase one's risk for *rurashka*. Patients suffering from *rurashka* experience the same symptoms already described for the other forms of *Jaki*. A person suffering from *rurashka* must be treated by a Quichua healer. *Rurashka* is considered a severe illness, and if left untreated, it can lead to death. For this illness, the treatment is multidimensional and includes the expulsion of evil spirits from the patient's body, the release of the person's spirit from the evil spirits, and care to relieve the patient from the intense emotional state.

We recommend that when Quichua patients present symptoms such as those listed previously, physicians seriously consider the possibility of *Jaki*.

UNDERSTANDING *JAKI* THROUGH PSYCHIATRIC RESEARCH

In a unique study conducted in the Andean region of Ecuador, it was shown that contrary to the common belief among Ecuadorian physicians, *Jaki* is not merely a primitive superstition. It is a real illness—a syndrome with depressive, somatoform, and anxiety features. Using a comparative transcultural psychiatric methodology, and following the *Diagnostic and Statistical Manual of Mental Disorders*, third edition, revision (DSM-III-R) criteria and administering a Quichua version of the Zung Depression Scale with proper cultural adaption, I was able to identify multiple psychiatric disorders among *Jaki* patients.[3] The somatic symptoms presented in order of frequency were: fatigue (64% of patients), migratory pain (52%), stomachache (50%), headaches (48%), loss of appetite (30%), and palpitations (20%), among others. It is worth noting that most *Jaki* patients were suffering from various types of pain.

With a proper, culturally sensitive interview, many psychological symptoms were disclosed. This is striking owing to the contrast to how Quichua patients

Table 28.1 FREQUENCY AND SEVERITY OF PSYCHIATRIC DISORDERS
AMONG *JAKI* PATIENTS*

Psychiatric diagnoses[†]	Patients (%)	Zung (mean)
Depressive disorders	82	65
Somatoform disorders	44	63
Anxiety disorders	40	59
Psychological factors affecting a physical condition	26	62
Adjustment disorders	10	54

* $N = 50$.
[†] More than one diagnosis per patient.

will almost exclusively prefer to show somatic symptoms to their *mishu* doctors. The most frequent psychological symptoms found were: sadness (84% of patients), worries (68%), frequent crying (48%), insomnia (46%), persecution ideas,(42%), feeling rejected (40%), and suicidal ideation (38%), among others.

Eighty-two percent of the 50 patients suffering from *Jaki* who participated in the study met the DSM-III-R criteria for depression and scored high on the Zung Depression Scale. In addition, 44% of the patients presented with somatoform disorders, and 40% had anxiety disorders (see Table 28.1).

These findings shed light on the nature of *Jaki*, a culture-bound pain and psychiatric syndrome of the Andes. Without more knowledge about *Jaki*, health professionals risk maintaining old biases, dismissing patients, and delivering poor-quality medical care. This is particularly important for Andean countries with a large Quichua- Inca population. These findings could also be useful for physicians in other countries around the world where Inca immigrants are present, such as Canada, the United States, and many European countries. Physicians working with Latino immigrants from South America, who are strongly influenced by the Quichua culture, may also find this information valuable. It is important to keep in mind that with appropriate culturally adapted psychometric tools, cultural sensitivity, and input from the Quichua people's theories of illness, the *Jaki* syndrome of the Andean region could be successfully managed by biomedically trained physicians.

CLINICAL RECOMMENDATIONS

To be able to diagnose a patient with *Jaki*, physicians should pay attention to the following cultural and linguistic issues during the medical encounter:

First, they should become aware of patients' health beliefs and theories of illness, as recommended by Kleinman.[9] This will help them reach a better understanding of the patients' condition, expectations, and preferences.

Second, physicians should demonstrate linguistic sensitivity by recognizing the expressions that patients use to convey their suffering. For instance, in the first moments of the clinical encounter, *Jaki* patients express solely physical symptoms to the physician. They abstain from talking about psychological distress altogether, even when asked to do so. The Quichua people consider illnesses in two broad categories: the "Quichua illnesses," which are treatable by a *Yachactaita* (Quichua healer), and the other diseases, such as serious injuries and a variety of chronic or acute diseases, which are treatable by a physician. Depending on the type of illness from which they believe to be suffering, patients will choose to consult either a healer or a physician. Because they consider the physician to be specialized in treating physical ailments, talking about emotional problems with a doctor is perceived as inappropriate and to be avoided. Hence, Quichua patients will only report physical symptoms to physicians.[10] Given these beliefs, how can we prime Quichua patients to share emotional symptoms? *Jaki* is frequently accompanied by complaints of physical pain. The physicians treating a Quichua patient should thus keep in mind that pain could be a psychological marker for *Jaki* and hence for depressive, somatoform, and anxiety disorders among the Quichua people of the Andes. A health professional working among Quichua patients should ask the patients to express their feelings and emotions by using a very specific phrase: *"Pinsamintuta charinguichu?"* ("Do you have sad thoughts, worries?"). This will trigger an abundant expression of worries and concerns if they are present.

Third, within a cross-cultural medical encounter, physicians should seek to improve mutual understanding. When conducting their interview, physicians could phrase their questions in various ways to ensure that their message is accurately transmitted to the patient. They should also avoid using highly technical jargon. In addition, to verify that they have in turn clearly understood their interlocutor, it could be useful for physicians to paraphrase their patient's statements. Lastly, the physician should be aware that information obtained from ad-lib interpreters without any formal training in medical terminology may not always be reliable.

Jaki is a complex and multidimensional illness. To improve clinical success, we suggest physicians who suspect that a patient is suffering from *Jaki* to rely on both the Quichua and Western medical systems for designing a treatment plan. Whenever possible, physicians should seek to work in collaboration with a *Yachactaita* (Quichua healer) in the making of diagnosis as well as in the preparation of a treatment plan, which could include, for example, antidepressants and the *Yachactaita*'s interventions. Such collaboration, in our experience, results in better patient satisfaction and clinical outcomes.

Furthermore, when treating Quichua patients, it is essential to be cognizant of the history of oppression and colonization that Indigenous Peoples have endured in the Americas because these experiences pervasively influence indigenous patients worldview, their attitude toward biomedically trained doctors, and their responses to treatment recommendations.

The basics reviewed here regarding how *Jaki* is experienced in the Andes will be crucial to physicians working with Quichua populations in order to navigate this culture-bound syndrome and provide culturally appropriate medical care. Likewise, the Quichua theory of illness regarding *Jaki* can serve as a model for physicians, elsewhere in the world, wishing to provide more culturally appropriate care to patients in a multicultural setting.

REFERENCES

1. Incayawar M, Bouchard L, Maldonado-Bouchard S. Living without psychiatrists in the Andes: Plight and resilience of the Quichua (Inca) People. *Asia-Pacific Psychiatry*. 2010;2(3):119–125.
2. Incayawar M, Maldonado-Bouchard S. The forsaken mental health of the Indigenous Peoples: A moral case of outrageous exclusion in Latin America. *BMC Int Health Human Rights*. 2009;9(1):27.
3. Maldonado MG. *Llaqui et Dépression: Une Étude Exploratoire Chez les Quichuas (Équateur)*. Montreal, Canada: Department of Psychiatry, McGill University; 1992.
4. Casagrande JB. Strategies for survival: The Indians of highland Ecuador. In: Whitten NE Jr, ed. *Cultural Transformations and Ethnicity in Modern Ecuador*. Urbana, IL: University of Illinois Press; 1981:260–277.
5. Briggs CL, Mantini-Briggs C. *Stories in the Time of Cholera: Racial Profiling During a Medical Nightmare*. Berkeley, CA: University of California Press; 2003.
6. Pernick MS. "They don't feel it like we do": Social politics and the perception of pain. In: *A Calculus of Suffering: Pain, Professionalism, and Anesthesia in Nineteenth-Century America*. New York, NY: Columbia University Press; 1985:148–167.
7. Clark EB. "The sacred rights of the weak": Pain, sympathy, and the culture of individual rights in antebellum America. *J Am History*. 1995;82(2):463–493.
8. Incayawar M. Indigenous Peoples of South America: Inequalities in mental health care. In: Bhui K, Bhugra D, eds. *Culture and Mental Health: A Comprehensive Textbook*. London, UK: Hodder Arnold; 2007:185–190.
9. Kleinman A. *Patients and Healers in the Context of Culture: An Exploration of the Borderland Between Anthropology, Medicine, and Psychiatry*. Berkeley, CA: University of California Press; 1980.
10. Bouchard L. A linguistic approach for understanding pain in the medical encounter. In: Incayawar M, Todd KH, eds. *Culture, Brain, and Analgesia: Understanding and Managing Pain in Diverse Populations*. New York, NY: Oxford University Press; 2013:9–19.

29

Taming Artificial Intelligence in Psychiatry and Pain Medicine

Promises and Challenges

USEF FAGHIHI, SIOUI MALDONADO-BOUCHARD, AND MARIO INCAYAWAR ■

INTRODUCTION

Artificial intelligence (AI) is revolutionizing many fields, from providing autonomous espionage airplanes to allowing companies to predict what products will be of interest to consumers. Image classification algorithms are already capable of detecting cancers from computed tomography scans.[1] Yet, although AI technology is helping many domains, it is not clear that it has done so in the medical field. More than half of US physicians suffer from burnout.[2] One of the causes of burnout repeatedly pointed out by physicians is the computerization of medicine. Instead of making their work simpler and more efficient, AI has added layers of paperwork. The complaints of physicians in this regard are many: added hours of work, often leaking into personal time at home during late evenings, completing paperwork; depersonalization, reduced doctor–patient interaction, with the computer sitting between them, and the physician's obligation to jot down in the electronic health record (EHR) all details at that critical moment; and rigidity of options for diagnostic tests and other tests imposed by the computerized system and the administrative hospital staff who decide its parameters.

In this chapter, we first discuss how new digital technology can help physicians with clerical and administrative tasks. We then discuss how AI can help physicians in better diagnosis and decision-making, and finally, we briefly touch on the current AI challenges in psychiatric and pain medicine practice, including limitations and dangers inherent to many of today's state-of-the-art AI systems.

SNAPSHOT ON ARTIFICIAL INTELLIGENCE

Artificial intelligence (AI) machines are ones that can learn and have the capacity to reason[3]; that is, *the capacity to explain and offer justifications for the actions one can take.*

AI can be divided into *narrow AI* and *strong AI*. Narrow AI focuses on producing provable results and commercial applications, such as voice recognition, image classification using artificial neural networks, computer vision, and data mining. *Strong AI* focuses on equipping machines with the capacity to reason and problem-solve.

Machine learning (ML) is a subdomain of AI that aims to give computers the ability to learn proficiency at a task without being explicitly programmed to do so. Early efforts in AI were dominated by AI systems that were painstakingly engineered by domain experts to possess the knowledge and processes necessary to perform their designated tasks. Most modern AI practitioners have eschewed this approach and have instead focused on applying powerful learning algorithms that can infer this knowledge directly from data (e.g., medical records and imaging).

ML can be subdivided into several dominant approaches, which include *supervised learning* and *unsupervised learning.* Supervised learning refers to a set of techniques that attempt to learn models (i.e., functions) from correctly labeled training data. When trained, these models typically perform either *classification* or *regression*. Classification outputs a discrete category value (e.g., "low" or "high" suicide risk based on patient age, gender, prior suicide attempts, and medical history[4]), whereas regression outputs a noncategorical, numerical value (e.g., predicting patient length of stay in psychiatric hospitals[5]). Unsupervised learning refers to a type of exploratory data analysis that attempts to learn patterns from *unlabeled* data; for example, Bansal et al.[6] found that local variations in the morphology of anatomical brain structures (visible by magnetic resonance imaging) could be used to identify clusters of individuals with similar neuropsychiatric disorders.

Deep learning (DL) is unique as opposed to the rest of ML because it is equipped with techniques that use multilayer artificial neural networks for training and

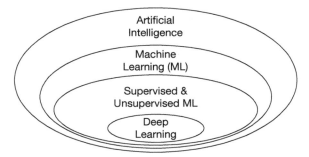

Figure 29.1. Relationship between artificial intelligence, machine learning, and deep learning.

predictions. The way DL works is that each node in a neural network has an input, a weight, and an output, which connect it to all other nodes in the next layer. DL techniques were created decades ago. However, these days, with the huge amount of data, increases in computational power of computers, and lower costs of computation, DL has become a buzzword because it can handle extremely large amounts of data.[7] DL can learn by itself (unsupervised) but lacks explainability (we will see why this is particularly important). Take a DL-based machine that must distinguish between guinea pigs, cats, and dogs. All these animals have fur, four legs, two ears, and so forth, but all these elements also have different properties. Guinea pigs have the shortest legs, and dogs have the longest. DL will distinguish these animals, but we will have no idea how.

Figure 29.1 portrays the relationship between artificial intelligence, machine intelligence, and deep learning.

SNAPSHOT ON ARTIFICIAL INTELLIGENCE ALGORITHMS

AI algorithms are similar to the decision tree presented in Figure 29.2, but whereas in the decision tree, the "if, then, else" conditions are predetermined by an expert, in an AI algorithm, the machine uses mathematical and statistical models to derive conditions on its own, without going through every condition before finding the answer. Various models exist. One example is the random forest model, an advanced decision tree. For a given problem, the random forest generates many potential decision trees (similar to that shown in Figure 29.2), and then through mathematical and statistical calculations (e.g., regression analyses), it derives the most appropriate decision tree. The details of these models are beyond the scope of this chapter. The reader is referred to Ho[8] and Barandiaran's[9] papers for more detailed information.

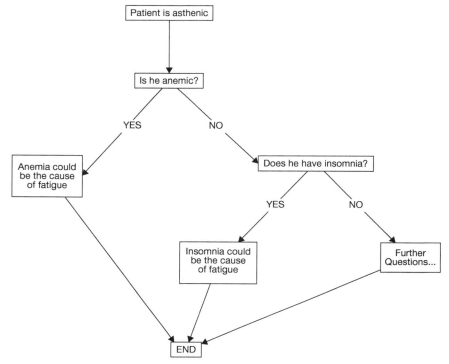

Figure 29.2. Example of a decision algorithm that could be used to create an artificial intelligence algorithm.

APPLICATIONS OF ARTIFICIAL INTELLIGENCE IN MEDICINE

Ideally, AI should help physicians improve the quality and quantity of their work. It should reduce physicians' time spent on burdensome tasks and assist in improving diagnosis and treatment. Many promising applications are being developed around the world aiming to address administrative issues, clinical decision-making, and patient clinical support, among others.

Artificial Intelligence and Precision Psychiatry

From an AI point of view, the process of detecting and identifying psychiatric disorders is more complex than that of "physical" diseases. To make a diagnosis, a psychiatrist must pay attention not only to quantifiable medical information but also, for example, to patients' emotions, chain of thoughts, and tone of voice—all pieces of information that are qualitative rather than quantifiable.

Most patient assessments are based on clinical observations and mental health practitioners' clinical experiences. In fact, patients may not be granted the same diagnosis if evaluated by different psychiatrists (interrater reliability).[10]

Part of the solution is to use AI in the effort to strengthen the quantitative aspect of psychiatry. Work is already underway in this direction. For example, Grisanzio et al.[10] applied an unsupervised machine learning (ML) algorithm to data obtained from 497 participants who were diagnosed with major depressive disorder, panic disorder, post-traumatic stress disorder, or no disorder (control participants). Unsupervised ML algorithms extracted Normative Mood, Anxious Arousal, General Anxiety, Melancholia, Anhedonia, and Tension as six major subtypes. These subtypes were found to have common characteristics in cognition, working memory, electroencephalogram, emotional resilience, and social functioning. Identifying subgroups in this manner may allow classification of patients based on common underlying mechanisms and provide patients with more appropriate treatment. Thus, ML has the potential to help psychiatrists find clusters of illness based on common biological, environmental, and psychosocial characteristics rather than only symptoms, as is the case now.

ML algorithms can also help psychiatrists save time during patient consultations. For instance, if a new patient completes a questionnaire on a laptop or phone before coming to the clinic, ML algorithms can produce an initial assessment of the patient. These algorithms can remember that in a patient of African or Middle Eastern origin, clozapine can cause harmless but higher than average neutropenia, and remind the mental health practitioner not to deprive the patient of effective treatment for schizophrenia (we provide more details on benign ethnic neutropenia later). ML algorithms, if applied to patients' medical histories, might also be capable of extracting misdiagnosed mental health problems or pharmacogenetics details that explain the unusual treatment responses related to patients' ethnicity.

Despite these steps forward, much computer science research is still needed in order to develop AI technology suitable to the mental health setting. At this point, one of the main challenges for computer scientists in developing such technology is natural language processing (NLP)—a subdivision of AI.[11] NLP-proficient AI technology is paramount for use in the mental health setting. At present, AI technology understands basic human conversation, but not its nuances; double meaning, subtle emotion, sarcasm, and other essential aspects of human talk are lost on AI. With the latest advances in NLP, researchers from IBM are now capable of predicting psychosis from patients' speech. Although the algorithm's accuracy to detect any psychosis is moderate (83%), NLP is capable of detecting the differences in speech patterns of high-risk patients who later may develop a full-fledged psychosis from those who may not.[12] Nonetheless, before adopting NLP for clinical purposes, this IBM algorithm should be tested with culturally diverse demographic groups. Although they do not suffer from depression, people from certain cultures and backgrounds may speak with a lower and softer tone, be less expressive, or use with more frequency certain words that convey negative emotions, which could cause algorithms to classify them as depressed. This brings out the fact that all algorithms and machines must be able to adapt to varying cultural and social norms, especially because these machines are more often than not designed for universal use.

Understanding patients' feelings and emotions is crucial in psychiatry. ML algorithms can now perform image processing, as well as emotion detection, but so far, only to passive data. That is, ML algorithms are applied to data that have already been gathered from patients. They have not been used in new face-to-face situations. However, in the real world, physicians face real patients who can change their tone of voice and facial expressions in response to the physicians' questions or reactions. People from different backgrounds and cultures express their emotions differently. It would be simplistic to say that during a conversation, a machine can detect patients' emotions from their speech. Some argue that a machine equipped with sensors capable of capturing patients' sensorimotor states, facial muscles, and other features could detect and interpret emotions. We suggest, however, that even this would not be enough to interpret emotions; it is paramount that machines factor in cultural and communication variables.

Despite the challenges and limitations of AI in psychiatry, it is worth noting the advances and efforts made in other aspects of medicine, which could eventually benefit all health practitioners, including mental health practitioners.

Artificial Intelligence for Clerical and Administrative Support Systems

More than half of the US physicians surveyed in 2014 suffered from symptoms of burnout according to Wright and Katz.[2] This is in large part attributed to the increased clerical burden imposed on physicians by EHR. For every hour a physician spends with a patient, the physician needs to spend about 2 hours working on EHR.[13] So far, one of the solutions in the United States to this problem has been the Ambulatory Process Excellence (APEX) physician assistance program.[14] However, not only are extra staff recruited to help physicians with EHR, but also rigorous training sessions for this new staff are required, leading to important costs in terms of money and time.[2]

Nonetheless, AI could be a promising tool to alleviate physicians' burnout. With the advances in NLP, ML algorithms can record the patient–physician conversations and help with EHR tasks[15]; Alexa, Siri, and Google Assistant already process language. Some specific software programs equipped with AI technology have already been used as virtual psychotherapists to help people with mental health issues.[16] Roughly speaking, conversational AI algorithms have access to databases containing different possible conversations that can occur in a therapy session between patients and psychotherapists. The algorithm is usually sensitive to some specific key words. If a patient uses those keywords, the algorithm will look for the answer in its database and reply to the patient. However, these artificial conversational algorithms are task-specific and therefore cannot replace a human therapist. When it comes to real-life conversations and problems, AI algorithms do not yet understand all forms of speech (varying accents and jargon) and less still all levels of meaning in a human conversation (e.g., understanding a poem). It is likely that within the next 5 to 10 years, AI technology will be able to fully understand human speech; as for the depth of meaning of human conversation, we do not have any clear solutions yet. Only when both speech and meaning are thoroughly grasped by AI will it be possible to personalize artificial conversational software to both physicians and patients.

Artificial Intelligence for Clinical Decision Support (Diagnostics and Precision Medicine)

In the past decade, the medical field has tried to redirect from a classical "standards of care," evidence-based approach to a personalized or precision medicine approach. In the first, decisions are based on group and population data from observational and clinical trials. In the classical approach, if physicians found a drug to be good for most of their patients with headaches, they would consider it to be a good treatment. In the evidence-based approach, physicians will consider results from studies with larger populations to guide their decisions. Individual patients with unusual responses to disease and treatments are bound to receive less-than-optimal care because the diagnoses and treatments applied to their case may not match the average. Technologies such as genomics, pharmacogenetics, biotechnology, and wearable sensors equipped with ML now allow us to gather data from patients for analysis and predictions. AI is poised to accelerate the development of individualized diagnosis and treatment and the shift toward a person-centered medicine.[17]

ML algorithms are capable of predicting the development of diseases such as hepatic steatosis.[18] Hepatic steatosis is diagnosed in part by ultrasonography. However, sonography exams vary in quality, and patients vary in physical dimensions, making for variation in interpretation of data. In one study,[18] the authors gathered data about age, gender, systolic blood pressure, diastolic blood pressure, abdominal girth, glucose A1C, triglyceride, HDL-C, SGOT-AST, and SGPT-ALT from 577 patients whose clinical diagnosis was known (positive or negative). Among others, the authors used an ML algorithm called Random Forest to determine which variables were most relevant in determining diagnosis. Roughly speaking, the first step in the Random Forest algorithm is taking a subset of the patients with hepatic steatosis. The algorithm begins learning by assessing one variable (e.g., age) and determining its association with all other variables (e.g., blood pressure, abdominal girth, gender) in the patients who have a positive diagnosis. The learning phase is complete when the strength of all these associations is established. The algorithm is then tested by applying the unseen data to the algorithm to measure its precision in classifying patients with the disease. This could be of great assistance in helping physicians make better diagnoses.

With the advances in genetics and AI, individualized treatments are becoming increasingly realistic and desired. One good example is that of clozapine, a frequently used drug for treatment-resistant schizophrenia. Clozapine can cause neutropenia in some individuals, and sometimes agranulocytosis. Thus, patients prescribed clozapine undergo regular blood tests in order to detect any drop in neutrophils and stop the treatment if needed. Importantly, treatment-resistant schizophrenia is more frequent in people of African descent than in the general population, and benign ethnic neutropenia is also more frequent in people of African descent and Middle Eastern descent. People with benign ethnic neutropenia have a level of neutrophils that falls below the threshold for neutropenia, but they are not more prone to infections; it is their normal physiological neutrophils level. When such individuals are treated for treatment-resistant schizophrenia, the clozapine treatment is often ceased too soon, owing to what is thought to be severe neutropenia. The consequence is that those patients are deprived of efficient medical treatment. Until recently, there was no way to know who had benign ethnic neutropenia, and treatment was ceased unnecessarily in numerous patients. However, now, with a genotyping analysis that is an ML algorithm, it is possible to identify individuals with benign ethnic neutropenia and apply a lower threshold for neutropenia to them.[19] In this example, ML can look at the history of patients with African and Middle Eastern descent and learn how their bodies react to clozapine. The algorithms could then remind the physicians about new patients with this profile. Physicians, as human beings, may forget this profile if they see it rarely, but AI will not.

These are a few examples of how advances in technology can assist health practitioners in considering individuals' genes, the environment in which they live, and their lifestyle in order to suggest personalized treatment. Given the massive amount of information (genes, combination of genetic variations, lifestyle, and environmental factors) and the vast number of diseases, it is impossible for a health practitioner to remember and track all the facts or variables during a consultation session with a patient. This is where a computer can be helpful when it comes to clinical decision-making.

Artificial Intelligence for Pain Patient Support (Continual Monitoring, Feedback, and Coaching)

One important challenge in a health care system is patients' compliance or participation. In the United States, only 70% of patients buy their new prescriptions, and only 70% of these take the medication as prescribed.[20] A better understanding of patients' behavior and their motivation could help physicians improve patients' adherence to treatment plans. It could also contribute to preventive medicine in general by helping physicians in motivating patients to improve health habits (e.g., eat health foods, exercise, don't smoke).

To improve patients' treatment compliance, gamification and AI techniques could be used. A dedicated software program could monitor patients' daily habits and motivate patients to report their progress or their problems with their current prescriptions. After receiving such reports from the software, physicians could adjust treatments to improve patient compliance.

Gamification techniques are already being used in specific areas of medicine, such as pain management. In the case of cancer treatment, which often induces considerable pain, it is difficult for the hospital team to know the pain level of their patients at all times and adjust medication accordingly. The Wasser Pain Management Centre in Toronto, Canada created Pain Squad[21] in order to monitor children's pain severity using gamification techniques. After chemotherapy, because of pain and fatigue, it was unrealistic to ask children to give a daily report about their pain. The app, which is very easy to use, sent an alert to children two times a day and asked them to report their pain. In addition, in order to encourage children to report their pain daily, the app used gamification techniques. The children were told that they were part of the Pain Squad, whose mission was to control pain. After having reported their pain for a certain time, they received virtual reward badges from TV series characters (a popular police TV show in Canada). This created some fun around the otherwise painful and bothersome experience. This way, health practitioners were able to monitor the degree of pain and the time of day or night at which it occurred. The app helped health practitioners come up with an individualized treatment for children. With the advances in technology, this type of app is becoming more common. For instance, one can easily buy Smartwatches to monitor one's blood pressure and heart rate automatically. This type of new user-friendly technology is making it easier than ever for individuals to report specific health metrics to their physicians or hospitals.

CURRENT LIMITATIONS OF ARTIFICIAL INTELLIGENCE

Explainability

There are domains in which we may not care how machines find solutions for us—for example, when social media platforms use AI to determine what products may interest you. If Facebook's AI algorithms determine that you will be interested in golf products when in fact you have never played golf and are not intending to do so, no human lives are lost. We can argue that it does not really matter that we do not understand exactly how the algorithm came to this erroneous conclusion. However, when it comes to medical diagnoses or treatment, the explainability of the machine's solution is essential. An error could put human lives at risk. In Europe, new medical apps are only approved if the solutions provided by the algorithms used can be explained.[22,23] In the United States, the Food and Drug Administration has not yet established such requirements, but the discussion is ongoing, and many believe it is only a matter of time.[24] The main concern is that of safety; because medicine deals with human lives, decisions based on computers should be verifiable by experts. To date, DL algorithms are lacking transparency; although they can find the solution, no one can explain how.

Rigidity

So far, DL algorithms are set up to look for specific criteria in datasets. If those criteria change, the DL output may be altogether different. Recently, DL algorithms obtained excellent results in image processing, such as finding cancerous cells in a computed tomography scan.[1] However, DL is vulnerable to adversarial attacks. For example, a DL algorithm trained to detect bananas sometimes grossly misclassifies them. When a user adds some pixels in the middle of an image that contains bananas, the DL algorithm may misclassify the banana as something else, for example, a toaster.[25] And we cannot yet explain how DL algorithms make these classification errors.

Empathy

An important aspect of diagnosis in depression disorder is to understand patients' feelings and emotions. To create intelligent machines, we need ML algorithms integrated into cognitive architecture, such as Learning Intelligent Decision Agent (LIDA),[26] which is biologically inspired by how the human brain works. LIDA agents' goal is to construct machines that can reason and think similarly to humans. DL also does not address cultural differences between patients, and it is not clear whether existing algorithms can be applied to people of different ethnicities and cultures.

Security

Security of patient data is crucial. With increased digitalization of health records come new potential breaches in security. Patient data must be protected from adversarial attacks (hackers). Where private and public health insurances are the norm, such as in the United States, health insurance companies' access to patient data can mean loss of insurance or increase in insurance cost for some individuals. On the other hand, the insurance companies require some patient health record information, such as for reimbursement purposes. More specifically, in the United States, if a patient has cancer, the insurance company can refuse to adhere the patient or even to pay their claims. It is worth reflecting, then, on who should have access to this data and when.

Feasibility

Change comes frequently and rapidly in AI. One can reasonably question whether hospitals are equipped or willing to keep up. Governments around the world are becoming increasingly aware of the importance of establishing a structural framework for AI technology in health care. International efforts are now deployed to support research and ethical discussions on this matter. For example, the Québec government (Canada) has funded the Observatoire International sur les Impacts Sociétaux de l'Intelligence Artificielle et du Numérique (OISIAN),* an international observatory on the social impacts of AI and digital technologies, which includes an international committee on health. Ideally, in the health care domain, consortiums such as OISIAN would receive the latest advances in AI, test them in a controlled health care setting, identify the problems with the new technology, and report them to the company that created it. After correcting the bugs and errors, the center would recommend them internationally. This would allow all countries to benefit from the advances in digital medicine.

* See https://observatoire-ia.ulaval.ca/.

CONCLUSION

When computers came into our lives, we expected that they would make life easier. Yet today, physicians are frustrated by extra work imposed on them by computers. Still, physicians are human, and humans are bound to make errors. They sometimes forget or are distracted, or are affected by fatigue or personal problems, and there is always a limit to their knowledge. AI could become a precious help to physicians in this respect: filling the gap where human limits are inevitable and giving them time for interacting with their patients humanely. In an ideal world, AI machines would be able to gather data not only from one physician but also from many throughout a country or worldwide, thus having extensive knowledge impossible for any physician to master. AI machines would not become fatigued. They would not make errors by distraction. They would help point out or bring out key clinical information to the physician in specific situations. However, all this comes at a cost: patients' information security. It is very difficult to assure patients that their data will be safe. At this point, many limitations remain with AI technology, such as reasoning or finding causes of events. We are a long way from an intelligent machine that can understand humans. Achieving such machines will only be possible when computer scientists and physician-scientists work together to find solutions adapted to medical reality.

REFERENCES

1. Mori Y, Kudo S-e. Detecting colorectal polyps via machine learning. *Nat Biomed Engineer.* 2018;2(10):713.
2. Wright AA, Katz IT. Beyond burnout: Redesigning care to restore meaning and sanity for physicians. *N Engl J Med.* 2018;378(4):309–311.
3. Russell SJ, Norvig P. *Artificial Intelligence: A Modern Approach.* Malaysia: Pearson Education Limited; 2019.
4. Walsh CG, Ribeiro JD, Franklin JC. Predicting risk of suicide attempts over time through machine learning. *Clin Psychol Sci.* 2017;5(3):457–469.
5. Pendharkar PC, Khurana H. Machine learning techniques for predicting hospital length of stay in Pennsylvania federal and specialty hospitals. *Int J Comput Sci Appl.* 2014;11(3).
6. Bansal R, Staib LH, Laine AF, et al. Anatomical brain images alone can accurately diagnose chronic neuropsychiatric illnesses. *PloS One.* 2012;7(12):e50698.
7. LeCun Y, Bengio Y, Hinton G. Deep learning. *Nature.* 2015;521(7553):436.
8. Ho TK. Random decision forests. *Paper presented at: Proceedings of 3rd International Conference on Document Analysis and Recognition;*1995.
9. Barandiaran I. The random subspace method for constructing decision forests. *IEEE Trans Pattern Anal Mach Intell.* 1998;20(8):1–22.

10. Grisanzio KA, Goldstein-Piekarski AN, Wang MY, Ahmed APR, Samara Z, Williams LM. Transdiagnostic symptom clusters and associations with brain, behavior, and daily function in mood, anxiety, and trauma disorders. *JAMA Psychiatry.* 2018;75(2):201–209.

11. Stark H. Artificial intelligence is here and it wants to revolutionize psychiatry. *Forbes.* https://www.forbes.com/sites/haroldstark/2017/10/30/artificial-intelligence-is-here-and-it-wants-to-revolutionize-psychiatry/. Accessed March 18, 2019.

12. Corcoran CM, Carrillo F, Fernández-Slezak D, et al. Prediction of psychosis across protocols and risk cohorts using automated language analysis. *World Psychiatry.* 2018;17(1):67–75.

13. Sinsky C, Colligan L, Li L, et al. Allocation of physician time in ambulatory practice: A time and motion study in 4 specialties. *Ann Intern Med.* 2016;165(11):753–760.

14. Lyon C, English AF, Smith PC. A team-based care model that improves job satisfaction. *Fam Pract Manage.* 2018;25(2):6–11.

15. Rajkomar A, Kannan A, Chen K, et al. Automatically charting symptoms from patient-physician conversations using machine learning. *JAMA Intern Med.* 2019;179(6):836–838.

16. Miner AS, Milstein A, Hancock JT. Talking to machines about personal mental health problems. *JAMA.* 2017;318(13):1217–1218.

17. Mesko B. *The Role of Artificial Intelligence in Precision Medicine.* London: Taylor & Francis; 2017.

18. Wu C-C, Yeh W-C, Hsu W-D, et al. Prediction of fatty liver disease using machine learning algorithms. *Comput Methods Programs Biomed.* 2019;170:23–29.

19. Legge SE, Pardiñas AF, Helthuis M, et al. A genome-wide association study in individuals of African ancestry reveals the importance of the Duffy-null genotype in the assessment of clozapine-related neutropenia. *Mol Psychiatry.* 2019:24(3):328–337.

20. Sauver JS. Nearly 7 in 10 Americans take prescription drugs: Mayo Clinic, Olmsted Medical Center Find. *mayonewsreleases.* June 19, 2013.

21. Stinson JN, Jibb LA, Nguyen C, et al. Development and testing of a multidimensional iPhone pain assessment application for adolescents with cancer. *J Med Internet Res.* 2013;15(3).

22. Schönberger D. Artificial intelligence in healthcare: A critical analysis of the legal and ethical implications. *Int J Law Inform Tech.* 2019;27(2):171–203.

23. O'Sullivan S, Nevejans N, Allen C, et al. Legal, regulatory, and ethical frameworks for development of standards in artificial intelligence (AI) and autonomous robotic surgery. *Int J Med Robot Comput Assist Surg.* 2019;15(1):e1968.

24. US Food and Drug Administration. Proposed regulatory framework for modifications to artificial intelligence/machine learning (AI/ML)-based software as a medical device (SaMD): Discussion paper and request for feedback. 2019. https://www.fda.gov/files/medical%20devices/published/US-FDA-Artificial-Intelligence-and-Machine-Learning-Discussion-Paper.pdf. Accessed April 18, 2020.

25. Brown TB, Mané D, Roy A, Abadi M, Gilmer J. Adversarial patch. *arXiv preprint arXiv.* 2017;171209665.

26. Faghihi U, Franklin S. The LIDA model as a foundational architecture for AGI. In: *Theoretical Foundations of Artificial General Intelligence.* Springer; 2012:103–121.

Tables, figures and boxes are indicated by *t, f* and *b* following the page number

For the benefit of digital users, indexed terms that span two pages (e.g., 52–53) may, on occasion, appear on only one of those pages.